GRILL
THIS
NOT
THAT!™

BACKYARD SURVIVAL GUIDE

BY DAVID ZINCZENKO
AND MATT GOULDING

RODALE.

© 2012 by Rodale Inc.

All rights reserved. No part of this publication may be reproduced or transmitted in any form
or by any means, electronic or mechanical, including photocopying, recording, or any other information
storage and retrieval system, without the written permission of the publisher.

Rodale books may be purchased for business or promotional use or for special sales.
For information, please write to:
Special Markets Department, Rodale, Inc., 733 Third Avenue, New York, NY 10017

Men's Health is a registered trademark of Rodale Inc.

Printed in the United States of America

Rodale Inc. makes every effort to use acid-free ♾, recycled paper ♺.

Book design by George Karabotsos

Photo direction by Tara Long

Cover photos by Jeff Harris / Cover prop styling by Roscoe Betsill
Hand modeling by Ashly Covington

All interior photos by Thomas MacDonald and Mitch Mandel/Rodale Images

Food styling by Diane Simone Vezza and Melissa Reiss

Illustrations on pages 129, 164, and 166 by Harry Campbell

Library of Congress Cataloging-in-Publication Data is on file with the publisher

ISBN-13: 978-1-60961-822-3 trade paperback
ISBN-13: 978-1-60961-934-3 direct mail hardcover

Trade paperback and exclusive direct mail edition published simultaneously in May 2012

Distributed to the trade by Macmillan

2   4   6   8   10   9   7   5   3   1   paperback
2   4   6   8   10   9   7   5   3   1   direct-mail hardcover

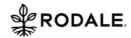

We inspire and enable people to improve their lives and the world around them.
www.rodalebooks.com

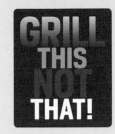
Dedication

To all the men and women who have
ever set fire to something, intentionally or not.
Here's how to harness your power
for the best purposes possible.
And to all of America's brave firefighters.
We're really, really sorry.

ACKNOWLEDGMENTS

Plenty of sizzling steaks and singed arm hairs went into making this book. So did a lot of long days and nights spent designing pages, checking facts, correcting punctuation, buying ingredients, crunching numbers, grating cheese, taking photos, and countless other efforts, both big and small. This book is the product of all those efforts—and all those people behind them that make this team the finest in the publishing industry. Thanks to all of you who were a part of this project, especially:

To Maria Rodale and the Rodale family, who have done as much to improve the way Americans eat as any other family in this country.

To George Karabotsos, whose vision and creativity continue to take these books in amazing new directions. And to his crew of rock star designers, including Laura White, Mark Michaelson, Courtney Eltringham, and Elizabeth Neal. If this series has proved anything, it's that this design team has no equal.

To Laura Perez, the world's most amazing sous chef. And to Clint Carter, Hannah McWilliams, and Cathyrne Keller, three individuals who make everything we do better.

To Debbie McHugh and Erin Williams, you two are the glue that holds these pages together.

To Tara Long, who has tamed many a fire to perform her acts of alchemy. And to the rest of the team that brings this food to life, including Diane Vezza, (Smokin') Joan Parkin, Tom MacDonald, Mitch Mandel, Troy Schnyder, Nikki Weber, and Melissa Reiss. No appetite is safe when you guys are at work.

To the talented and dedicated Rodale book team: Steve Perrine, Chris Krogermeier, Sara Cox, Jennifer Giandomenico, Wendy Gable, Keith Biery, Liz Krenos, Brooke Myers, Sean Sabo, Deri Reed, Sonya Vogel, and Jodi Schaffer. These books could not succeed without your incredible efforts.

And to our friends, family, and loved ones: There's no one we'd rather cook for.

—Dave and Matt

Check out the other bestselling books in the **EAT THIS, NOT THAT!**® and **COOK THIS, NOT THAT!**® series:

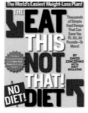

Eat This, Not That! for Kids! (2008)

Cook This, Not That! 350-Calorie Meals (2010)

Eat This, Not That! No-Diet Diet (2011)

Eat This, Not That! (2011)

Eat This, Not That! Supermarket Survival Guide (2012)

CONTENTS

"Feel the Burn"

You've heard it said hundreds of times, in spin classes and workout DVDs and gyms of every kind. If you want to lose weight, get in shape, and feel your best, you've got to "feel the burn." You have to "burn off calories," and "maximize your burn rate."

Well, that's all well and good, but it's not always fun. Wouldn't it be easier if, instead of feeling the burn, you could melt off pounds by applying the burn? And rather than burning off the calories from the foods you eat, what if you could burn the calories off before you eat them? And what if the only burn rates you had to worry about involved making sure you brought enough sunscreen?

Wouldn't that be a heck of a lot more fun?

It is. And that's what this book is all about. In the following pages, you're going to learn how to save hundreds, if not thousands, of calories at each meal, simply by using the easiest, most enjoyable, most tasty cooking method ever invented. You'll eat great, you'll look great—and you'll have a great time doing it.

Ready to get started?

In the beginning, there was fire.

Paleolithic man wouldn't have survived without it. He used it to heat his home, light his way, mold his tools. But most important of all, he used it to cook. The open flame tenderized his food, made it more appetizing, and even made it more delicious.

And if you've ever tried Woolly Mammoth Tartare...not good.

But besides making his food more palatable, the open flame made it healthier by melting off unwanted fat and making nutrients more accessible. Primitive man worshipped fire and kept it constantly burning, feeding it kindling and tending to it the way Taylor Lautner tends to his abs. And when wood wasn't plentiful, our ancestors used alternative fuels like weeds, moss, and even animal dung.

Nowadays, we're lucky enough not to have to cook with animal dung (although if we could actually harness all the animal dung tossed around in election campaigns, we'd have enough energy to power all of the Kardashian family hair dryers into eternity). Instead, we have grills: Eighty-two percent of American households own a grill, whether it's a propane-fueled combustion machine eating up a parking space in the garage or just a little bucket of charcoal hanging out on the terrace. And if you can learn to fire it up right, you'll discover that it just might be the most effective weight-loss tool in your arsenal. In fact, our research shows that you can save, in some instances, as many as 1,500 calories per meal just by choosing to grill dinner instead of driving to the local restaurant.

How's that, you ask? Isn't the backyard barbecue the sort of place for *King of the Hill*—type potbellied dads to gather 'round like priests worshipping at the altar of beer and hot dogs? Sure, it can be. But it can also be a perfect place to start stripping pounds from your body. When you drop a piece of meat on your grill, much of the fat bubbles out and burns up on the coals below. A study in the journal *Meat Science* found that grilling a pork chop could actually decrease its fat content by nearly a third!

Okay, sure, but there are plenty of "grilled" foods available at the chain restaurants that anchor your local mall. Why not just swing by one of those? Well, here's where things get tricky. In many cases, restaurant "grills"

are actually grill plates, or hot slabs of flat metal that lock fat in instead of cooking it out. Plus, restaurants routinely paint their meats with hot oil and clarified butter, effectively ramping up the fat count to flab-inducing levels. In fact, a USDA study found that people eat about 107 more calories each time they choose to eat out instead of eating at home.

But often, the reality is much worse. For instance, let's say you're hankering for a nice, meaty dinner—but you want to make sure you're eating healthy. So you'd naturally opt for chicken over red meat— if it's white meat, it's light meat, right? Well, in some cases that's true. But take a close look at some of those "healthier" alternative dishes out there. Outback's Alice Springs Chicken entrée might sound like a healthy choice, but wherever Alice Springs is, we think it's probably polluted with runoff from a lard factory. For the $14.49 you'll spend for that "healthy" option, you'll be getting 1,468 calories and a heart-stopping 2,220 milligrams of sodium— nearly two whole days' worth of salt! If you ask them to hold the Aussie fries, you're still getting 784 calories and a day's allotment of sodium. By comparison, you'll find a recipe on page 136 for something very similar: We call it Prosciutto Pesto Chicken. It comes in at only 230 calories, and has less than one-third the sodium. (And the ingredients will cost you about $1.83 a serving.) If you stayed home and grilled just once a week, a swap like this would save you 18 pounds this year alone! Just by eating the same food from your own backyard grill!

Oh, and did we mention you'll save a ton of time, money, and stress?

Beyond rescuing you from more than 18 pounds of flab every year, that chicken swap would also save you $12.66 per person. For a family of four making a swap like that just once a week, you're talking about putting—this sounds incredible, but it's true—an additional $2,633.28 in your pocket this year. Just by grilling once a week!

And that's before you factor in the hassle of loading everybody into the car, finding a parking spot, waiting out in the vestibule for that creepy little vibrator thing to light up, and then trying to feign interest in a restaurant you've probably been to a hundred times before—because all of these chains look exactly alike, whether you're dining in Austin or Augusta, Akron or Albany. So, instead of all the restaurant hassle and having to entertain the kids when they get fidgety, all you need to do is open the back door, arm the kids with some Super Soakers or a football, and call them when dinner's ready. Plus, there's no limited menu.

We've packed this book with 150 super-easy, super-delicious recipes so you can grill almost every night of the week.

And each one of these new foods will be something you selected yourself. You'll know exactly what's in it—something that can't be said about a plate from your local restaurant chain. Isn't it better to toss some fresh mushrooms on the grill and watch them sizzle, especially when you know that the canned kind often used in restaurants can legally contain up to 19 maggots and 74 mites in every 3.5-ounce can? Yikes! And wouldn't you rather be able to check the ingredients of your burger buns to make sure they're free of a dough strengthener called L-cysteine—a non-essential amino acid most often made from dissolved duck feathers or, sometimes, human hair? Blech! (Bet the waitress at your local diner can't tell you whether your entrée comes with a side of L-cysteine or not, huh?)

Is this book the best investment you've ever made, or what?

But you'll not only get leaner and richer—you'll get healthier, too!

New research has discovered that of all cooking methods, grilling is clearly the healthiest—better than frying (obviously), baking (hmm), and even nuking (really?). Consider what researchers are now saying about the magic of the grill:

You'll ingest less fat and calories. A 2011 study looked at how one kind of fish stacked up nutritionally depending on whether it was baked, fried, microwaved, or grilled. It was discovered that the lowest levels of fat and calories were found in the grilled fish.

You'll build more lean muscle. In the same study, researchers studied the amount of muscle-maintaining protein found in the fish. They found that the grilled fish actually had higher levels of protein than fish cooked by other methods! A second study, published in the *Journal of Medicinal Food*, looked at different ways of cooking five types of fish: In each species, the highest levels of essential amino acids—the building blocks of muscle—were found in the grilled samples.

You'll shrink your belly. The foods we recommend in *Grill This, Not That!* are designed predominantly to target belly fat—by keeping your belly full of smart, healthy choices that keep your resting metabolism revving and never let you go hungry. That means you'll be at the top of your game and burning fat all day, every day.

You'll boost your brain power. In a 2009 study from the journal *Food Chemistry*, researchers looked at the vitamin and mineral content in meat that was baked, grilled, microwaved, and fried. It found that grilling alone seemed to significantly increase the levels of vitamin B2, which is essential to a healthy nervous system.

You'll protect your heart. Grilling also increases levels of niacin, the researchers said. Niacin has been found to boost HDL, the "good" cholesterol that keeps arteries clear. And, in another shocker, all cooking methods significantly decreased the meat's level of vitamin B6—all except for grilling! By retaining the food's levels of B6, grilling helps to maintain normal levels of homocysteine, an amino acid in the blood. High levels of homocysteine have been linked to heart disease.

Okay, so let's be clear here: By grilling at home just once a week, you could strip more than 18 pounds off your belly; build lean, healthy muscle; and reduce your risk of heart disease. And you could do it all while saving enough money to buy four round-trip tickets to Paris.

Makes you think that maybe the backyard barbecue has gotten a bad rap, huh? Well that's about to change. It's time to forget about *King of the Hill*.

It's time to become *King of the Grill!*

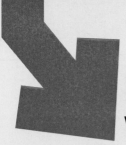

How to lose weight with this book

If you want to shed belly fat, there's only one formula you need to know, and, luckily for you, it's easier than anything you encountered in ninth-grade algebra.

The magic formula is this: Calories in – calories out = total weight loss or gain. This is the equation that determines whether your body will shape up to look more like a slender 1 or a paunchy 0, a flat-bellied yardstick or a pot-bellied protractor. That's why it's critical that you understand what sort of numbers you're plugging into this formula.

On the "calories out" side, we have your daily activities: cleaning house, lining up at the post office, hauling in groceries, and so on. Often when people discover extra flab hanging around their midsections, they assume there's something wrong with this side of the equation. Maybe so, but more likely it's the front end of the equation—the "calories in" side—that's tipping the scale. That side keeps track of all the fast-food value meals, Chinese buffets, and stuffed-crust pizzas you eat every day.

In order to maintain a healthy body weight, a moderately active female between the ages of 20 and 50 needs only 2,000 to 2,200 calories per day. A male fitting the same profile needs 2,400 to 2,600. Those numbers can fluctuate depending on height, age, and activity level, but they're reasonable estimations for most people. (For a more accurate assessment, use the calorie calculator at mayoclinic.com.)

Let's take a closer look at the numbers: It takes 3,500 calories to create a pound of body fat. So if you eat an extra 500 calories per day—the amount you'd take in by eating T.G.I. Friday's Pulled Pork Sandwich instead of the Spicy Asian Pork Burger in this book—then you'll earn 1 new pound of body fat each week. But here's the silver lining: If you currently make a habit of eating out at restaurants, and you start grilling in your backyard instead, then you can drop 52 pounds—or more—this year!

That's where this book comes in. Within these pages are nearly 150 flavorful recipes that save you as many as 1,500 calories over similar dishes constructed in the grease-stained restaurant kitchens of America. The more often you fire up your grill, the quicker you'll notice layers of fat melting away from your body! Check this out:

• **CHILI'S SMOKEHOUSE BURGERS** have more than 2,000 calories each! Our version—covered with bacon, dripping with sauce—still saves you 1,830 calories! (Check it out on page 90.)

• Despite the healthy-sounding name, **APPLEBEE'S ORANGE GLAZED SALMON** delivers 730 calories. Switch to the **CEDAR PLANK SALMON** on page 222 and save 490 calories. Make this or similar swaps a couple times a week and you'll shed 15 pounds this year.

• **ON THE BORDER'S DOS XX FISH TACOS WITH CHILI SAUCE** has 1,670 calories—before adding sides. Switch to our **GRILLED FISH TACOS WITH PICO DE GALLO** and you'll save an astonishing 1,350 calories a week. That's enough to burn off 9 pounds of flab in 6 months!

And here's the best news of all: While cooking on your grill shrinks your waistline, it also fattens your bank account. The food prepared by restaurants uses cheaper ingredients, yet it regularly costs two to four times as much as the meals you can prepare at home. So by making food yourself, you're saving both money and calories, and the more you fire up the grill, the more dramatic the savings. So go ahead: Get grilling!

America's
WORST
Grilled Foods

At the heart of the grill lies the key to a powerful convergence of flavor and nutrition, a fire that melts fat and delivers heaping quantities of smoke and sizzle, the world's greatest zero-calorie ingredients.

But a scorching Weber isn't always the weight-loss weapon we want it to be. Consider this: We've found dozens of grilled dishes in the restaurant world with more than 1,000 calories per serving, from salads with nutritional numbers that make double cheeseburgers seem healthy, to racks of ribs that pack more calories than 11 Krispy Kreme Original Doughnuts. Yes, it is possible to screw up food on the grill, as the biggest restaurants in the country continue to prove every day by choosing bad cuts of meat, coating them with sugary sauces, and serving them with a lousy supporting cast of side dishes—all tactics that compromise the inherent goodness of the grill.

To keep you from getting scorched next time you head out to dinner, we've identified the 20 worst flame-broiled foods in America. But it's not all bad news: We offer delicious alternatives that you can make at home for a fraction of the cost and calories, a strong reminder that the grill, when used responsibly, is a world-class weight-loss weapon.

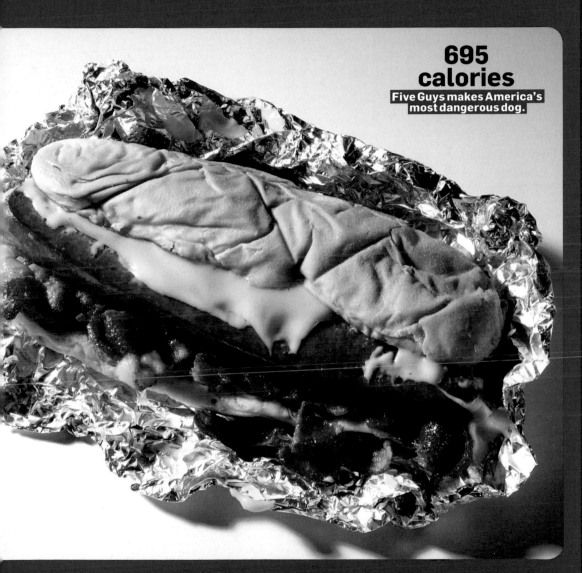

695
calories
Five Guys makes America's most dangerous dog.

WORST GRILLED HOT DOG

20 Five Guys' Bacon Cheese Dog
695 calories
48 g fat (22 g saturated)
1,700 mg sodium
Price: $4.75

Five Guys doesn't give you many options. Not in the mood for a burger? There's grilled cheese, a 1,474-calorie bag of French fries, or a hot dog with more than a full day's worth of saturated fat. You could eat two fully loaded dogs from a New York street vendor and still take in fewer calories and fat. Our favorite dog, a bacon-wrapped, teriyaki-glazed beauty, made with the high-quality, low-calorie franks from Applegate Farms, gives you all the decadence you need for less than half the calories.

Grill This Instead!
Teriyaki Dogs with Grilled Pineapple (page 98)
270 calories
9 g fat (3 g saturated)
880 mg sodium

Cost per serving: $1.65
Save 425 calories and $3.10!

WORST GRILLED WHITE FISH

19 IHOP's Grilled Tilapia Hollandaise
810 calories
46 g fat (13 g saturated)
1,890 mg sodium
Price: $9.99

An 8-ounce fillet of grilled tilapia contains just 6 grams of fat, so you know the calories in this dish aren't coming from the fish. For a better explanation of how one of the leanest pieces of protein ends up with more calories than a Wendy's Baconator, look no further than the sauce. Hollandaise is a butter- and egg yolk-based emulsion that clings to food like a blanket of molten fat. Along with packing an astounding 40 grams of fat, it also has the unique ability to make all food taste exactly the same.

Grill This Instead!
Swordfish with Smoky Aioli (page 242)
280 calories
14 g fat (2.5 g saturated)
490 mg sodium

Cost per serving: $4.04
Save 530 calories and $5.95!

WORST GRILLED LAMB

18 Outback Steakhouse's New Zealand Rack of Lamb
910 calories
56 g fat (29 g saturated)
2,197 mg sodium
Price: $19.99

We applaud Outback for being one of the only chain restaurants to serve lamb. In its best iteration, lamb is a lean, tender, tasty alternative to a steak. The rack is normally among the healthiest cuts of lamb, too—yet still, somehow, Outback manages to get this dish wrong, injecting their version with more than a full day's worth of saturated fat. Don't blame it on the lamb; blame it on the huge portion size and the rich red wine sauce poured liberally over the top.

Grill This Instead!
Balsamic Lamb Chops (page 184)
280 calories
21 g fat (8 g saturated)
435 mg sodium

Cost per serving: $3.66
Save 630 calories and $16.33!

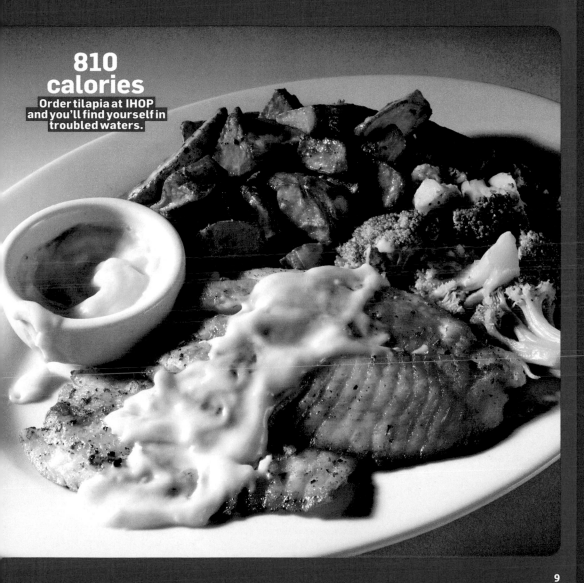

810
calories
Order tilapia at IHOP and you'll find yourself in troubled waters.

WORST GRILLED STEAK

17 Ruby Tuesday's Rib Eye (no sides)
912 calories
71 g fat
1,040 mg sodium
Price: $16.99

When it comes to a grilled steak, the cut of meat is everything. Opt for a sirloin, flank, or skirt steak and you're looking at a piece of beef that is predominantly protein, buffered by just enough fat to keep things interesting. On the flip side of the coin, rib eyes come from the most heavily marbled part of the cow, which means that along with rivers of fat, you also get a steak dense with calories. We're not sure where Ruby Tuesday gets its beef from, but its rib eye easily qualifies as the worst steak in the business.

Grill This Instead!
The Perfect Grilled Steak (page 168)
230 calories
7 g fat (2.5 g saturated)
620 mg sodium

Cost per serving: $2.61
Save 682 calories and $14.38!

WORST GRILLED FISH TACOS

16 Chevys Fresh Mex's Mesquite Grilled Fresh Fish Tacos
920 calories
27 g fat (8 g saturated)
2,400 mg sodium
Price: $10.89

There are tacos that are worse than these (though not many), but these land on the list by virtue of the gaping chasm between perception and reality. "Grilled fresh fish"—three healthier words have never lived together in the same menu blurb, and yet, Chevys nevertheless finds a way to deliver a plate that provides more than half of your day's calories and fat and nearly two full days' worth of sodium. It's a troubling turn of events to which we have only one response: Time to fire up the grill out back.

Grill This Instead!
Grilled Fish Tacos (page 238)
320 calories
13 g fat (2 g saturated)
490 mg sodium

Cost per serving: $2.89
Save 600 calories and $8!

WORST TURKEY BURGER

15 Ruby Tuesday's Avocado Turkey Burger
968 calories
61 g fat
1,601 mg sodium
Price: $8.99

This burger may sound like a nutritionist's dream dinner, but the truth is that it packs more calories than Ruby Tuesday's Classic Cheeseburger. Why? Because turkey alone does not a healthy burger make, especially when you consider that ground dark-meat turkey can contain as many calories as ground beef. Add to that the aggressive condiment treatment turkey burgers tend to receive and you start to see why it's not always the healthy alternative it pretends to be.

Grill This Instead!
Stuffed Meat Loaf Burgers (page 94)
460 calories
20 g fat (8 g saturated)
965 mg sodium

Cost per serving: $1.83
Save 508 calories and $7.16!

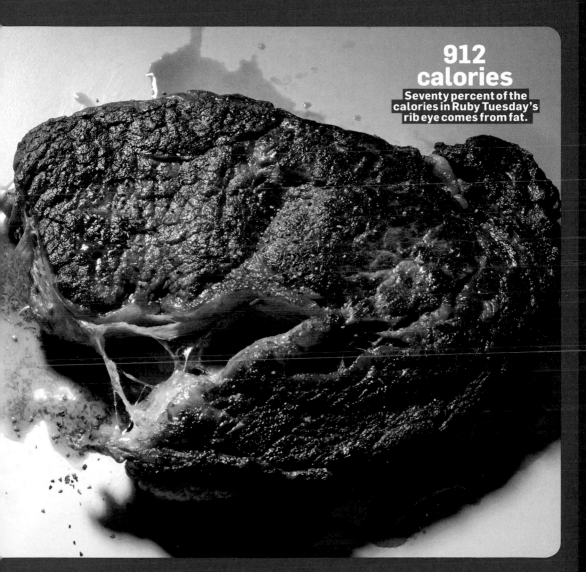

912
calories

Seventy percent of the calories in Ruby Tuesday's rib eye comes from fat.

WORST DRESSED-UP GRILLED STEAK
14 Outback's New York Strip (14 oz) with Blue Cheese Crumb Crust
989 calories
70 g fat (34 g saturated)
857 mg sodium
Price: $21.98

In an effort to squeeze a few extra bucks out of its customers, Outback offers diners the option of adding items like sautéed mushrooms, grilled scallops, and, worst of all, this blanket of bread crumbs and blue cheese. It turns an already hefty steak into a punishing proposition. Outback does offer a number of lean beef options (the small Outback Special and the 6-ounce Victoria's Filet are two excellent options), so go in with a game plan and you'll escape relatively unscathed.

Grill This Instead!
Strip Steaks with Blue Cheese Butter (page 196)
300 calories
20 g fat (10 g saturated)
510 mg sodium

Cost per serving: $2.92
Save 689 calories and $19.06!

WORST BARBECUE
13 T.G.I. Friday's Jack Daniel's Pulled Pork Sandwich
990 calories
35 g fat (11 g saturated)
2,710 mg sodium
Price: $7.89

A real pulled pork sandwich, like the kind they dish out in the barbecue shacks of eastern North Carolina, is a simple construction: steamed bun, a splash of vinegar-based sauce, maybe a bit of coleslaw. Friday's defies that formula by starting with a butter-packed brioche, then drowning the pork in sugary barbecue sauce and topping it all with fried onion strings. Somewhere out there a pitmaster is shuddering at the thought of this bastardized barbecue.

Grill This Instead!
Carolina Pulled Pork, Two Ways (page 186)
350 calories
16 g fat (5 g saturated)
650 mg sodium

Cost per serving: $1.31
Save 640 calories and $6.58!

WORST GRILLED SALMON
12 Red Lobster's Cedar Plank Salmon
1,050 calories
40 g fat (9 g saturated fat)
1,780 mg sodium
Price: $19.50

Red Lobster's fresh fish menu is one of the most admirable menu sections in the country: dozens of different types of seasonal fish, cooked over an open flame and served with an admirable selection of healthy sides. With that in mind, it's hard to figure out how they got this one so wrong. Sure, salmon is naturally loaded with health-boosting omega-3 fatty acids, but with a quadruple-digit calorie count and a full day's worth of sodium, you'd find a leaner meal in a 20-pack of Chicken McNuggets.

Grill This Instead!
Cedar Plank Salmon (page 222)
240 calories
9 g fat (1.5 g saturated)
470 mg sodium

Cost per serving: $2.91
Save 810 calories and $16.59!

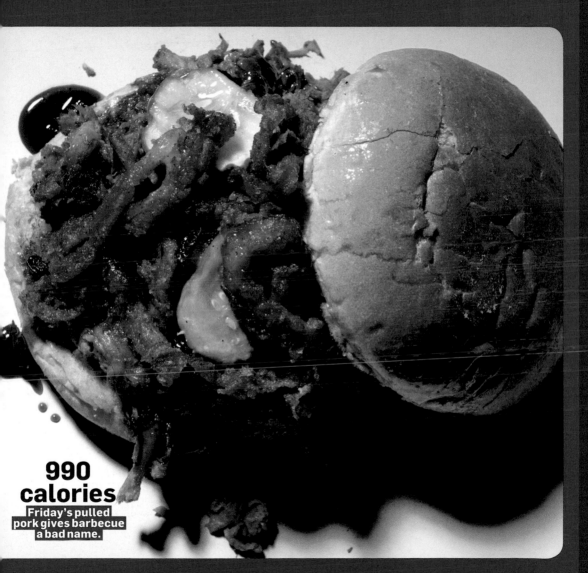

990 calories
Friday's pulled pork gives barbecue a bad name.

WORST GRILLED CHICKEN SANDWICH
11 T.G.I. Friday's Jack Daniel's Chicken Sandwich

1,140 calories
58 g fat (18 g saturated)
2,780 mg sodium
Price: $9.09

Jack Daniel's real name was Jasper Newton Daniel and he was a 5-foot, 2-inch pioneer of American distillery. He made a mean whiskey, but it's hard to imagine ol' Jasper being excited to know that his creation adorns some of America's worst grilled dishes, from steak to pork to chicken. He'd probably go on a bender if he ever found out that the Jack Daniel's Chicken Sandwich packs more calories than 17 shots of Jack Daniel's Tennessee Whiskey.

Grill This Instead!
Grilled Chicken & Pineapple Sandwich (page 88)
400 calories
11 g fat (6 g saturated)
640 mg sodium

**Cost per serving: $2.64
Save 740 calories and $6.45!**

WORST GRILLED CHICKEN
10 Romano's Macaroni Grill's Chicken Under a Brick

1,180 calories
18 g saturated fat
2,590 mg sodium
Price: $16

Macaroni Grill was smart to bring the long-held Tuscan tradition of cooking chicken under a brick to the shores of America. Unfortunately, the chicken put on about 700 calories, 10 grams of fat, and 2,000 milligrams of sodium on the journey. Save this one for the backyard, where the birds are lean, the bricks are abundant, and the beers are cheap.

Grill This Instead!
Chicken Under a Brick (page 158)
470 calories
28 g fat (8 g saturated)
780 mg sodium

**Cost per serving: $2.83
Save 710 calories and $13.17!**

WORST GRILLED SALAD
9 Chevys Fresh Mex's Grilled Chicken Fajita Salad

1,220 calories
90 g fat (23 g saturated)
1,480 mg sodium
Price: $12.19

Mexican-style salads are invariably clobbered with a blizzard of high-calorie add-ons such as sour cream and grated cheese. Don't be distracted by the words "grilled chicken" —this baby packs as much fat as 18 scoops of Breyers Original Strawberry ice cream. But the Mexican pantry has plenty of excellent ingredients to fill out a salad bowl that are both lean and deeply delicious. Don't believe us? Try our Blackened Chicken and Mango Salad.

Grill This Instead!
Blackened Chicken & Mango Salad (page 298)
440 calories
22 g fat (2.5 g saturated)
490 mg sodium

**Cost per serving: $3.69
Save 780 calories and $8.50!**

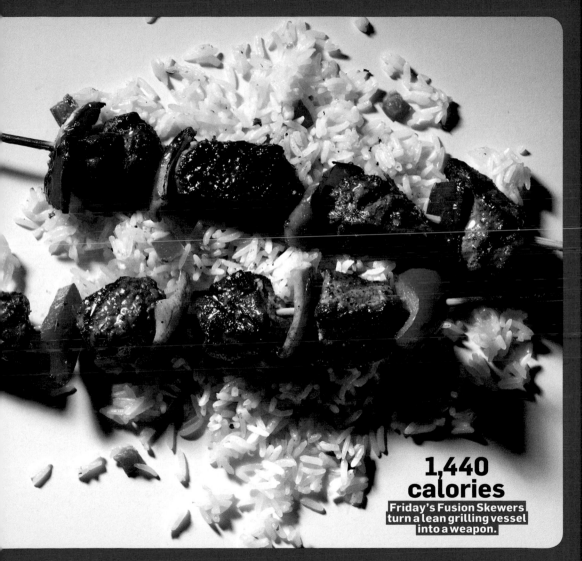

**1,440
calories**
Friday's Fusion Skewers
turn a lean grilling vessel
into a weapon.

15

WORST GRILLED FOODS

WORST GRILLED SAUSAGE

8 Olive Garden's Grilled Sausage and Peppers Rustica

1,320 calories
80 g fat (30 g saturated)
2,860 mg sodium

Price: $11.75

Olive Garden normally opts for the stovetop over the grill to concoct its line of pseudo-Italian fare, but here the chain proves that it's just as dangerous with a spatula as it is with a sauté pan. This dish boasts a solid foundation of grilled meat, fresh veggies, and antioxidant-rich marinara, but a huge pile of carb-heavy penne and an indecent amount of fatty pork sausage sabotage any shot for nutritional prudence. If it's sausage you seek, make sure it's chicken or turkey.

Grill This Instead!
Sausage & Peppers with Orecchiette (page 122)
520 calories
22 g fat (6 g saturated)
670 mg sodium

**Cost per serving: $2.23
Save 800 calories and $9.52!**

WORST FAJITAS

7 Applebee's Sizzling Steak Fajitas

1,410 calories
55 g fat (25 g saturated)
5,630 mg sodium

Price: $13.79

Picking this loser was no easy task; there are at least half a dozen viable candidates for the title of Worst Fajitas (Chili's, Chevys, and Baja Fresh among them), a reflection of just how easily corrupted an inherently good recipe can be when placed in the wrong hands. Applebee's comes out at the bottom of the pack not just because its sizzling platter edges out the others in the calorie department, but because it contains more salt than you'd find in 33 small bags of Lay's Potato Chips.

Grill This Instead!
Grilled Steak Fajitas (page 180)
430 calories
16 g fat (7 g saturated)
810 mg sodium

**Cost per serving: $3.86
Save 980 calories and $9.93!**

WORST SKEWERS

6 T.G.I. Friday's Mediterranean Black Angus Sirloin Fusion Skewers

1,440 calories
77 g fat (19 g saturated)
3,220 mg sodium

Price: $10.89

As you'll find in the pages to come, we're huge fans of the skewer. Just load one up with protein and vegetables and you're all but assured of a lean, tasty meal. Unfortunately, that equation only applies at home; in the bizarro restaurant world, a skewer more closely resembles a weapon than the means to a healthy dinner. Friday's Fusion Skewers are wrong for so many reasons, but most of all because they make a mockery of one of our favorite grilling vessels.

Grill This Instead!
Steak-and-Potato Skewers with Horseradish Steak Sauce (page 198)
440 calories
15 g fat (6 g saturated)
710 mg sodium

**Cost per serving: $2.74
Save 1,000 calories and $8.15!**

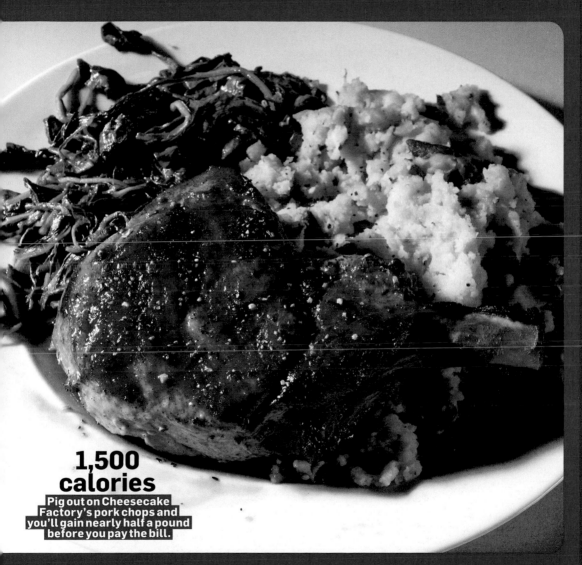

1,500 calories

Pig out on Cheesecake Factory's pork chops and you'll gain nearly half a pound before you pay the bill.

WORST GRILLED PORK

5 Cheesecake Factory's Grilled Pork Chops

1,500 calories
52 g saturated fat
2,441 mg sodium
Price: $18.95

Pork chops rule. Just ask Homer Simpson. Besides being drool-inducingly delicious, a loin chop can be surprisingly lean, containing a modest 5 grams of saturated fat per average serving. Unfortunately, Cheesecake Factory's servings are anything but average; they tend to feed their diners as if they were on the eve of a hunger strike. Through the combination of elephantine portion sizes and reckless cooking habits, this plate ends up with more than six times the saturated fat of our decadent goat cheese—stuffed chops.

Grill This Instead!
Stuffed Pork Chops (page 178)
410 calories
19 g fat (8 g saturated)
460 mg sodium
Cost per serving: $2.28
Save 1,090 calories and $16.67!

WORST GRILLED SHRIMP

4 Cheesecake Factory's Grilled Shrimp and Bacon Club Sandwich

1,740 calories
22 g saturated fat
2,608 mg sodium
Price: $13.95

Not only is this the worst shrimp dish we've seen, it's also America's worst sandwich. You'd think the latter would be reserved for a hulking cheesesteak or a foot-long submarine of sinful excess, but the diabolical minds responsible for Cheesecake Factory's menu manage to put two slices of bread around one of the world's leanest proteins and create a sandwich that contains as many calories as you'd find in nearly 4 pounds of cocktail shrimp.

Grill This Instead!
Shrimp Po' Boys (page 82)
370 calories
5 g fat (1 g saturated)
860 mg sodium
Cost per serving: $3.17
Save 1,370 calories and $10.78!

WORST GRILLED APPETIZER

3 Baja Fresh's Charbroiled Steak Nachos

2,120 calories
118 g fat (44 g saturated)
2,990 mg sodium
Price: $7.25

People don't always look to the grill when they think about appetizers, but as a toaster of bread, a melter of cheese, and a crisper of lean proteins, it is well suited for the task of kicking off a meal. But even genius devices can be used for dubious ends when left in the wrong hands. Baja Fresh, for all of its talk about fresh ingredients, is responsible for some of America's most caloric Mexican food: bulging burritos, catastrophic salads and fajitas, and nacho platters that would be dangerous if shared among an entire room full of eaters.

Grill This Instead!
Ham and Pineapple Quesadillas (page 260)
370 calories
18 g fat (10 g saturated)
620 mg sodium
Cost per serving: $1.77
Save 1,750 calories and $5.48!

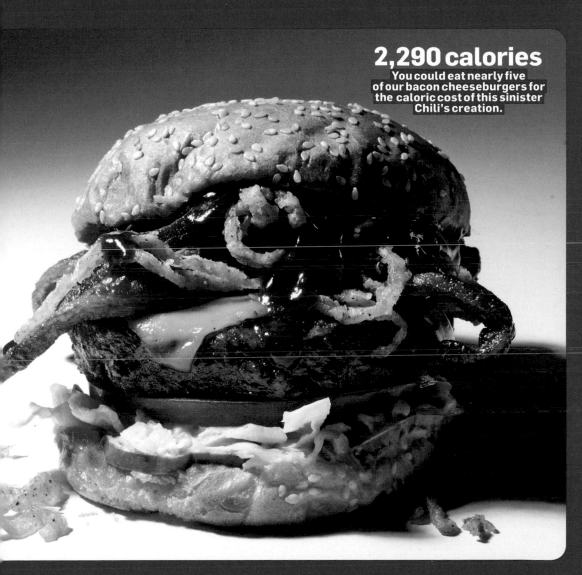

2,290 calories
You could eat nearly five of our bacon cheeseburgers for the caloric cost of this sinister Chili's creation.

WORST BURGER

2 Chili's Southern Smokehouse Burger with Ancho Chile BBQ

2,290 calories
139 g fat (46 g saturated)
6,500 mg sodium

Price: $9.69

The average American eats 150 burgers a year. That's an eye-popping reminder that for most people, burgers aren't an occassional indulgence, but a lifestyle. We stand by America's love affair with the burger, just as long as most of those burgers are coming from your backyard and not some dubious restaurant griddle glazed in a sea of molten beef fat. Unfortunately, we're afraid more burgers are consumed at places like Chili's than they are around the family dinner table, and that's a frightening prospect, because there is no worse place in America to eat a burger. Even the most basic Chili's option—the plain Oldtimer—will saddle you with more than 1,300 calories. What's most shocking about

the Southern Smokehouse, America's worst burger by a long shot, isn't that it alone will add two-thirds of a pound of pure body fat to anyone crazy enough to eat it, it's that you can have a burger with the exact same flavors (bacon, cheddar, sweet onions, barbecue sauce) at home for a fifth of the caloric cost.

Grill This Instead!
Cowboy Burgers (page 90)

460 calories
22 g fat (11 g saturated)
850 mg sodium

Cost per serving: $2.62
Save 1,830 calories and $7.07!

WORST GRILLED DISH IN AMERICA

1 Chili's Shiner Bock Ribs

2,310 calories
123 g fat (44 g saturated)
6,340 mg sodium

Price: $17.99

Eating ribs at a sit-down restaurant is risky business no matter where you've chosen to eat. The problem begins with the fact that baby back ribs are a naturally fatty cut. The danger

is only compounded by portion distortion and reckless sauce application, a killer combination that leaves even the "leanest" ribs packing quadruple-digit calorie counts. That's why the biggest restaurants in America—Applebee's, Friday's, Outback—all serve ribs with more than 1,500 calories per serving. Chili's adds insult to injury by rubbing their rendition with enough salt to preserve an entire hog. Even at home, there are only two ways to avoid the wrath of the ribs: Control your portion size (no more than half a rack per person) and keep the sauce slathering to a minimum.

Grill This Instead!
Classic Baby Back Ribs (page 182)

370 calories
15 g fat (4.5 g saturated)
870 mg sodium

Cost per serving: $2.93
Save 1,940 calories and $15.06!

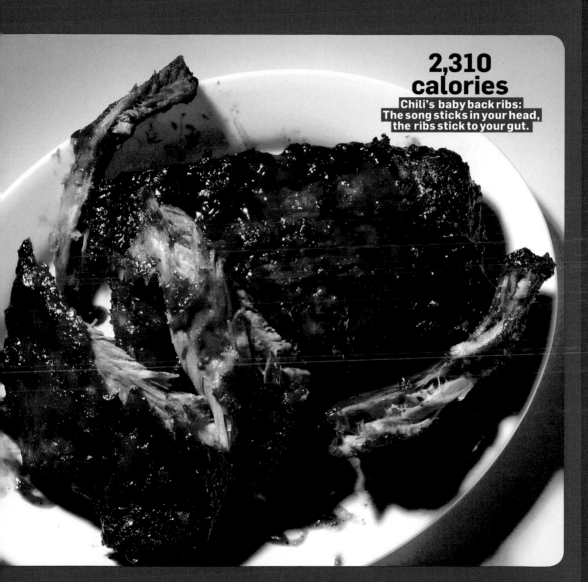

2,310 calories

**Chili's baby back ribs:
The song sticks in your head,
the ribs stick to your gut.**

THE BACKYARD BASICS

CHAPTER **1**

POP QUIZ:

What do these three things have in common?

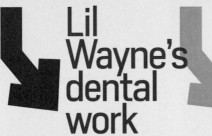

Lil Wayne's dental work

Every single episode of *Law & Order*

Super-easy weight loss

ANSWER: They all involve grills!

Of course, the part that's relevant to you—the weight-loss part—doesn't involve sweating out a confession from a perp or adding diamonds to a rapper's teeth. (Although both would seem to make overeating pretty impossible.) But a grill is the place where you can make healthy foods even healthier— and help those less-than-lean indulgences shed some of their sin. (In fact, a study in the journal *Meat Science* found that grilling a pork chop by conventional methods could actually decrease its fat content by nearly a third.)

That said, the starting line for any healthy diet is healthy ingredients. Yes, a cheeseburger is better for you when it's grilled rather than fried, but you can't turn a nutritional Paula Deen into a tasty Paula Patton just by tossing it on the grill. Using simple swaps that up your nutrition intake will make stripping away pounds easier.

Here's why: When you eat a meal packed with nutrients, your body doesn't send you out searching for MIA vitamins and minerals, driving you to eat more and more. In fact, the more healthy food you eat, the

less food you'll eat overall: In a 2006 study published in the *European Journal of Clinical Nutrition,* researchers found that participants who had fish for lunch ate 11 percent fewer calories at dinner than participants who had beef for lunch.

So, to make sure your pantry, fridge, and freezer are stocked with only the healthiest ingredients, we've broken down every major fire-friendly food brand in the supermarket, compared them all, and found the foods that should be picked for the grill— and some that should be kicked in the grill.

The BEST & WORST
Foods for the Grill

The path to healthy grilling starts off in the supermarket. Fill your cart with starch-riddled buns, sugary condiments, and calorie-dense dogs and sausages and you're undermining one of the world's greatest weight-loss weapons. To make sure your pantry is stocked with the best possible building blocks, we've raided the aisles and identified the most dangerous waistline saboteurs in the supermarket. More importantly, we've picked out 24 first-rate staples that no smart griller should be without.

BEEF HOT DOG

Eat This

**Applegate The Super
Natural Beef Hot Dogs**
(one frank)
70 calories
6 g fat (2 g saturated)
6 g protein
330 mg sodium

Applegate Farms uses lean,
preservative-free meat,
so you get real beef flavor
minus the hefty
saturated-fat load found
in other franks.

Not That!

**Oscar Mayer Selects
Angus Beef Hot Dogs**
(one frank)
180 calories
17 g fat (7 g saturated)
6 g protein
420 mg sodium

Angus beef is no leaner—
and arguably no tastier—
than regular beef, and these
franks pack nearly
three times the fat found
with Applegate Farms.

LIGHT HOT DOG

Eat This

**Hebrew National 97%
Fat Free Beef Franks**
(one frank)
40 calories
1 g fat (0 g saturated)
6 g protein
520 mg sodium

With no fillers and an
impressively low calorie
count, these uber-lean
dogs are a nutritious,
protein-packed addition to
your cookout.

Not That!

**Oscar Mayer Classic
Light Beef Franks**
(one frank)
90 calories
7 g fat (3 g saturated)
5 g protein
380 mg sodium

"Light" is a relative term
when it comes to shopping
for franks. Just one of
these low cal dogs has more
fat than half a dozen
of the Hebrew Nationals.

PORK SAUSAGE

Eat This

**Aidells
Cajun Style Andouille**
(one link)
160 calories
11 g fat (4 g saturated)
15 g protein
600 mg sodium

Aidells uses quality lean
pork in its sausages,
which translates into
better flavor, more protein,
and less fat.

Not That!

**Hillshire Farm
Smoked Bratwurst**
(one link)
240 calories
22 g fat (8 g saturated)
8 g protein
780 mg sodium

Fat crowds out protein in
these brats, accounting
for 83 percent of
the calories. We'll take Aidells
all summer long.

SPICY SAUSAGE

Eat This

**Al Fresco Chipotle
Chorizo Chicken
Sausage (one link)**
140 calories
7 g fat (2 g saturated)
15 g protein
420 mg sodium

These lean chicken links—
like all of Al Fresco's
sausage selections—pack
tons of flavor and a
generous portion of protein.

Not That!

**Hillshire Farm Hot &
Spicy Italian Style
Smoked Sausage**
(one link)
250 calories
22 g fat (8 g saturated)
8 g protein
670 mg sodium

To justify these sky-high
calorie and fat counts,
this link would need to
pack triple the protein.

The Best & Worst Foods

CHEESY SAUSAGE

Eat This

Johnsonville Chicken Sausage Chipotle Monterey Jack Cheese
(per link)
170 calories
12 g fat (4 g saturated)
13 g protein
770 mg sodium

Because this sausage is made with lean chicken, adding cheese doesn't take it over the calorie edge.

Not That!

Johnsonville Beddar with Cheddar
(per link)
200 calories
17 g fat (6 g saturated)
8 g protein
620 mg sodium

There's nothing better about these links: Extra calories, more fat, but only half the protein of the Johnsonville sausage.

VEGGIE BURGER

Eat This

Boca Bruschetta
(per patty)
90 calories
2 g fat (0.5 g saturated)
13 g protein
440 mg sodium

Plenty of protein and low calories—exactly what you want in a meat substitute. Try a double stack for a more powerful protein punch.

Not That!

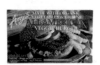

Amy's All American Veggie Burger
(per patty)
140 calories
3.5 g fat (0 g saturated)
13 g protein
390 mg sodium

Amy's patties pack 50 extra calories without providing any extra protein in return.

GUACAMOLE

Eat This

Wholly Guacamole
(per 2 Tbsp)
60 calories
5 g fat (1 g saturated)
1 g protein
90 mg sodium

With nothing but avocados and seven other simple ingredients, this dip's the closest you'll find to homemade guac at the supermarket.

Not That!

Mission Guacamole Flavored Dip (per 2 Tbsp)
40 calories
3 g fat (0 g saturated)
0 g protein
150 mg sodium

Oil, cornstarch, and "avocado powder" replace real avocados in this guacamole imposter.

HOT DOG BUN

Eat This

Martin's Famous Long Potato Rolls
(per bun)
130 calories
1.5 g fat (0 g saturated)
26 g carbohydrates
4 g fiber
200 mg sodium

Martin's mines the humble spud to pack these rolls with as much fiber and protein as you'll find in any hot dog buns on the market.

Not That!

Pepperidge Farm Classic Hot Dog Buns
(per bun)
140 calories
2.5 g fat (0.5 g saturated)
26 g carbohydrates
<1 g fiber
180 mg sodium

Bread products should have at least 2 grams of fiber per serving.

for the Grill

HAMBURGER BUN

Eat This

Martin's Potato Rolls
(per roll)
130 calories
1.5 g fat (0 g saturated)
25 g carbohydrates
3 g fiber
200 mg sodium
This isn't just one
of the lightest, most fiber-
and protein-rich buns
on the shelves,
it's also the tastiest.

Not That!

Arnold Select
White Hamburger Rolls
(per roll)
150 calories
2 g fat (0.5 g saturated)
30 g carbohydrates
1 g fiber
350 mg sodium
These refined buns give
you 15 percent
more calories and
67 percent less fiber than
the Martin's rolls.

TRADITIONAL BBQ SAUCE

Eat This

Stubb's Original
Bar-B-Q Sauce
(per 2 Tbsp)
30 calories
6 g carbohydrates
220 mg sodium
Robust flavor without a
ton of sugar or salt.
What more could you
ask for in a barbecue sauce?

Not That!

Kraft Original
Barbecue Sauce
(per 2 Tbsp)
60 calories
15 g carbohydrates
450 mg sodium
High-fructose corn syrup
is this sauce's
primary ingredient,
which is why it packs twice
as many calories
as the bottle of Stubb's.

SWEET BARBECUE SAUCE

Eat This

Jack Daniel's
Honey Smokehouse
(per 2 Tbsp)
45 calories
11 g carbohydrates
280 mg sodium
One of the few "honey"
sauces that won't
put you in a sugar coma.

Not That!

Famous Dave's
Sweet & Zesty
(per 2 Tbsp)
70 calories
17 g carbohydrates
320 mg sodium
With more than 3 teaspoons
of sugar per serving,
this condiment is better
suited for an ice cream
sundae than a rack of ribs.

ALL-PURPOSE MARINADE

Eat This

Lawry's
30 Minute Marinade
Steak & Chop
(per 2 Tbsp)
10 calories
0 g fat
1 g carbohydrates
780 mg sodium
The lemon juice and vinegar
base of this marinade
will tenderize your
meat and poultry without
adding a ton of sugar.

Not That!

KC Masterpiece
Steakhouse
(per 2 Tbsp)
60 Calories
2 g fat
7 g carbohydrates
660 mg sodium
KC Masterpiece goes heavy
on the high-fructose corn
syrup, which adds
unnecessary calories. Sugars
also convert to bitter-tasting
carbon when they hit the grill.

The Best & Worst Foods

Eat This

**McCormick Grill Mates
Applewood Rub
(per 2 tsp)**
15 calories
350 mg sodium

McCormick's line of rubs
is relatively low
in sodium, and this
Applewood option adds
smoky flavor and
a hint of sweetness to
chops, chicken, and steak.

Not That!

**Emeril's
All Natural Steak Rub
(per 2 tsp)**
0 calories
1,680 mg sodium

Would you like some steak
with your salt?

TERIYAKI SAUCE AND MARINADE

Eat This

**La Choy
Stir Fry Teriyaki
(per Tbsp)**
10 calories
3 g carbohydrates
105 mg sodium

This bottle is low in both
sugar and salt—a rare find
in the world of
store-bought teriyaki sauces.

Not That!

**La Choy Teriyaki
(per Tbsp)**
40 calories
10 g carbohydrates
570 mg sodium

Each tablespoon has almost
as much sugar as two
Oreo cookies and more salt
than three small bags of
Lay's Classic potato chips!

KETCHUP

Eat This

**Heinz Organic
Tomato Ketchup
(per Tbsp)**
20 calories
5 g carbohydrates
190 mg sodium

A study from the *Journal
of Agricultural and Food
Chemistry* found that organic
ketchup has nearly three
times the amount of lycopene,
a cancer-fighting antioxidant,
as conventional ketchup.

Not That!

**Heinz Tomato Ketchup
(per Tbsp)**
20 calories
5 g carbohydrates
160 mg sodium

This iconic condiment
from Heinz placed dead last
in a blind ketchup
taste test conducted for
*Eat This, Not That!
All-New Supermarket
Survival Guide.*

HONEY MUSTARD

Eat This

**Grey Poupon
Savory Honey Mustard
(per Tbsp)**
30 calories
3 g carbohydrates
15 mg sodium

Heart-healthy mustard
seeds are this bottle's
primary ingredient, and
unlike other brands,
Grey Poupon doesn't use
"honey" as an excuse to
load its mustard with sugar.

Not That!

**Inglehoffer
Sweet Honey Mustard
(per Tbsp)**
45 calories
6 g carbohydrates
135 mg sodium

When sugar and water
show up before
mustard seeds on the
ingredients list,
should it really
be labeled mustard?

for the Grill

MAYO

Eat This

Kraft Reduced Fat Mayonnaise with Olive Oil
(per Tbsp)
45 calories
4 g fat (0 g saturated)
95 mg sodium

By slashing the calories in half and adding heart-healthy monounsaturated fats, Kraft gives mayo a much-needed makeover.

Not That!

Hellmann's Real Mayonnaise
(per Tbsp)
90 calories
10 g fat (1.5 g saturated)
90 mg sodium

"Real" mayonnaise is one of the heaviest condiments around. One hundred percent of this bottle's calories come from fat.

DELI-STYLE CHEESE SLICES

Eat This

Sargento Reduced Fat Swiss
(per slice)
60 calories
4 g fat (2 g saturated)
7 g protein
30 mg sodium

Low-fat cheese will lighten your burger's caloric load, and Swiss has a fraction of the sodium of most other popular cheeses.

Not That!

Kraft Deli Fresh Sharp Cheddar
(per slice)
90 calories
8 g fat (5 g saturated)
5 g protein
140 mg sodium

You could eat two servings of Sargento's Reduced Fat Swiss and still not reach the saturated fat load of these Kraft slices.

PASTEURIZED CHEESE SLICES

Eat This

Kraft Singles 2% Milk Sharp Cheddar
(per slice)
45 calories
3 g fat (1.5 g saturated)
4 g protein
250 mg sodium

You'd be hard-pressed to find a cheese slice with fewer calories. Plus, it melts like a dream.

Not That!

Kraft Deli Deluxe Sharp Cheddar Slices
(per slice)
110 calories
9 g fat (5 g saturated)
6 g protein
450 mg sodium

These slices are labeled "Deluxe," but there's nothing superior about them: More calories, three times the fat, same flavor.

PICKLES

Eat This

Vlasic Reduced Sodium Kosher Dill Spears
(per 2 spears)
0 calories
0 g carbohydrates
450 mg sodium

Great straight out of the jar or as a burger topper, these spears are crispy, calorie-free, and not too salty.

Not That!

Vlasic Bread & Butter Spears
(per 2 spears)
75 calories
15 g carbohydrates
510 mg sodium

By adding high-fructose corn syrup, Vlasic turns an otherwise guilt-free condiment into an indulgence.

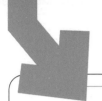

DIPPING SAUCE

Eat This

Peter Luger Steak Sauce
(per 2 Tbsp)
60 calories
0 g fat
14 g carbohydrates
250 mg sodium

Steak sauce is the perfect low-calorie meat condiment, and this full-flavored option from Brooklyn's famed chophouse can't be beat.

Not That!

Kraft Buttermilk Ranch Dressing & Dip
(per 2 Tbsp)
120 calories
12 g fat (2 saturated)
2 g carbohydrates
290 mg sodium

It's unfortunate ranch has become a default dip and sauce for so many; few condiments pack more calories and fat.

CHUTNEY

Eat This

Wild Thymes Mango Papaya Chutney
(per Tbsp)
15 calories
0 g fat
3.5 g carbohydrates
0 mg sodium

This jar contains only fruit, spices, and a touch of sugar. Perfect for pork, chicken, and lamb dishes.

Not That!

Kitchens of India Shredded Mango Chutney
(per Tbsp)
80 calories
0 g fat
18 g carbohydrates
50 mg sodium

Sugar's the first ingredient in this jar.

BEER

Eat This

Guinness Draught
(per bottle)
127 calories
10 g carbohydrates
4.2 percent alcohol

It's the lightest dark brew around, and it pairs nicely with grilled meat.

Not That!

Guinness Extra Stout
(per bottle)
153 calories
18 g carbohydrates
4.3 percent alcohol

Extra stout means extra calories. This beer's packed with flavor, but it'll add too much weight to your meal, especially if you have more than one.

LIGHT BEER

Eat This

Amstel Light
(per bottle)
95 calories
5 g carbohydrates
3.5 percent alcohol

Under 100 calories and refreshing, not watery—everything a light beer should be.

Not That!

Michelob Light
(per bottle)
123 calories
8.8 g carbohydrates
4.3 percent alcohol

This brew has far too many calories and carbs to bear the "light" label.

3 Grilling Buzzkills

It may be an inherently healthy cooking method, but grilling is not without its hazards. Here are three of the biggest health concerns that come with cooking over an open fire, along with strategies for cutting back on the risk.

1. Heterocyclic amines (HCAs)

What they are: Carcinogens that develop when the creatine, sugars, and amino acids in meat react to your grill's high temperatures.

Why they're bad: Several studies have linked HCAs with cancer development in animals, and a growing body of research supports a connection between HCA exposure and increased risk of colorectal, pancreatic, and prostate cancers in humans.

Chop your risk: *SPICE IT UP!* A 2011 study published in the *Journal of Food Science* revealed that adding antioxidant-rich spices like rosemary to beef patties before grilling can slash the production of HCAs up to 39 percent. Another way to reduce your risk? Turn down the heat—burnt meat contains higher concentrations of HCAs.

2. Advanced glycation end products (AGEs)

What they are: Toxic compounds that develop when animal proteins are heated at high temperatures. Grilled beef has been shown to contain the highest levels of AGEs.

Why they're bad: AGEs can increase oxidative stress and have been linked to the development of chronic diseases like diabetes and heart disease.

Chop your risk: *SOAK BEFORE YOU SEAR.* A 2010 study from the American Dietetic Association found that marinating meat in lemon juice or vinegar for 1 hour cuts AGE production in half.

3. Polycyclic aromatic hydrocarbons (PAHs)

What they are: Carcinogens that form when fat drippings burn at the bottom of your grill. The burnt fat produces PAH-rich smoke, which then penetrates whatever food you're grilling.

Why they're bad: Recent research has linked PAHs to an increased risk of a variety of cancers, including prostate cancer and renal cell carcinoma. A 2011 Polish study also found a correlation between prenatal PAH exposure and lower birth weight.

Chop your risk: *CUT THE FAT.* Lean meats produce less drippings and, therefore, less PAHs. Choosing propane over charcoal may also limit your PHA exposure, as charcoal grilling creates more smoke.

The GRILL
Glossary

To conquer the backyard, you'll first need to decode the loaded language of fire and smoke.

Barbecue

A style of cooking distinguished by indirect heat and low temperatures. Barbecuing typically takes place between 200 and 250°F, which is less than half the temperature reached with direct heat. At this low, steady temperature, tough muscle fibers break down and collagen slowly melts, giving you the rich taste and luscious mouthfeel characteristic of awesome barbecue. Barbecue sauce, while common, is not the defining characteristic of barbecue, and it often buries delicious smoke flavors under unnecessary sugars.

Beef, Prime

Only 2 percent of beef is rated Prime by the USDA, and most of that goes to restaurants willing to pay the premium. But let the restaurants have it; the rating system is based largely on marbling—i.e., fat—and Prime is the fattiest of all the grades. Falling just below Prime is Choice, and just below that is Select. Lower grades are considered less flavorful, but they're also cheaper and less caloric.

Caramelization

A reaction in which sugar browns and develops delightfully bitter flavors. A similar reaction is known as the Maillard reaction, and it occurs when small quantities of sugars or carbohydrates are cooked alongside proteins. In most cases, it's the Maillard reaction—not caramelization—that's responsible for the flavorful crust created when you sear meat.

Dry Rub

Similar to a marinade, a dry rub utilizes seasonings, spices, and other adjuncts to add flavor to food. Since it contains no liquid, it has to be rubbed onto the meat. Whereas marinades are great for softening muscle tissue, rubs are better for creating complex and flavorful crusts.

Grilling, Direct

Cooking directly over flame. This is the simplest and most common type of grilling, and it's best for thin and fast-cooking pieces like steaks, burgers, vegetables, and individual cuts of chicken.

Grilling, Indirect

A technique that moves food away from the flame, allowing it to cook slowly, as in an oven. The easiest method for the home griller is banking, which means heaping charcoal along one side of the grill, placing the food on the opposite side, and closing the lid. You should also slide in a small pot of water to keep the meat from drying out. Indirect grilling is ideal for large or tough cuts of meat like ribs, briskets, and whole chickens.

Grilling, Plank

A faster and simpler variant of smoking that places the meat directly on a flat piece of wet wood, and then places the plank directly above the flame.

Marinade

Liquid used to add flavor to and help tenderize meat before cooking. The best marinades pair big-flavor ingredients with some sort of acid like vinegar or citrus, which breaks down tissues for more tender meat.

Searing

Cooking meat over high heat to create a thick and flavorful external crust. (However, as we discuss on the next page, searing does not "seal in the juices.") With thinner pieces of meat, the inside can reach doneness while the outside sears, but with thicker cuts, you'll want to finish cooking over low heat after the crust forms. For the best possible crust, pat your protein dry before cooking.

Smoking

A type of indirect grilling that infuses meats, fish, and vegetables with the roasted notes of woods like oak, mesquite, and hickory. Smoked foods can be cooked entirely over wood, or a combination of charcoal or gas and wet wood chips.

Grill Myths DEBUNKED

These popular beliefs may be making your food worse. We hope to relieve you of them once and for all.

MYTH 1
Searing locks in the juices.

This may be the most persistent cooking myth of all time, propagated at every opportunity by self-anointed grill masters and television "chefs" alike. Amazingly enough, research has been out for many years disproving this theory, particularly by the king of all kitchen scientists, Harold McGee, author of *On Food and Cooking*. McGee's studies have shown that, if anything, searing actually decreases the amount of moisture in the end product.

Searing still has its place on the grill: High heat causes rapid browning, which amplifies the flavor and texture on the surface of your meat or fish. But for the best of all worlds (i.e., moist, tender meat inside paired with a deeply browned, almost-crunchy exterior), turn the process on its head, starting first with a low, steady flame, then finishing with serious heat. By reversing the order of operations, the browning will occur more rapidly (since the surface of the meat will already be quite warm after time on the grill), resulting in juicier, more evenly cooked meat inside.

MYTH 2
Flip your meat once and only once.

This is another misguided maxim that holds a lot of currency with the talking heads on the Food Network. Research done by Harold McGee found that flipping meat frequently helps meat cook both more evenly and more rapidly, cutting cooking time by as much as 40 percent overall. McGee recommends flipping every 15 seconds, but even flipping the meat once every minute could help improve the quality of your food.

That being said, there is a fine line between careful flipping and destructive manipulating. Grilling is still mainly a spectator sport, an exchange between meat and fire that demands minimal human interference. Get too aggressive with the food on the grill and you can puncture your meat, sacrificing all of those precious juices to the fire below.

MYTH 3
Hotter is better.

Not necessarily. While grill marks and deeply browned crusts on meat, fish, and vegetables are attractive to the eye and tasty to the palate, high-heat cooking isn't always the path to grilling enlightenment. Try a fillet of salmon cooked over a low, steady flame—taste how the fish gently flakes and melts like warm butter across your palate—and you'll see the other side of the coin.

As a general rule for choosing the heat of your grill, think about the size of what you're cooking: For a thin cut of steak like flank or skirt, you'll need high heat if you want to develop a crust on the meat without overcooking the inside. But try to cook a big piece of meat—a brisket, a leg of lamb, a tri-tip—over high heat and you'll end up with a burnt exterior and a cold center—not exactly good eats.

As for chicken with the skin on, cooking over high heat is an invitation for flare-ups, those aggressive fire spikes that will char your chicken to smithereens before the meat closest to the bone is fully cooked. Medium-low should be your go-to temperature.

MYTH 4
All of that grill buildup is extra flavor for your food.

That crusty stuff clinging to your grate? That's not flavor; that's dirt. Carbonized fat and protein, to be specific, and not only does it add an unpleasant bitter note to your food, it can also be a health hazard, since these burnt particles have been shown to be carcinogenic.

Always keep a wire grill brush beside your grill. The best time to clean the grate is when it's hot, so just before you load up the grill with goodies, take 30 seconds to scrape it clean.

MYTH 5
Thermometers are for suckers.

Know what's really for suckers? Cutting into a piece of meat to see if it's done and losing all the delicious juices. Do what the pros do and keep a thermometer close at hand for careful monitoring of your food's internal temperature.

Still, thermometers can provide escape routes for swirling juices, too, so don't go poking holes in that nice steak as if it were a voodoo doll. Better to wait until the meat looks close to being done, then insert the thermometer in the thickest part of the cut and leave it there until you hit your target temperature. With time and practice, you can learn when a steak or a burger is done by touch, but better to be safe than to eat a piece of raw—or scorched—meat.

MYTH 6
Food is best hot off the grill.

That first juicy bite is the stuff food dreams are made of, but if you cut into a piece of protein directly off the grill, every bite that follows will be drier and more disappointing than the last. When meat and fish are hot, the muscle fibers contract, leaving all those savory, swirling juices with no way to be reabsorbed into the flesh. Cut into meat or fish too soon and those juices go leaking out onto your plate or cutting board. By waiting for the temperature of the meat to cool, you allow the muscle fibers to reabsorb all of those juices, which ensures a moist, flavorful steak, chop, chicken breast, or fish fillet.

So, how long do you have to wait before diving in? Depends on how thick the food is. Think 5 to 7 minutes for burgers, chicken breasts, and pork chops, 10 minutes for a thick steak, and at least 15 minutes (and up to 30) for whole chickens, turkey breasts, and large cuts of meat like pork shoulder and brisket.

MYTH 7
Grilling is a warm-weather pastime.

Unless you live in northern Minnesota, grilling can be a year-round affair. According to a 2008 study conducted by Weber, 57 percent of grill owners grill all year round. One major benefit of uncooperative weather is that it teaches you to work more efficiently. Here's the best way to grill when you don't feel like lingering outside: Fire up the grill, return to the kitchen to do prep work while the heat builds, then return with everything you need for the grill on a cutting board or baking sheet. Be sure to keep the lid closed to speed up the cooking.

If you do happen to live in northern Minnesota, or if you just don't feel like going outside on a frosty January evening, a grill pan provides many of the same advantages of the real thing (high heat, nice grill marks) without the need to leave your kitchen.

8 Ways to Up Your Grill Game

From professional tricks to overarching outdoor techniques, these savvy strategies will produce healthier, more delicious results every time you fire up the grill.

Cook Food Perfectly Every Time.

Everything else is just frosting on the cake. Your steaks can come from pampered bovine royalty and be showered with black truffles and molten foie gras, but if they're not properly cooked, then they're barely worth eating. People have their own tastes and should grill accordingly, but for us perfect means a rosy medium-rare with burgers and steaks, a hair beyond medium for pork and salmon, and until that last bit of pink disappears from the chicken and not a minute more.

More than anything, this book is about teaching you how to cook food simply, but expertly. We try to highlight as often as possible the tricks and tips—big and small—that will help you turn something as basic as a chicken breast or sirloin steak into something memorable. For more on how to cook every type of protein to your desired level of doneness, see "Is It Done Yet?" on page 70.

Adopt a New Salt Strategy.

A great marinade is a marvelous thing, and we discuss the technique at length later in Chapter 6, but there is an even simpler way to instantly improve your grilling: salting. Salt is the single most important ingredient in the kitchen, yet we give so little thought to how best to employ it. A shower of salt right before grilling is the default approach we all use, but that means only the surface of the meat or fish is seasoned. There are two simple techniques you can employ to make sure your food is seasoned all the way through.

The first is called curing, which is a term normally reserved to describe the process of seasoning and drying hams or sausages. Salt will slowly, steadily extract water from meat, both preserving it and concentrating its flavors. For something like prosciutto, the curing process might last 18 months, but try salting a whole chicken the night before you cook it, or a handful of pork chops a few hours ahead, and you'll be amazed at how juicy and flavorful they emerge from the grill.

The second is brining, a tactic used everywhere in the food industry—from the greatest high-end restaurants to the largest cold-cut manufacturers—to impart moisture and flavor to meat, particularly pork and poultry, before cooking. Despite its ubiquity outside of the home, few cooks ever use it in their kitchen. But try it once and we promise you'll be convinced.

HERE'S A BASIC BRINE RECIPE:

Combine 8 cups of water with ½ cup kosher salt and ½ cup light brown sugar. Heat just enough to dissolve the salt and sugar, then cool completely before using. Working with this as your base, you can flavor the brine in dozens of different ways: Apple juice, honey, chile peppers, whole garlic cloves, bay leaves, orange peels, peppercorns, rosemary, and many more flavor builders are common additions to brines.

Immerse the food in the brine and refrigerate. Remember that size and brining time are directly related. Shell-on shrimp can be brined for 30 minutes, pork chops and chicken parts for an hour or two, and whole chickens, turkeys, and pork shoulders can soak overnight.

3 Go High and Low.

Whether gas or charcoal is your fuel of choice, there's a huge strategic advantage to having more than one temperature zone on your grill. Having hotter and cooler sides of your grill allows you to sear and to slow cook over the same surface. It also allows you to cook big, tough pieces of meat via indirect heat (try cooking a pork shoulder or a brisket over a direct flame and you'll need jaw replacement surgery when you're finally done chewing). Here's how to set up your grill to maximize its potential.

For a charcoal griller, it means banking: Build your charcoal fire (for the easiest, safest way to do that, see page 35), and when the coals have burned down and are ready for grilling, use a long metal spatula to "bank" your charcoal against one side of the grill, leaving the other side either empty, or with a few scattered lumps to maintain a low heat. When cooking big cuts of meat, place them on the cool side of the grill and close the top.

If gas is your weapon of choice, then a two-fire zone is simple: Turn one or two of the burners on high and leave one on low— or, if you're cooking something for a long time, leave the burner off entirely.

4 Bring Smoke to the Fire.

Few home cooks have the time and patience to smoke a brisket, pork shoulder, or rack of ribs over hardwood for 8 hours, but by using a small wood-chip tray or even a foil packet with a normal grill setup, you can infuse your foods with that rich barbecue flavor with minimal effort.

Choose the right wood for your meal in the same way you'd choose a wine: The stronger the dish, the more intense the wood flavor can be. Here's a rundown of the most common woods used for smoking:

HICKORY: Well-loved among barbecue barons for its assertive aroma, hickory is the chip of choice for pulled pork and baby back ribs.

MESQUITE: Another intense wood, mesquite works best with pork chops, chicken wings, and burgers.

OAK: The preferred wood of the beef masters of Texas is oak, used to smoke brisket and sausages.

APPLE AND ALDER: These lighter-scented woods are best used for more delicate proteins like chicken breast and salmon fillets, or when you only want the faintest whisper of smoke in your finished product.

HERBS: Spiking your fire with fresh and dried herbs can add an extra layer of complexity to your grillables. Rosemary creates an intense aroma best for beef and lamb. Thyme gives off a moderate smoke well suited for pork chops and grilled chicken. For fish, try a handful of tarragon.

Soak the chips in hot water: The heat opens up the wood fibers, helping the water penetrate more deeply, which in turn creates more smoke for your grill.

Wet wood can go directly onto a charcoal fire. For a gas grill, use a small wood-chip box, like the one we recommend on page 69. Or make a smoker packet by wrapping the soaked chips in a foil packet poked with holes all over so that the smoke can escape. Whether using the box or the packet, it goes directly over the fire just before you begin cooking.

Become a Spice Master.

There is no faster, healthier, cheaper way to bring flavor to your food than a skillfully deployed spice rub. A few pinches can transform a chicken breast from boring to brilliant. And given that most common spices are essentially calorie-free vessels for powerful antioxidants, it's a markedly more nutritious way to season your food than relying on heavy sauces and dressings.

A true grill master develops his or her own specific spice blends and you should, too. Salt (kosher), sugar (light brown), and black pepper (fresh cracked, please!) are good starting points, but from there you can tweak however you see fit. Cumin, chili powder, and cayenne pepper have become common constituents in the American spice rack, but to really turn up the heat on your food, try out new grill-friendly spices: crushed fennel seed for pork; cracked coriander on meaty fish fillets like mahi-mahi; ground chipotle or ancho powder for steaks. Make big batches of spice rubs to have on hand at all times; covered, they keep in your cabinet for up to 3 months. (Check out a few of our favorite rubs at the end of this chapter.)

Over time, spices' essential oils fade, and with them goes the flavor you're looking (and paying) for. To avoid the outrageous markup on bottled spices, refresh your rack at stores like Whole Foods and ethnic markets where you can buy spices from bulk containers that allow you to control for quantity. Fifteen grams of cardamom or cumin or coriander will cost you about a quarter of what a normal supermarket charges for a small bottle and will last for months. Plus, high turnover ensures you're getting potent spices—not something that's been sitting on a shelf since the Reagan era.

Create Your Own Sauces.

Sauces are kitchen game-changers, capable of lifting mediocre meals to heroic heights. But why pay $5 for a bottled sauce made primarily with high-fructose corn syrup when high-quality sauces can be improvised on the spot from common pantry items? The important thing is to always think about balance when making a sauce: If it's too spicy, a hit of sweetness will help cool things off; if it's too salty, a splash of acid from vinegar or citrus will cut through the sodium and liven the sauce up. Mix and match members from each major flavor group below and it's hard to go wrong.

SWEET: Ketchup, honey, brown sugar, molasses, maple syrup, hoisin

SALTY: Soy sauce, Worcestershire, fish sauce, miso paste, peanut butter

SOUR: Vinegar (red or white wine, balsamic, rice wine, or apple cider are your best bets), lemon, lime, orange

SPICY: Dijon mustard, chipotle peppers, cayenne pepper, Tabasco, chili sauces like sriracha

Thickness is paramount. You want a sauce that's substantial enough to cling to meat and fish but not so thick that it's gloppy or smothering. Shoot for the consistency of ranch dressing. Keep in mind when applying sauces that sugars burn quickly, so if you have a particularly sweet sauce, or a large piece of meat that will take time to cook, don't apply the sauce until the final stage of cooking. For more on improvising first-rate sauces, check out the Sauce Matrix on page 218.

Mop Up the Competition.

This one comes straight from the competitive barbecue circuit, where pitmasters are desperate for tricks and techniques that will help them stand out in a crowded field. Mopping is essentially basting over an open flame, the constant application of liquid helping to soften tough connective tissue as well as adding a layer of flavor to the final product.

Mops can be made from just about any liquid imaginable—beer, booze, vinegar, oil, juice—usually accompanied by a few supporting cast members to help build flavor. You can buy a special mopping tool from barbecue stores, but save your money and just use a brush instead. Generally speaking, mops are best reserved for bigger cuts of meat like whole chickens, brisket, and pork shoulder, but that doesn't mean individual servings of meat and fish wouldn't also benefit from the same treatment. Here are a few of our favorite mops:

FOR BEEF: 1 (12 oz) Guinness draught, 2 Tbsp Worcestershire sauce, 2 Tbsp honey

FOR PORK: 1 cup cider vinegar, ½ cup vegetable or canola oil, Tabasco to taste

FOR CHICKEN: 1 cup orange juice, ½ cup vegetable or canola oil, 2 cloves minced garlic, 2 Tbsp chipotle pepper puree, 1 Tbsp dried oregano

Grill This *and* That!

If all you're cooking on that big, hot surface are a couple of steaks or chicken breasts, then you're wasting a lot of heat—and an easy opportunity to cook the rest of your meal at the same time. It's a time-crunching, money-saving measure that will not only help lower your monthly gas or electric bills, but also open up your grill repertoire to a world of new flavors.

Next time you have a pork chop or sirloin or salmon fillet to cook, plan at least one other element of your meal around the grill. Skewers of mixed vegetables are just a starting point: You can also sear lettuce for salads (yes, firm heads of lettuce like romaine love a bit of face time with the grill—check out the Sizzling Caesar Salad on page 286), roast oysters for appetizers, or grill fruit for dessert. With a bit of practice, the only time you'll need to head inside is to fetch another drink.

The Backyard
BUILDING
BLOCKS

Use these versatile sauces, salsas, dressings, and rubs to instantly elevate your grilling game.

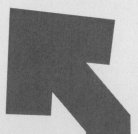

Classic Barbecue Sauce

Forget the high-fructose corn syrup–laden supermarket sauces: You have everything you need for a killer batch of homemade sauce in your pantry. Consider this your barbecue-sauce blueprint; from here, you can adjust with ingredients like molasses, honey, beer, hot sauce, or anything else that excites your taste buds.

You'll Need:

2 Tbsp butter
1 small onion, minced
1 cup ketchup
2 Tbsp brown sugar
2 Tbsp apple cider vinegar
1 Tbsp Worcestershire sauce
½ Tbsp dry mustard
½ tsp paprika (preferably smoked)
½ tsp garlic powder
⅛ tsp cayenne
Black pepper to taste

How to Make It:

In a medium saucepan, melt the butter over low heat. Add the onion and sauté until soft and translucent. Stir in the ketchup, brown sugar, vinegar, Worcestershire, mustard, paprika, garlic powder, cayenne, and a few pinches of black pepper. Simmer over low heat for 15 minutes until you have a thick, uniform sauce.

Makes about 1½ cups; keeps in the refrigerator for up to 2 weeks.

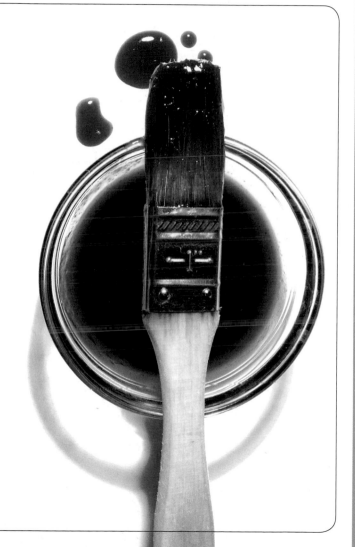

NC Vinegar Sauce

In eastern North Carolina, barbecue means finely chopped whole hog dressed in a spicy vinegar-based sauce. It's a distinctive flavor used to cut through the intensity of the smoked pork without masking its flavor the way thicker barbecue sauces do. It's our favorite way to eat pulled pork.

You'll Need:

2 cups apple cider vinegar
½ Tbsp red pepper flakes
1 Tbsp sugar
1 Tbsp hot sauce
Salt and black pepper to taste

How to Make It:

Combine all of the ingredients in a sauce pan over low heat. Heat until the sugar dissolves. (You can also heat this in the microwave for 30 seconds.) Cool completely before using.

Makes about 2 cups; keeps for 2 weeks in the refrigerator.

SC Mustard Sauce

Cross the border into South Carolina and suddenly pulled pork is served with a mustard sheen. Barbecue hounds will debate which is better until pigs fly, but there's only one person's opinion that matters: yours. This sharp sauce also goes well on grilled chicken and smoked baby back ribs.

You'll Need:

1 cup yellow mustard
    cup ketchup
¼ cup light brown sugar
2 Tbsp apple cider vinegar
Pinch cayenne pepper
Black pepper to taste

How to Make It:

Combine the ingredients in a sauce pan over low heat. Heat until the sugar dissolves. (You can also heat this in the microwave for 30 seconds.) Cool completely before using.

Makes about 1 cup; keeps for 2 weeks in the refrigerator.

Pico de Gallo

This chunky, fresh tomato salsa comes together with about 3 minutes' worth of knife work, yet it adds a complex trio of sweet, heat, and acid to everything from sandwiches to grilled fish.

You'll Need:

2 lb Roma tomatoes, seeded and chopped
1 small red onion, diced
1 jalapeño pepper, seeded and minced
½ cup chopped cilantro
Juice of 1 lime
Salt to taste

How to Make It:

Combine the tomatoes, onion, jalapeño, cilantro, and lime juice in a mixing bowl. Season with salt.

Makes about 3 cups; keeps for 3 days in the refrigerator.

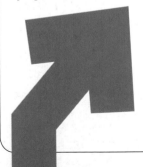

Grilled Chipotle-Lime Salsa

This is a smoky, spicy, all-purpose salsa, great on any of the Mexican-inspired recipes in the book (fish tacos, fajitas, etc.) or, of course, with a bag of tortilla chips.

You'll Need:

1½ lb Roma tomatoes, halved and seeded
2 (¼"-thick) slices from a medium red onion, skewered with a toothpick
Juice of 1 lime
1 clove garlic, minced
1 chipotle pepper
½ cup chopped cilantro
Salt to taste

How to Make It:

Preheat a grill or grill pan over high heat. When hot, grill the tomatoes and onion, turning, for about 10 minutes, until both are lightly charred and the tomato skins are blistered. Combine the tomatoes and onion in a blender or food processor along with the lime juice, garlic, and chipotle pepper and pulse for 10 seconds, until pureed but not perfectly smooth. Stir in the cilantro and season with salt.

Makes about 2 cups;
keeps in the refrigerator for up to 10 days.

Mango Salsa

This is deceptively simple to make for something that tastes so good. Especially awesome with blackened fish and chicken. Try folding in a cubed avocado for a tasty, creamy-sweet dynamic.

You'll Need:

2 fresh mangoes, peeled, seeded, and diced
1 small red onion, minced
½ cup chopped cilantro
1 jalapeño pepper, seeded and minced
Juice of 1 lime
Salt to taste

How to Make It:

Combine the mangoes, onion, cilantro, jalapeño, and lime juice in a mixing bowl. Season with salt.

Makes about 2 cups;
keeps in the refrigerator for up to 3 days.

Chimichurri

Chimichurri, an herb-based sauce from Argentina, is used to adorn and enhance a variety of different dishes—grilled meats and fish above all. After some careful reflection, we've decided that chimi is pretty much the world's greatest condiment, turning mediocre food good and making good food great. Once you make it, you'll have a hard time not painting it on everything you come across: sandwiches, grilled vegetables, eggs.

You'll Need:

2 Tbsp water
½ tsp salt
1 cup fresh parsley leaves, finely chopped
3 Tbsp red wine vinegar
2 cloves garlic, minced
Pinch red pepper flakes
3 Tbsp olive oil

How to Make It:

Combine the water and salt in a bowl and microwave for 30 seconds. Stir until the salt thoroughly dissolves, then mix in the parsley, vinegar, garlic, and pepper flakes. Slowly drizzle in the olive oil, whisking to incorporate. You can use the chimichurri now, but it's best to let the flavors marry for 20 minutes or more.

Makes about 1 cup;
keeps in the fridge for 3 days.

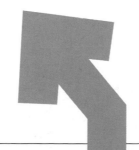

Grill This!

Peanut Sauce

Spicy peanut sauce is a vital grill staple throughout Southeast Asia. Classically, it doubles as a marinade and a dip for skewers of grilled chicken—but beef, pork, and shrimp all take well to its rich, spicy embrace.

You'll Need:

1 can (13.5 oz) light coconut milk
¾ cup creamy peanut butter
¾ cup sugar
2 Tbsp Thai red curry paste
2 Tbsp apple cider vinegar or white vinegar
1 Tbsp soy sauce
1 Tbsp minced fresh ginger
½ cup water
Juice of 1 lime

How to Make It:

Combine the coconut milk, peanut butter, sugar, curry paste, vinegar, soy sauce, ginger, and water in a medium saucepan. Simmer over low heat, stirring occasionally, for 10 minutes. Remove from heat and add the lime juice. Allow to cool completely before using.

Makes about 2 cups; keeps in the fridge for up to 1 week.

Green Sauce

Inspired by the epic Peruvian chicken restaurants of Northern Virginia, this all-purpose sauce is good slathered on sandwiches, drizzled over thick-sliced tomatoes, and used as a dip for grilled shrimp. And, of course, served alongside pieces of juicy grilled chicken.

You'll Need:

1 cup cilantro
Juice of 2 limes
¼ cup mayonnaise
¼ cup plain Greek yogurt
1 jalapeño pepper, stem removed (if you want a less incendiary sauce, remove the seeds as well)
2 cloves garlic, chopped

How to Make It:

Combine the cilantro, lime juice, mayonnaise, yogurt, jalapeño, and garlic in a food processor. Pulse until the ingredients form a smooth, light green puree.

Makes about 1½ cups; keeps in the fridge for up to 1 week.

Tzatziki

Though this Greek-style yogurt sauce matches perfectly with a charred lamb chop, it also can—and should—be applied to grilled chicken, pork, and fish on a regular basis.

You'll Need:

1 cucumber, peeled, halved, and seeded
1 cup plain Greek yogurt (we like Fage)
Juice of 1 lemon
2 Tbsp olive oil
2 cloves garlic, finely minced
2 tsp minced fresh dill
Salt and black pepper to taste

How to Make It:

Grate the cucumber with a cheese grater, then use your (clean!) hands to wring out all the excess water. Combine the cucumber with the yogurt, lemon juice, olive oil, garlic, dill, and a good pinch each of salt and pepper.

Makes about 1½ cups; keeps in the fridge for 5 days.

Honey-Dijon Vinaigrette

This is not just a great all-purpose salad dressing, it's also an easy way to brighten up slices of grilled chicken or a plate of asparagus.

You'll Need:

1 shallot, minced
¼ cup red or white wine vinegar
½ Tbsp Dijon mustard
½ Tbsp honey
½ cup olive oil
Salt and black pepper to taste

How to Make It:

Combine the shallot and vinegar in a mixing bowl and let sit for 10 minutes. Stir in the Dijon and honey, then slowly drizzle in the olive oil, whisking to fully blend the oil and vinegar into a uniform dressing. Season with salt and pepper.

Makes about 1 cup; keeps in the refrigerator for up to 1 week.

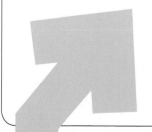

Pesto

You can buy perfectly fine pesto in the refrigerated section of most supermarkets (we like Cibo), but it will never taste as good as a homemade batch—which, by the way, takes all of 3 minutes to make. It works equally well as a marinade as it does for a post-grill dipping sauce. To keep it extra fresh and green, float a thin layer of oil on top of the pesto before refrigerating—the oil will keep the basil from oxidizing and turning dark. Try substituting arugula for the basil for a peppery alternative.

You'll Need:

2 cloves garlic, chopped
2 Tbsp pine nuts
3 cups fresh basil leaves
¼ cup grated Parmesan
Salt and black pepper to taste
½ cup olive oil

How to Make It:

Place the garlic, pine nuts, basil, and Parmesan, plus a few pinches of salt and pepper, in a food processor. Pulse until the basil is chopped. With the motor running, slowly drizzle in the olive oil until fully incorporated and a paste forms.

Makes about 1 cup; keeps for 2 weeks in the refrigerator.

Guacamole

Many American versions of guacamole include ingredients like cumin, sour cream, and (gasp!) mayo. But guac is really at its best with just a few carefully balanced ingredients: garlic (preferably chopped into an oily paste), a good pinch of salt, and a squeeze of lemon or lime. And of course, perfectly ripe Hass avocados. Use that as your base; everything else—onion, jalapeño, cilantro, tomato—is just a bonus.

You'll Need:

2 cloves garlic, peeled
Kosher salt to taste
¼ cup minced red onion
1 Tbsp minced jalapeño
2 ripe avocados, pitted and peeled
Juice of 1 lemon or lime
Chopped fresh cilantro (optional)

How to Make It:

Use the side of a knife to smash the garlic against the cutting board. Finely mince the cloves, then apply a pinch of salt to the garlic and use the side of your knife to work the garlic into a paste (the salt will act as an abrasive). Scoop the garlic into a bowl, then add the onion, jalapeño, and avocado and mash until the avocado is pureed, but still slightly chunky. Stir in the lemon juice, cilantro (if using), and salt to taste.

Makes about 2 cups; keeps in the refrigerator for 2 days.

Grill This!

Grilled Garlic

Raw garlic can be harsh and overpowering. Overcooked garlic can be acrid and off-putting. But slow-cooked garlic, roasted over the open flame of the grill, is like savory candy—sweet and inviting with its mellow garlic flavor. Fold into sauces or salad dressings (especially Caesar), or simply spread on slices of grilled bread, perhaps with a bit of crumbled goat cheese and a drizzle of olive oil.

You'll Need:
1 head garlic
Olive oil for coating

How to Make It:
Preheat a grill over medium heat. Use a sharp knife to cut off the very top of the garlic head, revealing just the tips of the individual garlic cloves. Place the head in the center of a piece of aluminum foil, drizzle with a bit of oil, then fold the foil to enclose the garlic. Place on the grill and cook, lid closed, for about 30 minutes, until the cloves are very soft and lightly caramelized.

To use the garlic, simply squeeze the bottom of the bulb until the soft individual cloves pop out.

Keeps in the refrigerator for up to 1 week.

Romesco

This Catalan condiment is used throughout Spain as a dip for vegetables and a sauce for grilled meats and fish. It's at its best when served alongside lightly charred asparagus spears, tuna steaks, or a few slices of sirloin.

You'll Need:
3 Tbsp olive oil
2 slices bread, torn into small pieces
2 Tbsp chopped almonds
2 cloves garlic, chopped
1 tsp smoked paprika
½ (12 oz) jar roasted red peppers
1 Tbsp red wine vinegar or sherry vinegar
Salt and black pepper to taste

How to Make It:
Heat 1 tablespoon of the olive oil in a medium sauté pan set over medium heat. Add the bread crumbs, almonds, garlic, and paprika and sauté for about 5 minutes, until the bread is lightly golden and crunchy. Transfer to a blender and add the remaining 2 tablespoons olive oil, the red peppers, vinegar, and a sprinkle of salt and pepper; puree until smooth. The romesco should have the texture of apple sauce; if you need to thin it out, stir in a tablespoon or two of water.

Makes about 1½ cups; keeps in the refrigerator for up to 1 week.

All-Purpose Barbecue Rub

Nearly all competitive barbecue teams have their own special spice blend, used for smoked chickens and racks of ribs and whole pork shoulders. This one is ours.

You'll Need:
¼ cup brown sugar
¼ cup salt
2 Tbsp paprika (preferably smoked paprika)
2 Tbsp black pepper
1 Tbsp garlic powder
1 Tbsp cumin
1 tsp cayenne

How to Make It:
Mix all of the spices together in a bowl or plastic storage container.

Makes about ¾ cup; keeps in your spice cabinet for up to 2 months.

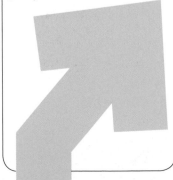

Southwestern Rub

Smoke and fire combine in this Tex-Mex-style spice blend, a perfect one-two punch for pork tenderloins, chicken legs, and skirt steak. Use about 1 tablespoon for every pound of meat (the same ratio functions for the other rubs here as well).

You'll Need:
1 Tbsp salt
1 Tbsp black pepper
1 Tbsp smoked paprika
1 Tbsp ancho or chipotle chile powder
½ Tbsp ground cumin
¼ Tbsp garlic powder
⅓ tsp cayenne pepper

How to Make It:
Mix all of the spices together in a bowl or plastic storage container.

Makes about 6 tablespoons; keeps in your spice cabinet for up to 2 months.

Moroccan Spice Rub

Rub this on a leg of lamb and grill it until it's tender and juicy and you'll be transported to the markets of Marrakesh. Or coat a fillet of salmon or halibut with this blend and serve it over a heap of steamed couscous.

You'll Need:
1 Tbsp paprika
1 Tbsp cumin seeds, roughly chopped, or 1 Tbsp ground cumin
1 Tbsp coriander seeds, roughly chopped, or 1 Tbsp ground coriander
½ Tbsp black peppercorns
1 tsp cinnamon
1 tsp ground nutmeg
¼ tsp cayenne pepper

How to Make It:
Mix all of the spices together in a bowl or plastic storage container.

Makes about ¼ cup; keeps in your spice cabinet for up to 2 months.

Magic Blackening Rub

Coat meat, fish, or vegetables with this potent blend of seasonings and cook over high heat until it transforms into a dark, savory crust.

You'll Need:
1 Tbsp paprika
1 Tbsp salt
2 tsp black pepper
2 tsp ground cumin
2 tsp garlic powder
2 tsp onion powder
1 tsp dried oregano
½ tsp cayenne pepper

How to Make It:
Mix all of the spices together in a bowl or plastic storage container.

Makes about ⅓ cup; keeps in your spice cabinet for up to 2 months.

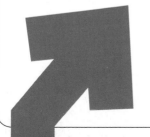

THE GRILL MASTER'S GEAR GUIDE

GRILL
THIS
NOT
THAT!

The Grill Master's GEAR GUIDE

Imagine going in for heart surgery and discovering once you're on the table that there are none of those precise scalpels and flashy medical tools on hand; all the doctor has to work with is a dull pocketknife and a bottle of whiskey to ease the pain (his).

Or imagine you've been invited to a rock concert, only to discover that there are no Marshall amps or Stratocasters to be found; the only instruments the band has are a half-dozen kazoos, a rusty cowbell, and a gallon drum of Justin Bieber's hair gel.

Not good, right?

It doesn't matter if your heart's in the hands of Dr. Oz or if your ears are in the hands of Ozzy Osbourne—without the right tools, even the most skilled medicine man can't heal; without the right instruments, even the wildest rocker can't rock.

And even the best chef can't cook.

It doesn't matter if you're some wild genetic mix of Mario Batali, Julia Child, and the Hamburglar; you're not going to be able to whip up a great meal—and strip away a great deal of calories—without the right tools.

Fortunately, we've tried, tested, and accidentally tipped over just about every kind of grill on the planet, as well as the myriad accoutrements of the grill game. So whether you're a weeknight warrior or a total grill geek, this comprehensive guide highlights the best equipment for every type of cook.

SEAR Factor

Whether you're a weeknight warrior or a fair-weather griller, this comprehensive guide highlights the best equipment for every type of cook.

If you've spent any time shopping for grills, then you understand the frustration. What was once little more than a metal clamshell with gridiron teeth has grown to resemble a Michael Bay creation outfitted with multiple burners, drawers, knobs, and levers. Some of those accessories might serve you well, but they can just as easily blind you from the basic goal of finding a grill that cooks honest food without bleeding your bank account dry. Ultimately the grill you buy should fit your needs and lifestyle, and this guide is designed to help you match your personality to your equipment. With the right grill, you'll be more likely to cook the recipes in this book, and that's your first step toward a leaner, tastier lifestyle.

30
Percentage of grillers who own more than one grill

53
Percentage of grill owners who cook out at least a few times per week during the grilling season

31
Percentage of grill owners who cook out more than they did the previous year because "they're trying to eat healthier"

THE NATURALIST

You don't mind getting your hands dirty, and when you go camping, you're the one tossing logs on the fire. Your pantry contains no pre-sweetened oatmeal packages, and you'd rather eat beans from a can than microwave a frozen dinner. For you, grilling is an art and, for the most part, you'd rather invest a little extra time than risk a subpar meal.

The Grill Type: CHARCOAL

Charcoal grills have three things going for them: They're cheap, they generate high heat, and they give your food a more pronounced smoky flavor. The downsides are that charcoal is messy and you have to factor in 20 minutes to heat the grill. What's more, studies indicate that by burning fat, charcoal grills are responsible for creating more carcinogenic polycyclic aromatic hydrocarbons (PAHs). You can reduce your risk by trimming fat and marinating (the acids in marinade further reduce carcinogens).

Make the Most of It: When building a charcoal fire, always have a hot zone and a cool zone. The hot zone should have 75 to 100 percent of the charcoal collected on its side of the grill. And the zone should occupy the same space on the grill every time, that way you know instinctually where you can sear steaks and where you can move a chicken leg that's burning because of flare-ups.

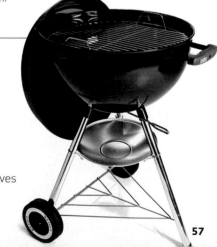

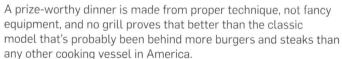

OUR PICKS

WEBER ONE-TOUCH SILVER 18.5"
$79, Weber.com
A prize-worthy dinner is made from proper technique, not fancy equipment, and no grill proves that better than the classic model that's probably been behind more burgers and steaks than any other cooking vessel in America.

CHAR-GRILLER OUTLAW
$159, CharGriller.com
More than 1,000 square inches of hot gridiron spread over two shelves makes this the best value for high-volume grilling. Plus the elongated barrel makes it easy to bank coals for indirect cooking.

THE PRAGMATIST

To you, grilling should be every bit as convenient as other methods of cooking. Sure you enjoy the sizzle of a steak against hot iron, but you have no intention of planning your day around a meal. You want to cook, eat, and get on with life.

The Grill Type: GAS

Barbecue buffs often belittle gas grills for producing food they deem inferior. They argue that gas doesn't generate smoky flavors, and that the grates of the gridiron rarely get hot enough for a proper sear. But today's gas grills are more powerful, versatile, and affordable than ever, capable of charring a chicken breast and slow-cooking a pork shoulder with nearly equal ease. Cooking on a gas grill is quicker and cleaner than the charcoal alternative, and if that's what it takes to keep you grilling, then by all means crank the propane.

Make the Most of It: There's no smoke better than that from wood chips, and you don't need charcoal for that. Wood-chip boxes and planks are both viable options (see pages 68 and 69), but for something even more low-tech, wrap a handful of soaked wood chips in aluminum foil and puncture it several times with a fork (to let the smoke escape). Place it over the flame before you cook and you'll notice a serious upgrade in the flavor of your food.

OUR PICKS

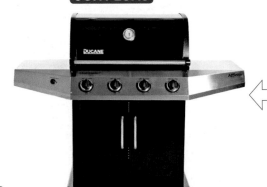

CHARBROIL K6B 6-BURNER GAS GRILL (with side burner)
$375, Charbroil.com
You won't find another grill with this combination of power and surface area for under $500.

DUCANE AFFINITY 4100
$410, Ducane.com
In a *Men's Health* field test, the Affinity 4100 heated twice as quickly as more expensive propane grills. Credit the burners' 48,000 BTUs of heating power.

THE GRILL GEEK

The perfect caramel-colored shell of a steakhouse rib eye gives you goose bumps, but you're equally impressed by the fall-from-the bone tenderness of slow-cooked ribs. In general you leave little to chance, and you approach grilling as equal parts science and art.

The Grill Type: CERAMIC

The hefty price tag keeps most people away from a ceramic grill—especially considering that most of the models appear to be little more than rudimentary orbs with vents at top. But don't be misled: These grills provide optimal control over cooking temperature, capable of holding a sirloin-searing 700°F heat just as steadily as a pulled-pork-perfect 250°F. They're also more efficient and durable than steel grills, and because they lock in heat so well, the outer surface remains cooler to the touch.

Make the Most of It: Stick with natural lump charcoal. Fumes from lighter fluid—soaked briquettes can linger and give subsequent meals a chemical-like aftertaste. And once the coals are lit, use the top and bottom vents to control temperature. Wide-open vents increase airflow for a warmer fire, while barely open vents create the lower temperatures necessary for slow-cooking barbecue.

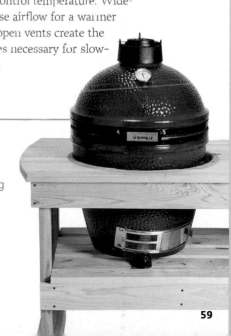

OUR PICKS

BIG GREEN EGG
$750 for a medium model with stand
($633.29 for the egg, $121.95 for the stand), BigGreenEgg.com
Egg Heads worship at the altar of this funky green grill, swearing by its ability to do it all, from searing to smoking. The medium-size model offers 177 square inches of cooking space, while the pricier extra-large model goes up to 452 inches.

PRIMO OVAL XL
$1,099, PrimoGrill.com
It's the only ceramic charcoal grill made entirely in America, and it features a massive 680-square-inch cooking surface.

THE HOST

"The more, the merrier" is an expression you use often, and when you grill, you expect neighbors, family, and friends to swing by. You think food should be the main attraction at a good party, and you're entirely comfortable commanding a grill with a beer in one hand and an 18-inch spatula in the other.

The Grill Type:
MULTI-FUNCTION

This is the Swiss Army knife of grills, complete with multiple burners and all the gadgetry necessary to prep sides and appetizers. If you're willing to invest the money, the drawbacks here are few— many multi-function grills provide all the amenities of a kitchen aside from the sink and dishwasher. But here's our advice for shopping on a budget: Don't sacrifice quality for extra bells and whistles. You're better with one really strong burner than half a dozen weak ones.

Make the Most of It: Don't neglect the side burner. Use it to warm beans, roast brussels sprouts, or fry bacon. Keep a sauce on simmer and it will thicken while your steak cooks, or sauté onions and peppers for instant fajitas. Think of the extra hot pad as the ideal alternative for anything that doesn't cook well on the grill.

OUR PICKS

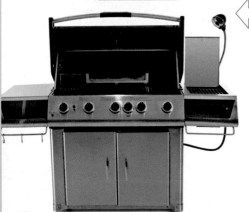

VERMONT CASTINGS 501 SIGNATURE SERIES GRILL
$2,199, VermontCastings.com
You can buy bigger, brasher, pricier grills, but with Vermont Castings' combination of power, versatility, and special features, we're not sure why you would want to. High-quality cast-iron grates, a built-in smoker box, and a 20,000-BTU rotisserie burner make this one of the best grills on the market today.

WEBER GENESIS E-330
$819, Weber.com
The porcelain-enameled cast-iron grates create even distribution for the 38,000 BTUs of heat coming off the main burners and 12,000 BTUs on the side.

THE GRILL DISCIPLE

You bow down at the altar of barbecue. Your fixation on smoky, tender meat borders on religious, and more than once you've traveled out of your way in pursuit of perfect barbecue. You are patient about grilling—perhaps even Zen-like—and you're willing to rise before the sun to begin prepping an evening feast with friends.

The Grill Type: SMOKER

A smoker is easily the best option for daylong cooking projects, and the meat it produces is more tender than anything you'll cook on a traditional grill. That said, if you're not committed to planning entire days—and sometimes weekends—around a cookout, then you're probably better off with a basic gas or charcoal grill.

Make the Most of It: The low, slow heat of the smoker works best on large pieces of meat—think ribs, brisket, pork shoulder, a whole chicken. But when you go to purchase wood, beware of the price gouge. Many stores will charge you a few bucks for a couple handfuls of wood chips, and you'll probably need a couple bags just for one big job. Look for better prices at your local lumberyard. If they don't sell wood chips in bulk, save some cash by purchasing untreated cedar and chopping or slicing it into chunks.

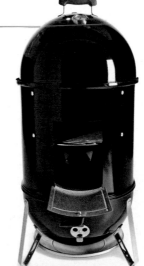

OUR PICKS

BRINKMANN PROFESSIONAL CHARCOAL GRILL
$380, Brinkmann.net
Constructed entirely of steel, the Brinkmann Pro is a tank among grills, and it's the best solution for grillers who want to dabble with smoke. The side-mounted chamber functions as a smoker box, but also works to cook smaller meals while using less charcoal or wood.

WEBER SMOKEY MOUNTAIN COOKER ⇨
$299, Weber.com
Smoking made simple: The Smokey's bullet-shaped housing holds two 18.5-inch gridirons, a top mounted thermostat, and an easy-access door for adding water and wood chips without letting all that precious heat escape.

THE TRAVELER

Your Coleman cooler gets more use than your DVD player, and your weekends are reserved for camping, tailgating, and family gatherings in the park. You're not fussy about food, but when it comes down to it, you'd much rather eat a hand-pressed burger hot off the grill than a prefab factory burger coming at you through a drive-thru window.

The Grill Type: PORTABLE

The upside is obvious: These grills go wherever you want them to. They also store easily in the closet, so they're great for people who don't have dedicated outdoor space for grill storage. That said, a grill that's built to travel is certainly not going to provide the biggest cooking area, and you won't find one that gets as hot as a well-built standing model.

Make the Most of It: Find the grill that best suits your needs. If it's too small you won't be able to use it, and if it's too big you won't want to lug it around. Our favorite models are those that maximize gridiron surface area without being overly bulky, and we appreciate firmly attaching lids that make them easy to carry.

OUR PICKS

LODGE LOGIC SPORTSMAN GRILL
$140, Lodgemfg.com
This throwback hibachi-style grill sports thick cast-iron grates that can sear a steak better than most full-size grills. It's heavy, but also small enough to fit in your fireplace for rainy-day grilling.

WEBER GO-ANYWHERE CHARCOAL GRILL
$50, Weber.com
The rectangular design makes good use of surface area, and when you travel, the grill's legs fold over the lid to hold it firmly in place. It's available in both charcoal and gas models.

THE WEEKNIGHT WARRIOR

Sure, you'd grill outside every day if you could. But that's not happening with your schedule. You barely have time to cook, let alone keep a grill clean and shuffle food in and out of the house as you slog over to the Weber. You're okay sacrificing barbecue's smoky flavor so long as you can still preserve some of the magic of the grill.

The Grill Type: GRILL PAN

Technically it's not a grill, but it does mimic some of the effects. The grill pan's running grooves create authentic-looking grill marks, and they allow some fat to drip out. That's ideal for thin cuts of steak, burgers, and pork chops, but it's useless if you're tying to obtain the indirect heat needed for ribs or brisket.

Make the Most of It: A panini press goes for about $150, but a good grill pan can produce the same crispy, melty sandwiches for no extra cost to speak off. Set the grill pan over medium heat, stack your bread with meat, cheese, and vegetables

(we suggest grilled chicken, roasted peppers, and fresh mozzarella for your maiden panini voyage), then use a light weight to press the sandwiches down; a pot filled with a bit of water works perfectly. Once the first side is crisp, flip the sandwiches and repeat.

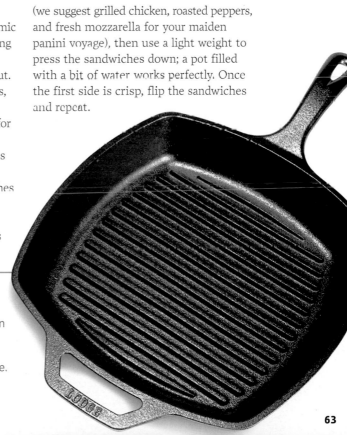

OUR PICK

LODGE LOGIC SQUARE GRILL PAN
$30.95, Lodgemfg.com
There are plenty of nonstick grill pans on the market, but nothing handles high temperature as well as cast iron. And nobody makes cast iron as well as Lodge. Consider this the closest thing to a grill that fits into your cupboard.

USE THIS,
Not That!

The essential
tool kit for the
savvy griller

To Build the Fire

Use This!

**NATURAL LUMP
CHARCOAL**

OUR PICK

BIG GREEN EGG NATURAL LUMP CHARCOAL
$27.99 for a 20-lb bag, bbqislandinc.com

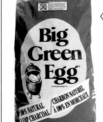

Not That!

**BRIQUETTES
(like from
Kingsford)**

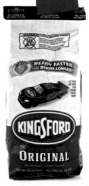

Lump charcoal is a simple product created by burning wood
in the absence of oxygen. Briquettes, on the other hand,
are bound together with starch, laced with lime,
and often soaked in lighter fluid. Lump coal may cost a little
more, but for our dollar, it's worth the extra money.
Among the many reasons the world's greatest pitmasters
choose lumps over briquettes: They light faster, provide
better temperature control, and produce less ash to clean.

*To test your grill
heat, place your
hand 3 inches
above the grilling
surface and
count, "One
Mississippi, two
Mississippi…"
until you have
to pull away.
Less than
3 Mississippis is
high heat; 5 to
6 is medium;
10 to 12 is low.*

To Light the Grill

Use This! | Not That!

CHIMNEY | **LIGHTER FLUID**

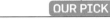

OUR PICK

WEBER RAPIDFIRE CHIMNEY STARTER
$17.99, Weber.com

Lighter fluid is a petroleum-derived chemical, but if that alone doesn't freak you out, pay close attention next time you eat food that was cooked over lighter fluid–soaked coals. Notice the tinge of a metallic, chemical aftertaste? That's the result of lighter fluid. No thanks. The speed, ease, and purity of chimney starters is slowly making lighter fluid a thing of the past, and we couldn't be happier. Pick one up on weber.com for $18.

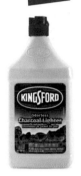

Stuff wadded paper—old newspaper is perfect—in the bottom of the chimney, and fill the top half with coals. Light the paper, and as it burns it will ignite the coals above. When they begin to glow, slowly lift the chimney off the grill. Angle the mouth of the chimney down toward the grill, give it a shake, and the hot coals will spill out into your grill. Now start cookin'.

To Tenderize the Meat

Use This! | Not That!

MEAT MALLET | **MEAT TENDERIZER WITH BLADES**

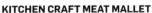

OUR PICK

KITCHEN CRAFT MEAT MALLET
$12.99, Amazon.com

The classic meat tenderizer, a metal mallet with a textured striking surface, is a perfect tool. But in an ill-conceived attempt to innovate, manufacturers have begun producing blade-style tenderizers: meat-mangling weapons that impale your steak with dozens of steel spikes. The result is a mushy hunk that falls somewhere between whole and ground meat. A few thwacks with the mallet (or failing that, a heavy pan) is all the tenderizing your steak needs.

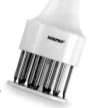

Avoid the packaged grill tool sets offered by so many companies these days. They're expensive and invariably include one or more tools you'll never use (like the dreaded fork). If forced to cook for the rest of our lives with only one tool, we'd take tongs, hands down.

To Flip the Steak

Use This!

Not That!

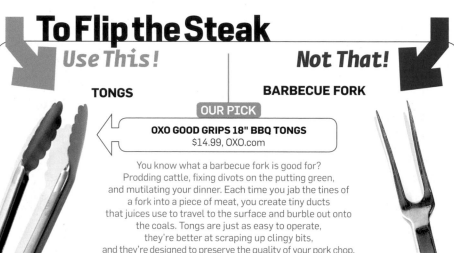

TONGS

BARBECUE FORK

> **OUR PICK**
> **OXO GOOD GRIPS 18" BBQ TONGS**
> $14.99, OXO.com

You know what a barbecue fork is good for?
Prodding cattle, fixing divots on the putting green,
and mutilating your dinner. Each time you jab the tines of
a fork into a piece of meat, you create tiny ducts
that juices use to travel to the surface and burble out onto
the coals. Tongs are just as easy to operate,
they're better at scraping up clingy bits,
and they're designed to preserve the quality of your pork chop.

To Spread the Sauce

Use This!

Not That!

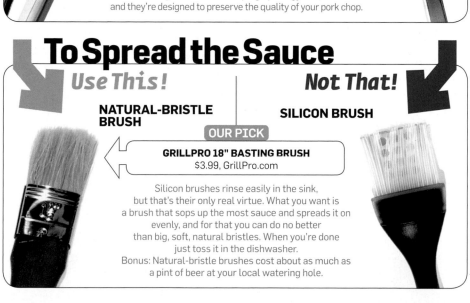

NATURAL-BRISTLE BRUSH

SILICON BRUSH

> **OUR PICK**
> **GRILLPRO 18" BASTING BRUSH**
> $3.99, GrillPro.com

Silicon brushes rinse easily in the sink,
but that's their only real virtue. What you want is
a brush that sops up the most sauce and spreads it on
evenly, and for that you can do no better
than big, soft, natural bristles. When you're done
just toss it in the dishwasher.
Bonus: Natural-bristle brushes cost about as much as
a pint of beer at your local watering hole.

To Roast the Chicken

Use This!

BEER CAN

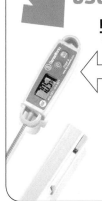

Not That!

VERTICAL CHICKEN ROASTER

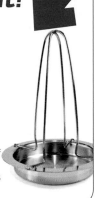

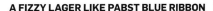

OUR PICK

A FIZZY LAGER LIKE PABST BLUE RIBBON

Sure you can buy fancy wire scaffolding to prop a chicken up on your grill, but what's the point? It's just one more bulky piece of equipment taking up space in your cupboard. Besides, a beer can is better since it serves both to prop up the chicken and to provide a moist cooking environment. Simply crack open the can, drink half of the suds, then lodge the can in the open cavity of the chicken. Now use the protruding end of the beer can as a stand. Your bird remains upright and stays moist from beer simmering inside.

To Test the Doneness

Use This!

MEAT THERMOMETER

Not That!

KNIFE

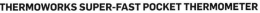

OUR PICK

THERMOWORKS SUPER-FAST POCKET THERMOMETER
$24, ThermoWorks.com

Slicing open a steak to peek inside will give you a good indication of doneness, but it will also decimate an otherwise pristine piece of meat. So do like the pros and use a thermometer. Touch and appearance can serve as rough indicators, but ultimately it's the internal temperature that determines the doneness of meat. For more on how to know when your meat is perfectly cooked, see "Is It Done Yet?" on page 70.

Thermometers run the price and tech spectrum, from $4 basic probes to instant thermometers that would make Steve Jobs proud. Our favorite of the high-end camp is Taylor's Waterproof Dual Temperature Thermacouple and Infrared Thermometer, which measures up to 626°F in one second. ($99; Taylorusa.com)

5 KILLER Grill Gadgets

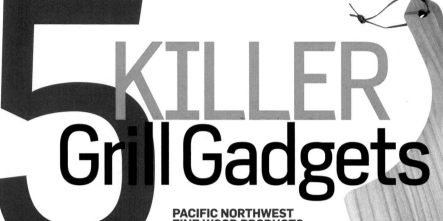

PACIFIC NORTHWEST FINE WOOD PRODUCTS CEDAR BARBECUE PLANKS

Set of 6, $17.95

PacificNorthwestPlanks.com

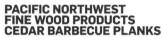

Even easier than a wood-chip box? Planks—slices of wood that you set directly on the grill with steaks or fish on top. Pacific Northwest's are thick enough to use a few times, but they'll still cost you more than the wood chips you load into a wood-chip box. Save some cash by asking your local lumberyard if they carry untreated cedar shingles. If they do, stock up. You're essentially getting the same product for a fraction of the cost.

2 MR. BAR-B-Q PLATINUM PRESTIGE STAINLESS STEEL WOK TOPPER

$19.90, MrBarBQ.com

Asparagus spears and portobello caps can go directly on the grill grates, but unless you want to lose smaller vegetables to the fire, you'll need some protection. This perforated grill basket exposes vegetables directly to the flames without the risk of sacrificing anything to the grill gods. Use it to cook chopped vegetables, roast the skins off small peppers, or add a nice char to green beans. Mr. Bar-B-Q backs this one with a lifetime warranty, but we're guessing you won't need it.

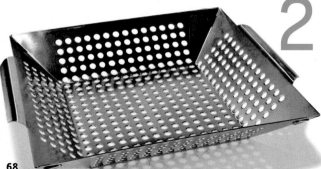

4

CHAR-BROIL CAST-IRON SMOKER BOX

$15.99, CharBroil.com
A wood-chip box is the easiest way to earn big smoky flavor without investing in a dedicated smoker grill. Just load it with soaked wood chips, set it over the flame, and let the smoke permeate your food. This cast-iron version from Char-Broil will handle the heat with ease and cost you less than a steakhouse rib eye.

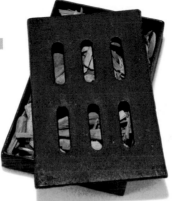

5 Gadgets to Avoid

1. BURGER PRESS
Pressing ground beef too firmly gives you tough, rubbery patties. For juicy burgers that melt in your mouth, there's no better compression contraption than two human hands.

2. SMOKING GUN
In order for smoke to permeate food, you need time and heat. Using a "gun" to blast smoke at a cooked brisket won't provide more than a fleeting scent.

3. RIB RACK
Propping your ribs vertically saves a little space on the grill, but you can achieve the same effect by wrapping them in aluminum foil and stacking them directly on the grill.

4. ROTISSERIE SHISH KEBAB WHEEL
A chicken is a large, tricky piece of meat that benefits from the rotation of a rotisserie. A kebab? Drop it on the grill, give it a good high-heat sear, and enjoy. Let's not make this fussy.

5. HOT DOG BASKET
A basket designed to holster your dogs while they cook. The purpose? We don't know either.

3

ITALIAN VILLA PIZZA PEEL

$14.99, Amazon.com
Several recipes in this book show you how to cook pizza directly on the grate of your grill, but transferring a pie on and off a hot gridiron can be tricky. Forgo the blistered knuckles by purchasing a pizza peel, the pie-shoveling device preferred by pros from New York to Naples. The price tag here is modest, and the stubby handle makes it ideal for grillwork.

5

CHARCOAL COMPANION 13" NONSTICK GRILLING KABOB SKEWERS

$6.98, Amazon.com
Skewers are perhaps the most underutilized of all cooking implements. They're the grilling equivalent of the one-pot meal, allowing you to balance a meal's worth of meats and vegetables on a single scrap of metal and requiring very little cleanup effort. Opt for metal over wood and you can skip the soaking step, and with flat skewers like these, you don't have to worry about foods spinning around and cooking unevenly.

Is It DONE Yet?

When it comes to grilling, it's the most important question of all. Here's how to get it right every time.

We've all been there before: You go down to the market, carefully pick out a beautiful piece of beef, shell out $15 a pound for it, and return home to lovingly cook it. But by the time you sit down to eat, it looks like a hockey puck and tastes like leather. You owe it to yourself, your dining mates, the butcher, and the cow to cook that steak as skillfully as possible.

To avoid any major grilling mishaps, it's essential to always have a thermometer on hand—especially for bigger cuts of meat. But with enough practice, you can turn your finger into a divining rod capable of properly judging steaks, burgers, and chops with a single touch. We've broken it down for you both ways, with the empirical data of doneness as well as the keys and clues that will help sharpen your tactile instincts.

Fish

Target Temperatures:
MEDIUM: 130°F
MEDIUM-WELL: 140°F
WELL-DONE: 170°F

The thickest part of any fish fillet should flake with gentle pressure from your fingertip. Or use this great chef trick: Insert a metal skewer (or the tip of a paring knife) into the thickest part of the fillet. After three seconds remove it and touch it to the base of your thumb (where the skin is especially sensitive). If it's warm to the touch, it's perfectly cooked; if it's hot, it's overdone. When cooking salmon, watch out for white spots that form on the surface; those deposits of coagulated protein mean your salmon is overcooked.

Shrimp

Target Temperatures:
SHRIMP ARE TOO SMALL FOR THERMOMETERS.

Shrimp go from raw to perfect to dry all in a matter of 3 minutes, so look alive! Luckily, there are a few visual clues to guide you:

The translucent flesh will turn the lightest shade of pink and the tails will begin to slowly curl inward. You want your shrimp to look more like Js than Cs, so once the tails begin to curl, they're done.

Pork

Target Temperatures:
MEDIUM: 145°F
MEDIUM-WELL: 155°F
WELL: 165°F

Great restaurants cook their pork to medium, with a light pink center, and if you know that your pork comes from a reputable source, you can follow suit. For those squeamish about seeing pink in their pork, aim to cook it to 155°F; go much above and you'll see why so many people complain about pork being dry.

Chicken

Target Temperatures:
MEDIUM-WELL: 155°F
WELL: 165°F

A perfectly cooked boneless,

skinless chicken breast will feel firm and bouncy to the touch, like a tennis ball. For chicken cooked on the bone, look for the juices that escape to run clear, meaning the last of the pink by the bones has been cooked off. If the meat on the drumstick begins to pull away from the bone, it probably means it's overcooked.

Beef and Lamb

Target Temperatures:
RARE: 125°F
MEDIUM-RARE: 135°F
MEDIUM: 145°F
MEDIUM-WELL: 155°F
WELL: 170°F

People's taste for red-meat temperature runs from nearly mooing to burnt to a crisp, so much of what you're looking for is a personal judgment call.

Some experts swear by the thumb method, which works by touching the tip of your thumb with the tips of your other fingers. As you work your way from index

finger to pinkie, the fleshy base of your thumb firms up, representing the various degrees of doneness. This method works for all meat.
Index Finger: RARE
Soft and squishy, like a pink sponge
Middle Finger: MEDIUM-RARE
Firm but yielding, like a Nerf football
Ring Finger: MEDIUM
Barely yielding, like a racquetball
Pinky Finger: WELL
Hard yet springy, like a tennis ball

Burgers
(Beef, Turkey, Etc)

Target Temperatures:
RARE: 125°F
MEDIUM-RARE: 135°F
MEDIUM: 150°F
MEDIUM-WELL: 155°F
WELL: 160°F

Burgers, especially ones made from lean cuts like sirloin or buffalo, are fickle creatures, going from juicy to arid in a matter of a minute. If it's the former you seek, the center of the burger should feel firm, but easily yield. Once the patty begins to feel springy, you've entered the medium-well stages of doneness.

GRILL
THIS
NOT
THAT!

BURGERS &
SANDWICHES

THE PERFECT
Grilled Burger

There are burgers, and then there are burgers, those juicy, beefy objects of our desire that linger around on our taste buds and our memories long after we've devoured them. What follows is the formula to ensure every burger you grill falls into the second camp. Use these tips and techniques for all the burgers in this chapter, and for all the burgers you make from this day forward.

Use only the freshest ground beef.

Ideally, that means grinding your own at home. If you have a KitchenAid mixer, you can buy a grinding attachment ($65), one of the greatest investments a burger hound can make. Make sure both the attachment and the beef are very cold before grinding on the coarsest setting. The easy alternative to grinding at home is asking the butcher to do it for you at the store. Purchase a whole chunk of brisket (or, failing that, chuck or sirloin) and ask him to grind it and wrap it up.

Don't overwork the meat.

The worst thing you can do to a burger, besides overcook it, is overpack it. No kneading, massaging, punching, or hard-packing necessary. Bring the meat loosely together, just enough to hold its shape, and leave it at that.

Salt at the last moment.

Salt the meat before you form the patties and the sodium chloride will work to break down protein strands, creating a dense texture closer to sausage than the loose, tender ideal you're looking for. Always salt your burgers seconds—not minutes—before grilling.

Cook the patties over a steady heat.

After testing a dozen different cooking methods, we came up with one clear path to juicy, medium-rare results: Form the patties and let them sit at room temperature for 15 minutes before cooking; in our tests, allowing the temperature of the chilled meat to rise made for more even cooking results. After 15 minutes, cook the burgers, with the lid up, over a medium flame—enough heat to give the patties a nice char, but not so much that you cook the outside before the center of the burger reaches a perfect pink.

You'll Need:

1 lb freshly ground brisket

Salt and black pepper to taste

4 slices American cheese

4 potato buns, lightly toasted

1 large, very ripe tomato

1 yellow onion, thinly sliced

Lettuce

Sliced pickles

- Form the beef into four equal patties, being careful not to overwork the meat. Allow the meat to sit at room temperature for at least 15 minutes before cooking (about as much time as it takes for the grill to heat up).

- Preheat a grill or grill pan over medium heat. Just before cooking, season the burgers all over with salt and pepper. Place on the grill and cook for 4 minutes, until light grill marks have developed. Flip the patties, cover with the cheese, and continue grilling for 3 to 4 minutes, until the center of a burger feels firm but yielding, like a Nerf football, and an instant-read thermometer inserted in the thickest part of a burger registers 135°F.

- Serve the burgers on the buns with tomato, onion, lettuce, pickles, and any other condiments you like. Makes 4 servings.

Grill This!
The Burger Matrix

Beef will always be our first love when it comes to burgers, but anything that can be formed into a patty and inserted in a bun has the potential to be something special. Turkey and salmon are two common alternatives, but ground chicken, tuna, bison, and lamb all can be shaped into out-standing burgers. Avoid the temptation to overdress the burger: A balance among bun, patty, and condiments is at the heart of every great burger recipe.

Four Quick Recipes

Burgers by their very nature are prime canvases for creative cooking. Consider these a mere jumping-off point. Choose your toppings carefully and cook your burger skillfully and you can't go wrong.

CHOOSE A PROTEIN

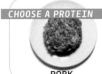
PORK

CHICKEN

LAMB

BISON

CHOOSE A BUN

SESAME-SEED BUN

DELI FLATS

With the exception of lettuce leaves, these restrained pockets from Pepperidge Farm are the lightest option, packing about 100 calories apiece.

POTATO ROLL

CHOOSE A CHEESE

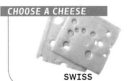
SWISS

SHARP CHEDDAR

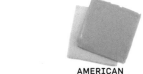
AMERICAN

CHOOSE VEGETATION

ROASTED PEPPERS

AVOCADO

RAW OR GRILLED ONIONS

GRILLED PINEAPPLE

CHOOSE CONDIMENTS

Mix together two parts ketchup, two parts mayo, one part regular mustard, and a scoop of finely chopped pickles.

SPECIAL SAUCE

GUACAMOLE

Much like pesto, this garlicky herb sauce pairs great with any type of patty. See the recipe on page 47.

CHIMICHURRI

THE ALOHA BURGER
Turkey + English muffin + Swiss + grilled onions + pineapple + teriyaki

THE BIG KAHUNA
Chicken + sesame bun + pepper-Jack + salsa + guacamole + jalapeños

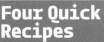

76

To form tuna or salmon patties, chop 1 pound of meat very finely and combine with 1 egg, ½ cup bread crumbs, and any seasonings you want to add.

TUNA

SALMON

Make your own veggie patties by pureeing ½ pound mushrooms, 1 cup black beans, ¾ cup bread crumbs, 1 egg, and a few shakes of Worcestershire food processor.

VEGGIE

Burger Basics

Rule 1
Lightly pack your patties. Overwork the meat and you'll have a dense, tough burger, rather than a light, juicy one.

Large, foldable leaves like Bibb and red leaf lettuce are your best options.

LETTUCE

ENGLISH MUFFINS

We don't normally love upscale buns like focaccia or ciabatta, but they pair well with tuna and salmon burgers.

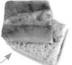

"FANCY" ROLL

Rule 2
Only use produce that tastes great on its own. A tomato flown in from halfway around the world that tastes like wet cardboard isn't doing your burger any favors. Neither is that brown lettuce in the refrigerator.

While crumbled cheeses like feta, goat, and blue don't melt as well as the other options here, they pair well with burgers that are dressed with bold condiments.

BLUE

PEPPER-JACK

When grating cheese for burgers, always use the smallest holes—that way the cheese melts more quickly and covers the burger more thoroughly.

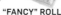

MOZZARELLA

Rule 3
Match the intensity of the meat with the condiments. A tuna burger with blue cheese isn't going to win anyone's heart, but ground bison dusted with spices and topped with crumbled blue is a winning combination.

SAUTÉED MUSHROOMS

PICKLES

LETTUCE

TOMATOES

Rule 4
Bun-to-burger ratio is key: You don't want a huge bun dominating your burger. Not only does it throw off the balance, it also invites unwanted calories. Lightly toast the inside parts of the bun only: The contrast between soft, warm top and crunchy inside is what a good bun is all about.

A.1. OR OTHER STEAK SAUCE

TERIYAKI SAUCE

You can use the Pico de Gallo recipe on page 46, or turn to your favorite bottled salsa.

SALSA

BLACK AND BLUE
Bison + potato roll + blackening spices + blue cheese + sautéed mushrooms + A.1.

THE FANCY PANTS
Tuna + focaccia + roasted peppers + arugula + chimichurri

Lamb Burgers
with Roasted Red Pepper Spread

Beyond beef, lamb may be our favorite protein for making burgers. Its rich, mildly gamy flavor takes well to smoke and char, just as it takes well to heady spices and boldly flavored condiments like this goat cheese-red pepper spread.

You'll Need:

- ½ cup bottled roasted red peppers
- ¼ cup fresh goat cheese
- ¼ cup plain low-fat Greek yogurt
- 1 clove garlic, smashed and peeled
- 1 lb ground lamb
- ½ tsp fennel seeds
- ¼ tsp ground coriander
- ¼ tsp ground cumin
- Salt and black pepper to taste
- 4 slices yellow onion, skewered with toothpicks
- 4 potato rolls
- Bibb Lettuce or arugula

If your market doesn't sell ground lamb, ask the butcher to grind a pound of lamb leg or shoulder meat.

How to Make It:

- Preheat a grill or grill pan over medium-high heat. In a food processor, combine the peppers, goat cheese, yogurt, and garlic. Pulse until thoroughly pureed and uniform in color.

- Combine the lamb with the fennel seeds, coriander, and cumin. Gently mix with your hands, then form into four equal patties. Just before grilling, season both sides of the patties with salt and pepper.

- Grill the burgers for 4 to 5 minutes per side, until firm but still giving to the touch (like a Nerf football). At the same time, grill the onion slices for 3 to 4 minutes per side, until soft and lightly charred. While the burgers rest, lightly toast the insides of the buns.

- Divide the red pepper spread among the buns. Place lettuce on the bottoms of each, top with a burger, then crown with the grilled onions and bun tops.

Makes 4 servings

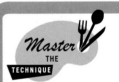

Master
THE
TECHNIQUE

Toasting spices

Preground spices like cumin, coriander, and fennel lose much of their punch during the processing. To maximize flavor, buy whole seeds and grind them yourself. First, warm the spices in a dry stainless-steel pan set over medium-low heat until the volatile oils begin to release and fill the kitchen with a deep aroma. Transfer to a clean coffee grinder and pulse. Do this just before cooking to ratchet the flavor of your food up a few notches.

Per Serving:
$3.03

490 calories
28 g fat (10 g saturated)
580 mg sodium

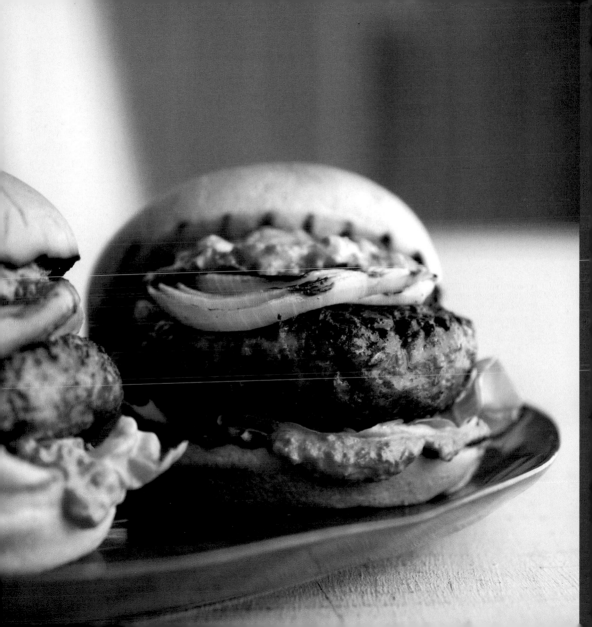

Steak Tortas

The *torta* may be the greatest sandwich you've never heard of. Born in Mexico, a culinary culture blessed with amazing meat preparations and world-class condiments, the pillowy sandwich comes stuffed with an embarrassment of culinary riches: grilled meat and onions, fresh avocado, salsa, chiles, a swipe or two of refried beans. It's everything we love about burritos, but on a roll that packs a fraction of the calories of a large tortilla.

You'll Need:

- 1 lb flank or skirt steak
- ½ tsp cumin
- ⅛ tsp cayenne pepper
- Salt and black pepper to taste
- 1 medium red onion, sliced into ¼"-thick rings and skewered with toothpicks
- 4 crusty rolls, lightly toasted
- ½ cup low-fat refried beans, warmed
- 1 avocado, peeled, pitted, and thinly sliced
- 1 cup shredded Jack cheese
- Pico de Gallo (page 46)
- Hot sauce for serving (optional)

How to Make It:

- Preheat a grill or grill pan over high heat. Season the steak all over with the cumin, cayenne, and salt and black pepper. Grill the steak, turning, for about 10 minutes, until a nice char has developed on the outside, the flesh feels firm but yielding to the touch, and an instant-read thermometer inserted into the thickest part of the steak registers 135°F. While the steak cooks, grill the onions, turning, for about 10 minutes, until caramelized and soft. Allow the steak to rest for at least 5 minutes, then slice into thin pieces against the natural grain of the meat.

- Spread the roll bottoms with a thin layer of refried beans, then pave each with avocado slices and grilled onions. Top with the steak slices, cheese, and pico de gallo, then the roll tops. Serve with hot sauce if you like.

Makes 4 servings

Mexicans will eat their tortas with whole chipotle peppers on top, but a less-incendiary alternative would be a few pickled jalapeños or a hit of hot sauce.

Per Serving:	
$4.74	450 calories 22 g fat (7 g saturated) 570 mg sodium

MEAL MULTIPLIER

Tortas can be made with dozens of different fillings playing the lead role. These are some of our favorites:

- Grilled chicken breast marinated in lime juice, cilantro, and chipotle pepper
- Grilled portabella mushroom caps
- Al pastor–style pork (see Tacos al Pastor, page 190)
- Tequila-Jalapeño Shrimp (page 230)

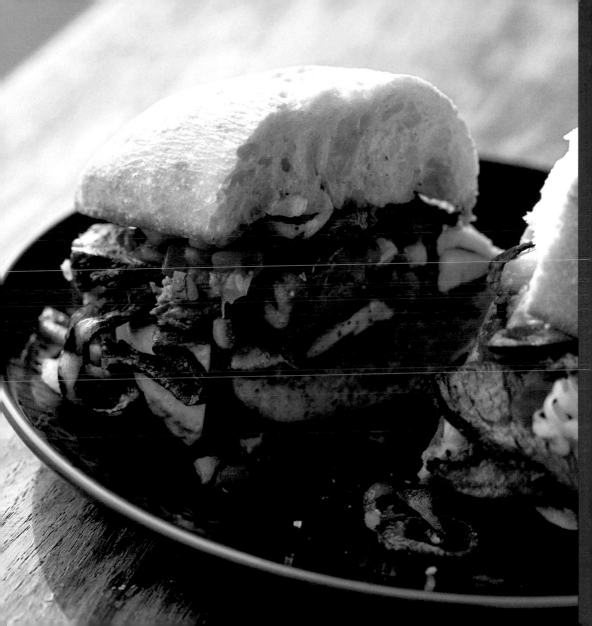

Shrimp Po' Boys

The po' boy is a New Orleans classic, a hearty grab-and-go lunch for the blue collar and white tablecloth sets alike. The blueprint is simple: A long crusty roll is split, layered with a generous amount of traditional sandwich fixings, then piled high with everything from cold cuts to fried oysters. We ratchet up the classic flavors by pairing Old Bay-spiked grilled shrimp with remoulade, a tartar-like sauce that binds the sandwich together. Nothing po' about that.

You'll Need:

- 2 Tbsp Worcestershire sauce
- 2 Tbsp olive oil mayonnaise
- 1 Tbsp grainy mustard
- 1 Tbsp ketchup
- 2 Tbsp chopped pickles
- 1 lb medium shrimp, peeled and deveined
- 1 tsp Old Bay Seasoning
- ⅛ tsp cayenne pepper
- Salt and black pepper to taste
- Metal skewers, or wooden skewers soaked in water for 30 minutes
- 1 large French loaf or baguette
- 1 large tomato, sliced
- 4 cups shredded iceberg lettuce
- ½ yellow onion, thinly sliced

How to Make It:

- Preheat a grill or grill pan over high heat. For the remoulade, combine the Worcestershire, mayonnaise, mustard, ketchup, and pickles in a mixing bowl and stir together. Set aside.

- Season the shrimp with the Old Bay, cayenne, salt, and black pepper and thread onto the skewers. Grill for 1 to 2 minutes per side, until pink and just firm.

- Cut the bread in half horizontally and scoop out a bit of the bread from the top and bottom halves. Slather the bread with the remoulade, then dress with the tomato slices, lettuce, onion, and shrimp. Cut into 4 sandwiches and serve.

Makes 4 servings

Traditional po' boy bread is actually a hybrid of a French loaf and a baguette: crunchy crust with a pillowy interior. A French loaf is probably the best compromise in most American markets.

Per Serving:
$3.17

370 calories
5 g fat (1 g saturated)
860 mg sodium

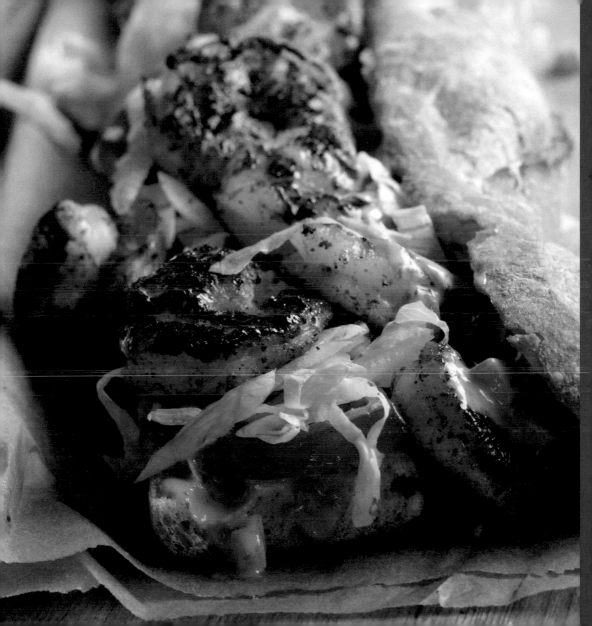

Spicy Asian Pork Burgers

For the purists who say that a burger must be made from beef and topped with the same predictable toppings, we say lighten up! The burger is an ingenious delivery system for protein and produce and its general awesomeness should not be limited to ground chuck and American cheese. This pork patty, infused with garlic and ginger and dabbed with chili mayo, is delicious testament to the versatility of the burger.

You'll Need:

½ **English cucumber,** thinly sliced

½ **cup rice wine vinegar**

Salt to taste

1 **lb ground pork**

2 **cloves garlic, minced**

1 **Tbsp minced fresh ginger**

2 **scallions, thinly sliced**

2 **Tbsp mayonnaise**

1 **Tbsp Asian-style chili sauce like sriracha**

4 **sesame seed hamburger buns, lightly toasted**

¼ **cup hoisin sauce**

How to Make It:

- Preheat a grill or grill pan over medium heat. Combine the cucumber, vinegar, and a few pinches of salt in a bowl and set aside.

- In a large mixing bowl, combine the pork, garlic, ginger, and scallions. Gently shape the meat into 4 equal patties. Season the burgers on both sides with salt and grill the burgers for about 5 minutes per side, until nicely browned on the outside and firm to the touch.

- Combine the mayonnaise and sriracha and spread on the bottom buns. Top with the burgers and then a small pile of cucumbers. Spread the bun tops with the hoisin and place on top of the burgers.

Makes 4 servings

Per Serving:
$2.39

490 calories
28 g fat (10 g saturated)
770 mg sodium

SECRET WEAPON

Sriracha

If you've read any of our cookbooks before, you'll know that we're addicted to this stuff, but so is anyone who's ever squirted it onto a hot dog or stirred it into a barbecue sauce. It's made primarily from pureed red chilies, but sriracha is more than just firepower: It adds a touch of sweetness, acidity, and garlic bite to raw and cooked dishes alike. Many of the recipes in this book call for sriracha or some form of Asian chili sauce. Our favorite brand has a red rooster on the label; these days, you can find it in nearly every supermarket in America.

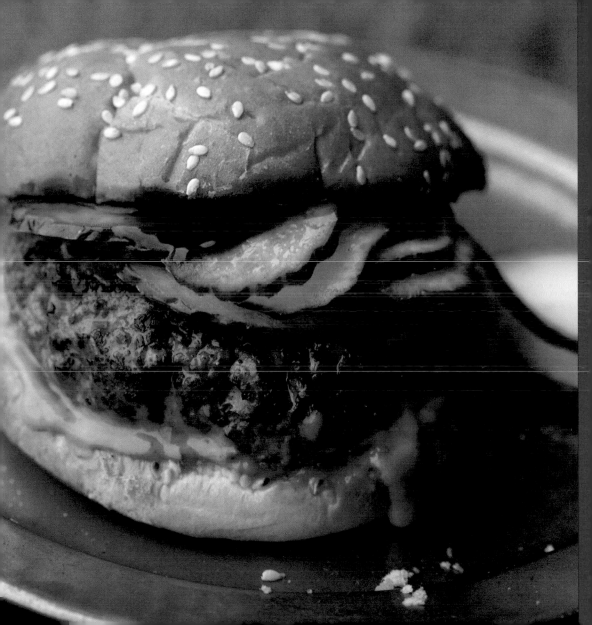

Grilled Pork Sandwiches
with Broccoli Rabe

This sandwich is inspired by the roast pork sandwiches of Philadelphia, which live in the long, greasy shadow cast by the city's handheld titan, the cheesesteak—despite being vastly superior (and considerably healthier).

You'll Need:

- 4 cloves garlic, minced
- 1 tsp chopped fresh rosemary
- 1 tsp fennel seeds, roughly chopped
- 3 Tbsp olive oil
- 1 lb pork tenderloin
- Salt and black pepper to taste
- 1 bunch broccoli rabe, bottom half of stems removed
- ½ tsp red pepper flakes
- ½ cup jarred roasted red peppers
- 4 slices sharp provolone
- 4 seeded hoagie rolls

How to Make It:

- Combine half of the garlic, the rosemary, and fennel seeds in a mixing bowl with 2 tablespoons of the olive oil. Season the pork all over with salt and pepper and combine in a sealable plastic bag with the rosemary mixture. Seal and refrigerate for at least 1 hour (or up to 6 hours).

- Bring a pot of salted water to a boil. Add the broccoli rabe and cook for about 7 minutes, until just tender. Drain. Heat the remaining 1 tablespoon olive oil in a large sauté pan. Add the remaining garlic and the red pepper flakes and sauté for 2 minutes. Add the broccoli rabe and cook for 3 minutes, until very tender. Season with salt and pepper.

- Preheat a grill over medium-high heat. Remove the pork from the bag and grill, turning occasionally, for about 12 minutes, until the surface is lightly charred and firm but gently yielding to the touch, and an instant-read thermometer inserted into the thickest part of the meat registers 150°F. Rest the pork for 5 minutes before slicing into thin rounds.

- Divide the pork, broccoli rabe, peppers, and provolone among the hoagie rolls. Place the sandwiches on the grill and cook for about 2 minutes per side, until the bread is lightly toasted.

Makes 4 servings

Per Serving:
$2.88

510 calories
23 g fat (8 g saturated)
660 mg sodium

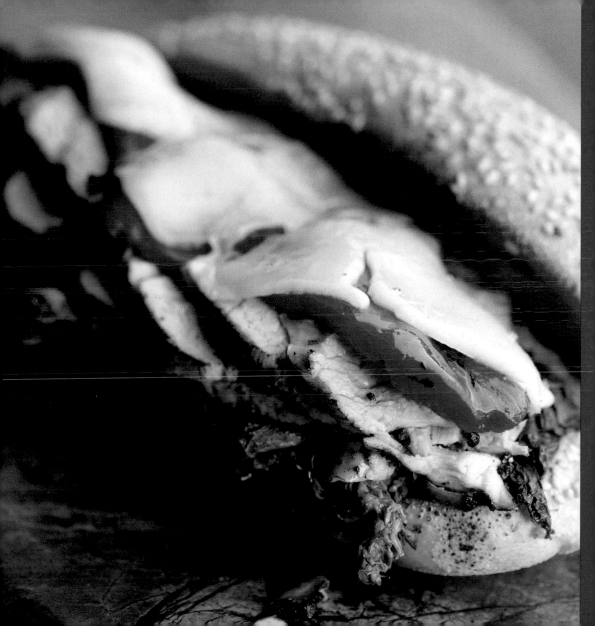

Grilled Chicken & Pineapple Sandwich

Not even the relatively healthy genre of grilled chicken sandwiches is a safe bet when you seek sustenance away from home. That's because restaurants go long on the oil and the dressing, producing high-fat, high-sodium sandwiches. Our version is a spicy-sweet combination of teriyaki-glazed chicken, juicy grilled pineapple, and fiery jalapeños —a chicken sandwich to end all fatty chicken sandwiches.

You'll Need:

- 4 **boneless, skinless chicken breasts** (4–6 oz each)
- ½ cup **teriyaki sauce**
- 4 slices **Swiss cheese**
- 4 **pineapple slices** (½" thick)
- 4 **whole-wheat buns**
- 1 **red onion, thinly sliced**
- **Fresh sliced or pickled jalapeños to taste**

Whole-wheat buns are often made with a small percentage of whole grains and a surplus of sugar. Settle on a brand with 3 grams of fiber and fewer than 130 calories per bun.

How to Make It:

- Combine the chicken and the teriyaki sauce in a resealable plastic bag and marinate in the refrigerator for at least 30 minutes and up to 12 hours.

- Heat a grill or grill pan over high heat. Remove the chicken from the marinade and place on the grill; discard any remaining marinade. Cook for 4 to 5 minutes on the first side; flip and immediately add the cheese to each breast. Continue cooking until the cheese is melted and the chicken is lightly charred and firm to the touch.

- While the chicken rests, add the pineapple and the buns to the grill. Cook the buns until they're lightly toasted and the pineapple until it's soft and caramelized, about 3 minutes per side. Top each bun with chicken, red onion, jalapeño slices, pineapple, and a bit more teriyaki sauce, if you like.

Makes 4 servings

Per Serving: **$2.64**	400 calories 11 g fat (6 g saturated) 640 mg sodium

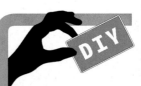

Teriyaki Sauce

There are a few decent teriyaki sauces in the supermarket aisles, but making a superior version at home requires just a few basic pantry items and about 10 minutes of your time. In a small pan, combine ½ cup reduced-sodium soy sauce with ¼ cup brown sugar, a clove of minced garlic, a tablespoon of grated ginger, and a tablespoon of cornstarch dissolved in a bit of water. Simmer for 5 minutes until thickened and you've got homemade teriyaki.

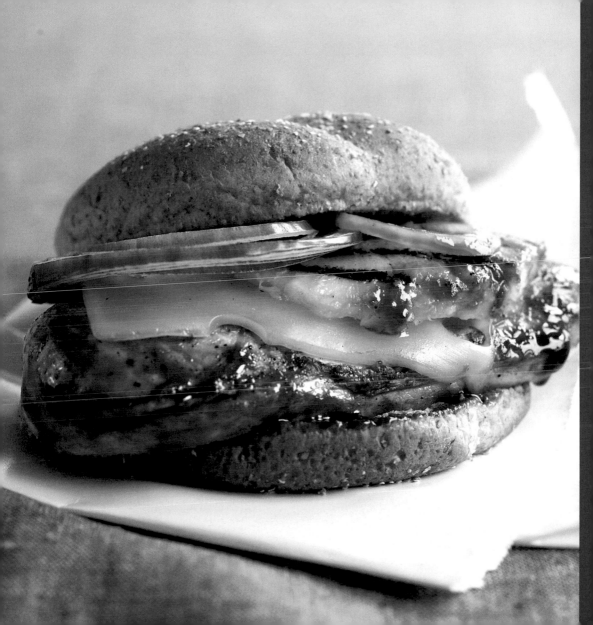

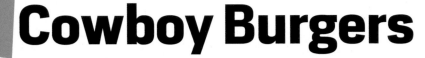

Cowboy Burgers

We're not afraid to admit when a fast-food joint has a good idea. The inspiration for this burger comes from a Carl's Jr. classic, the Western Bacon Cheeseburger, a how-can-it-not-be-delicious comingling of beef, barbecue sauce, and fried onions. Problem is, the small version of Carl's burger packs 740 calories and a full day's worth of saturated fat. This version uses naturally lean bison and replaces the breaded onion rings with sweet grilled ones.

You'll Need:

- 1 lb ground bison or beef sirloin
- 1 medium red onion, sliced into ¼"-thick rings and skewered with toothpicks
- ½ Tbsp finely ground coffee
- 1 tsp chipotle or ancho chile powder
- Salt and black pepper to taste
- 4 slices sharp Cheddar
- 4 sesame seed buns, lightly toasted
- 6 strips bacon, cooked until crisp and halved
- 4 Tbsp Classic Barbecue Sauce (page 45 or store-bought)

How to Make It:

- Gently form the beef into 4 patties, being careful not to overwork the meat. Let the patties rest for 15 minutes.

- Preheat the grill or grill pan over medium heat. Grill the onion slices, turning, for about 10 minutes, until soft and lightly charred. Just before cooking the patties, season them on both sides with the coffee, chile powder, and salt and pepper. Grill the patties alongside the onions for about 4 minutes, until nicely browned. Flip, top with the cheese, and continue grilling for 3 to 4 minutes longer, until the centers of the patties are firm but gently yielding to the touch and an instant-read thermometer inserted into the thickest part of a burger registers 135°F.

- Place the burgers on the bun bottoms, top with onions, bacon, and barbecue sauce.

Makes 4 servings

We have no idea if cowboys actually eat burgers, but if they did, they would taste an awful lot like this one.

Normally we're not huge fans of heavily spiced burgers, but the coffee here adds a roasted depth to the burger that pairs beautifully with the barbecue sauce and bacon.

Per Serving:
$2.62

460 calories
22 g fat (11 g saturated)
850 mg sodium

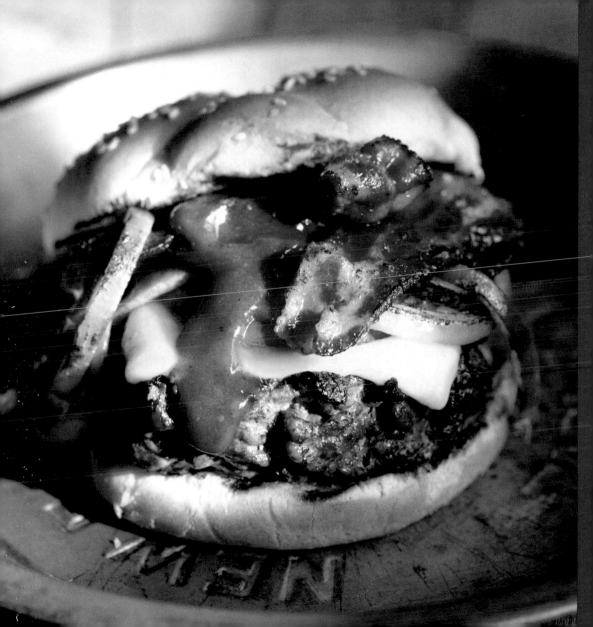

Italian Sausage Sandwiches

Ground chicken and turkey make for heroic sausage, capable of capturing all of the rich flavors of pork sausage for about half the calories. They've become an indispensable part of our grilling pantry. Sausage and peppers is a classic pairing that can never be wrong, whether eaten alone, slathered with spicy mustard, or covered in tomato sauce and a thin layer of bubbling cheese.

You'll Need:

- 4 **Italian-style chicken or turkey sausages**
- 1 **large green bell pepper, stemmed, seeded, and quartered**
- 1 **yellow onion, sliced into ¼"-thick rings and skewered with toothpicks**
- 4 **sesame seed hoagie rolls, split**
- ½ **cup Tomato Sauce (page 110) or store-bought marinara sauce, heated**
- ¾ **cup shredded Provolone or mozzarella cheese**

Pork sausage can be substituted, but add about 120 calories to the nutrition numbers.

How to Make It:

- Preheat a grill or grill pan over medium heat. When hot, place the sausages, peppers, and onions on the grill. Cook the sausages, turning, for about 12 minutes, until lightly charred and crispy on the outside and cooked all the way through. Cook the onions and peppers for about 5 minutes per side, until soft and caramelized.

- Preheat the broiler. Chop the onion rings in half and slice the peppers. Place each sausage inside a hoagie roll and top with onions and peppers. Spoon on enough marinara to cover and top with the cheese. Place the hoagies under the broiler and cook for about 3 minutes, until the cheese is fully melted and the top of the rolls are lightly toasted.

Makes 4 servings

Per Serving:
$1.89

490 calories
16 g fat (5 g saturated)
890 mg sodium

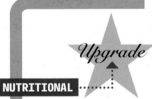

Upgrade

NUTRITIONAL

As much fun as it is to eat this dish with your hands, the roll is by no means necessary. Like nearly every sandwich in this chapter, the flavors and ingredients are strong enough to stand on their own. By serving the sausage straight off the grill, swaddled in peppers, onions, and tomato sauce (and maybe a grating of Parmesan cheese), you'll save 150 calories and still have something hugely satisfying to sit down to. (It will, however, require a knife and fork.)

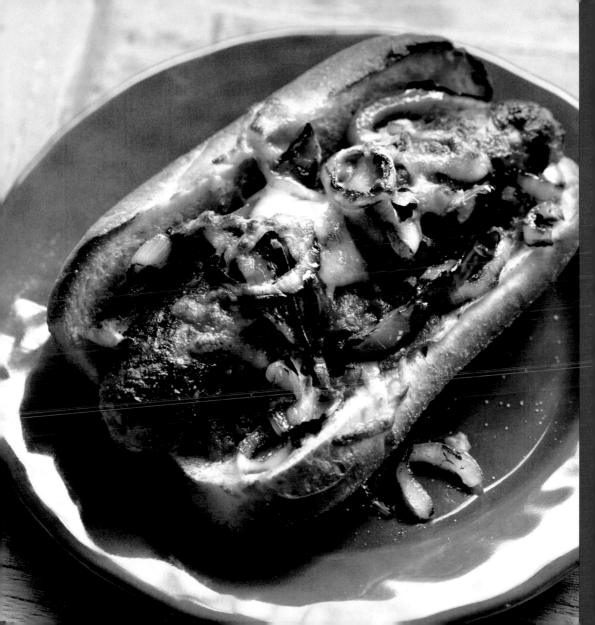

Stuffed
Meat Loaf Burgers

Much like Thanksgiving turkey, the best part about making meat loaf is the sandwiches the next day. But why not skip right to the good stuff? The good stuff here means a turkey patty infused with the classic flavors of meat loaf (ketchup, Worcestershire, caramelized onion), then stuffed with a molten pocket of smoked Gouda cheese. It's not your mama's meat loaf, but that's the whole point.

You'll Need:

- 1 tsp butter
- 1 large yellow onion, diced
- 1 clove garlic, minced
- ½ cup ketchup
- ¼ cup chicken stock
- 1 Tbsp Worcestershire sauce
- 1 tsp dried thyme
- 1 lb ground turkey
- 1 egg
- ½ cup bread crumbs
- ¾ cup shredded smoked Gouda
- 4 potato buns, toasted

How to Make It:

- Melt the butter in a large sauté pan or cast-iron skillet over medium heat. Add the onion and garlic and cook for about 5 minutes, until the onion is soft and translucent. Add the ketchup, stock, Worcestershire, and thyme. Simmer for about 10 minutes, until the liquid has reduced enough to cling to the onions. Allow the mixture to cool for at least 10 minutes.

- Combine the turkey, egg, bread crumbs, and half of the onion mixture in a mixing bowl. Gently mix together. Form four patties, making a very large indentation in the center of each. Fill each indentation with Gouda, then carefully fold the meat over the top of the cheese and reshape the patties.

- Preheat a grill or grill pan over medium heat. Grill the burgers for about 5 minutes per side, until lightly charred on the outside and cooked all the way through. Place on the buns and top with the remaining onion mixture.

Makes 4 servings

Per Serving:
$1.83

460 calories
20 g fat (8 g saturated)
965 mg sodium

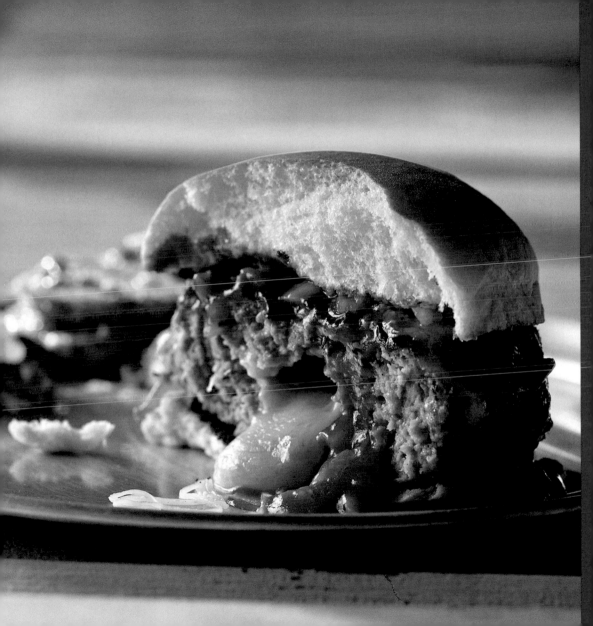

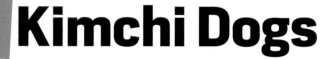

Kimchi Dogs

Once upon a time, on the corner of Ludlow and Stanton on New York's Lower East Side, a young cook named Sam would spend every weekend night cooking a full menu of classic street food. Sam's claim to fame? Every item could be topped with kimchi, spicy pickled cabbage that is the cornerstone of Korean cuisine and serves as a perfect foil to burgers and hot dogs (think sauerkraut). A decade later, North American streets are flooded with food trucks and sidewalk vendors doing the same, but we'll always remember Sam as the guy who pioneered this funky combination.

You'll Need:

4 cups thinly sliced Napa cabbage

Juice of 1 lime

1 Tbsp olive oil mayonnaise

1 Tbsp toasted sesame seeds

½ Tbsp sesame oil

Salt and black pepper to taste

4 all-beef hot dogs (we like Applegate Super Natural Uncured Beef Hot Dog)

4 potato hot dog buns, lightly toasted

½ small onion, minced

½ cup kimchi

How to Make It:

- Preheat a grill or grill pan over medium heat. In a large mixing bowl, combine the cabbage, lime juice, mayonnaise, sesame seeds, sesame oil, and salt and pepper. Toss until the cabbage is evenly coated.

- Grill the hot dogs, turning, for about 10 minutes, until the skin is lightly charred. Place in the buns and top each with minced onion, kimchi, and the cabbage mixture.

Makes 4 servings

Find kimchi in the international section of large supermarkets, in Asian grocery stores, or online at AsianFoodGrocer.com.

Per Serving:
$1.79

260 calories
9 g fat (2.5 g saturated)
830 mg sodium

SECRET WEAPON

Kimchi

"Fermented cabbage" doesn't do much as a description to endear kimchi to first-time eaters, but this Korean staple, with its bold balance of chili spice and vinegar tang, has a profound ability to turn skeptics into life-long devotees. It's most often made by pickling Napa cabbage with red chiles, garlic, ginger, and a host of other rotating ingredients. It's an amazing foil to grilled foods, either as a topping for burgers, a stuffing for cheesy quesadillas, or pureed and served alongside a steak or slices of pork tenderloin.

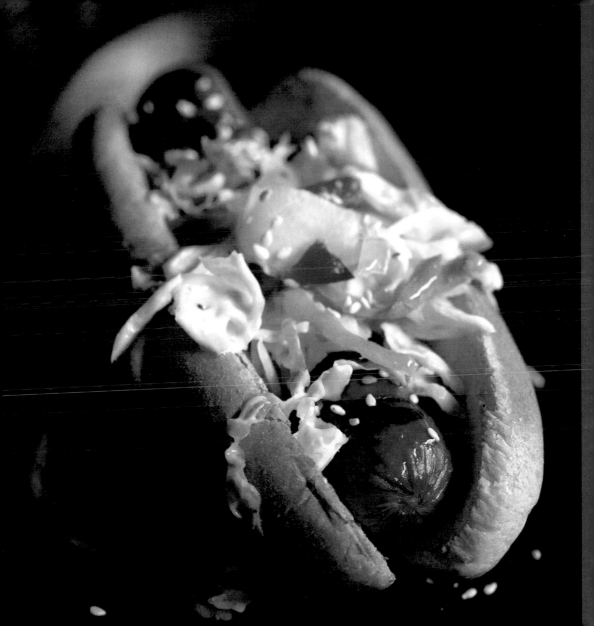

Teriyaki Dogs
with Grilled Pineapple

A bacon-wrapped dog might seem a little extreme, and perhaps it is, but sometimes we all need to cut loose, and 35 calories' worth of smoked pork is a fine way to do so in our book. As the bacon sizzles and the fat melts away, it forms a tight, crispy skin around the dog, which matches up perfectly with the sweetness of the teriyaki glaze and grilled chunks of pineapple. The jalapeños are there to bring some heat to the equation, but a squeeze of chili sauce or a shake of Tabasco would have the same effect.

You'll Need:

- 4 all-beef hot dogs (we like all dogs from Applegate Farms)
- 4 slices bacon
- 2 thick slices peeled fresh pineapple
- ¼ cup teriyaki sauce
- 4 potato hot dog buns, lightly toasted
- Pickled jalapeño peppers, or thinly sliced fresh jalapeños (optional)

How to Make It:

- Preheat a grill or grill pan over medium heat. Wrap each hot dog with a slice of bacon, stretching the bacon so that it covers the dog as tautly as possible (you may end up using less than a full slice—simply cut off any unused end).

- Place the hot dogs and the pineapple slices on the grill and cook, turning and basting both occasionally with the teriyaki sauce, for 10 to 12 minutes, until the bacon fat has rendered and the meat is browned and crispy and the pineapple flesh is soft and has nice grill marks.

- Chop the pineapple into bite-size pieces, discarding the tough core. Place the dogs in the toasted buns and top with the pineapple, jalapeños (if using), and another swipe of teriyaki sauce.

Makes 4 servings

Per Serving:
$1.65

270 calories
9 g fat (3 g saturated)
880 mg sodium

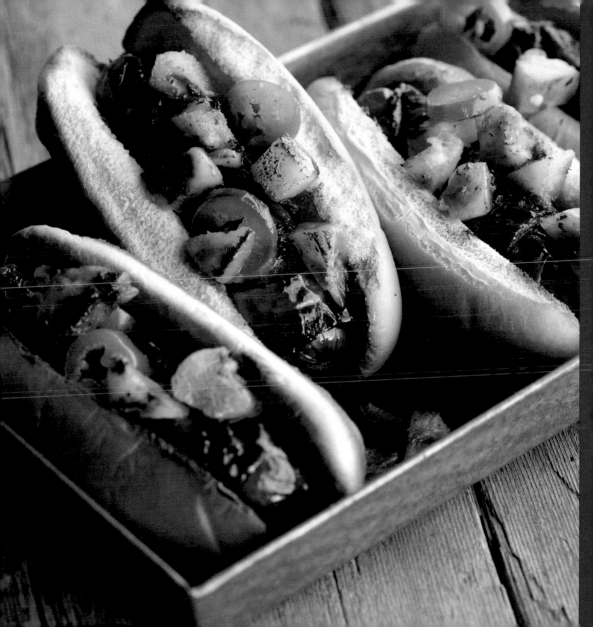

Teriyaki Salmon Burgers

Burger patties can be made out of anything that can be ground up and bound together, from bison to black beans to ostrich. It's a fine line between gimmicky and gourmet, but a few proteins are particularly well-suited to stand in for beef in the burger-making business: lamb, turkey, tuna, and salmon. The latter takes well to sweet and spice, the better for cutting through the healthy fats that abound in salmon. Be mindful of the cooking time, though, because overcooked salmon is a drag. Think of salmon like ground beef: It's best when cooked to medium, so that the fish emerges juicy and tender rather than dry and chewy.

You'll Need:

- 1 lb salmon, finely chopped
- 1 egg
- ½ cup bread crumbs (preferably panko), plus more if needed
- 4 scallions, thinly sliced
- 1 Tbsp soy sauce
- Asian-style chili sauce like sriracha to taste
- 2 Tbsp teriyaki sauce, plus more for serving
- 4 whole-wheat sesame seed buns, toasted
- 1 cup Asian Slaw (page 340)

How to Make It:

- Preheat a grill or grill pan over medium heat. Combine the salmon, egg, bread crumbs, scallions, soy sauce, and chili sauce in a bowl and mix thoroughly. Use your hands to gently form 4 patties. The patties will be very moist, but if the mixture is too loose to form patties, stir in more bread crumbs until it firms up enough to shape.

- Brush the tops of the burgers with about half the teriyaki sauce and place on the grill, sauce side down. Grill for about 4 minutes, until the meat firms up and easily pulls away from the grill. Brush the tops with the remaining teriyaki sauce and flip. Continue grilling for 4 minutes longer, until the burgers are cooked all the way through.

- Divide the burgers among the buns, brush with a bit of additional teriyaki sauce, and top with generous piles of the slaw.

Make 4 servings

Per Serving:
$3.13

350 calories
11 g fat (2 g saturated)
910 mg sodium

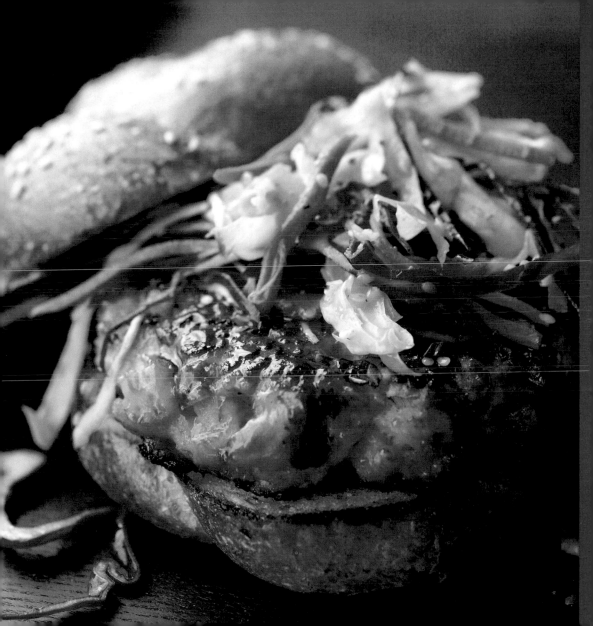

Cubano Sandwiches

People routinely invest hundreds of dollars in a fancy panini press when they have the world's largest crispy-sandwich maker sitting idly by outside. That's right, a hot grate and a little bit of weight is all you need to transform a cold sandwich into a crispy, melty marvel. We put the grill into action here, first using it to cook the pork tenderloin, then using the hot grate and a few foil-wrapped bricks to press the sandwich—the amazing Miami staple known as a Cubano—into cheesy submission.

You'll Need:

- 1 lb pork tenderloin
- ½ Tbsp chili powder
- Salt and black pepper
- ¼ cup deli-style mustard
- 1 baguette, cut in half lengthwise, or 4 soft hoagie rolls
- 12 pickle slices
- 4 slices Swiss cheese
- 4 slices deli ham

How to Make It:

- Preheat a grill or grill pan over medium heat. Rub the pork tenderloin with the chili powder and a few pinches each of salt and pepper. When the grill is hot, cook the tenderloin, turning, for 10 to 12 minutes, until just cooked through. Allow the tenderloin to rest for at least 5 minutes, then slice into ¼"-thick pieces.

- Spread the mustard on the bottom half of the baguette, top with the pickles, tenderloin slices, Swiss, ham, and the other half of the baguette. Cut into four equal sandwiches.

- Place the sandwiches directly on the grill grate and place something heavy over them (a cast-iron skillet or a brick wrapped in a foil both work great); this will help flatten and crisp them up the same way a panini press does. Cook for 2 minutes per side, until the bread is toasted and the cheese is melted.

Makes 4 servings

Per Serving:
$2.97

380 calories
11 g fat (5 g saturated)
680 mg sodium

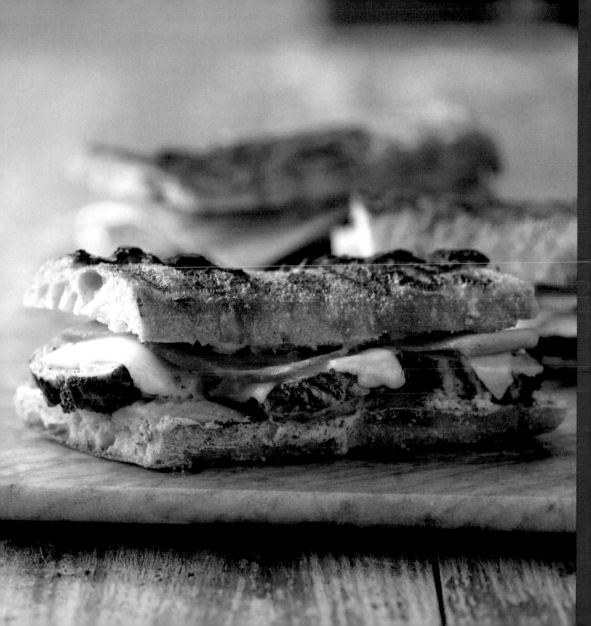

Cheesesteak Sandwich

The famous sandwich from Philly is a nutritionist's nightmare: mounds of greasy beef and fried onions; a massive, oil-soaked hoagie roll; and to top it all off, a viscous deluge of Cheez Whiz (that's right, traditional cheesesteaks are made with Whiz). But we want you to have your steak and eat it, too, so we came up with this version, which relies on a lean flank steak, a whole-wheat roll, and a yogurt-based blue cheese sauce. It's a bit fancier than the sandwich from the City of Brotherly Love, but to our tastes, it's also better.

You'll Need:

2 Tbsp plain Greek-style yogurt (we like Fage 2%)

2 Tbsp olive-oil mayonnaise

¼ cup crumbled blue cheese

16 oz skirt or flank steak

Salt and black pepper to taste

1 yellow onion, sliced and skewered with toothpicks

2 cups arugula

2 tomatoes, sliced

4 whole-wheat or sesame-seed rolls

How to Make It:

● Combine the yogurt, mayonnaise, and blue cheese. Set aside.

● Heat a grill or grill pan over high heat. Season the steak with salt and pepper and cook for 3 to 4 minutes per side, until the steak is firm but still gives with gentle pressure. While the steak cooks, grill the onions, turning, until soft and caramelized, about 10 minutes. Allow the steak to rest for at least 5 minutes before slicing into thin strips.

● Divide the arugula and tomatoes among the rolls. Top with the steak and grilled onions and drizzle each sandwich with the blue cheese mayo.

Makes 4 servings

Diffuse the caloric heft of mayo-based condiments by cutting the goop with 50 percent Greek yogurt.

Per Serving:
$5.00

400 calories
14 g fat (4 g saturated)
730 mg sodium

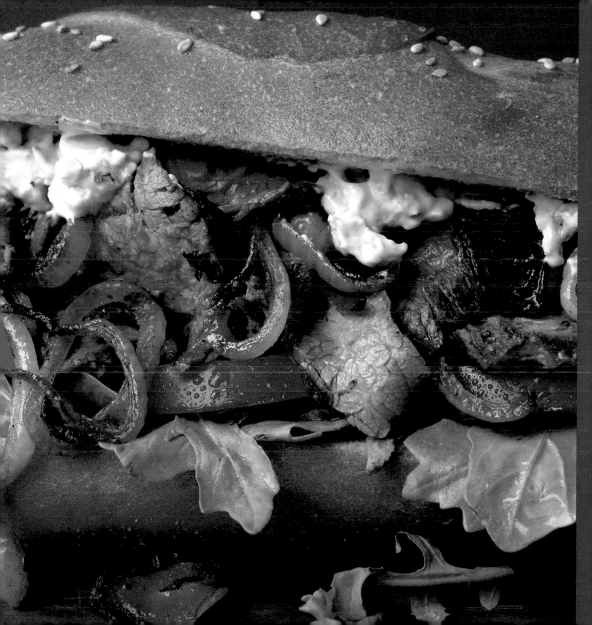

PIZZA & PASTA

CHAPTER **4**

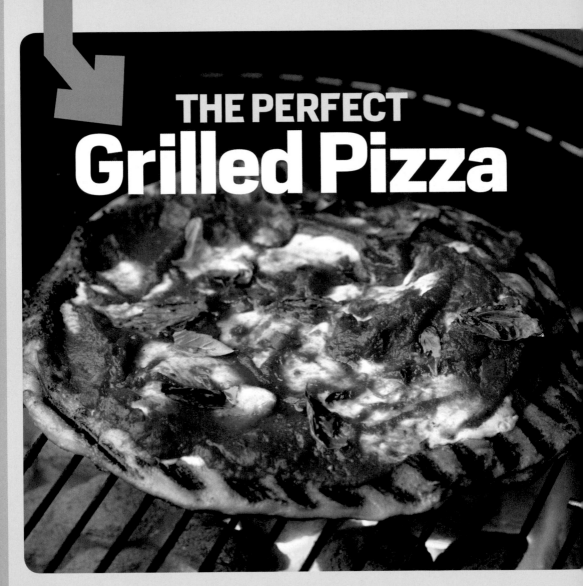

THE PERFECT
Grilled Pizza

After a decade of cooking pizzas in every device possible—from a toaster oven to a 1,000°F, centuries-old oven in Italy—one immutable truth has emerged: Short of owning a $5,000 hand-built oven imported from Naples, nothing captures the magic—the blistered crust, the smoke-perfumed sauce and cheese—of real wood-fired pizza quite like a grill can. Master this technique and you will be putting out pies that will be the envy of even the finest local pizzerias.

Ease up on the toppings.

Pizza is about the union of bread, sauce, and cheese—a harmony totally disturbed by a thick blanket of melted dairy. There's also a structural-integrity element at play here: Because wood fired pizzas are thinner than classic American chain pizza, they aren't built to support a barrage of toppings. Use just enough sauce to lightly blanket the dough (about three good spoonfuls), and scatter just enough cheese to cover about half the surface area of the pizza—about 3 ounces per pizza. As the cheese melts, it will spread out and cover the perfect amount of pizza real estate.

Use two kinds of heat.

If using charcoal, bank all of the hot coals onto one side of the grill. If using gas, turn the left burners all the way up and the right burners all the way down. Start the pizza over high heat, effectively searing the raw dough to create a charred, puffy crust and suffuse the whole pie with smoke. When you flip it, move it over to the cooler side of the grill. The lower temperature will give you ample time to top the pizza and close the lid. Keep the lid closed as much as possible: A closed grill functions as both a grill and an oven, charring the bottom of the crust while melting the cheese and crisping the toppings.

Have all your ingredients ready.

In Naples, pizzas cook in under 90 seconds. These pies take a few minutes longer, but they grill up very quickly all the same. Because of the unique cooking process, one that requires quick action and careful monitoring, you'll need to have your sauce, cheese, and other toppings fully ready to go when you start grilling. As soon as you flip the pizza, start in with the toppings: cheese first (so it melts easily from the heat of the crust), then sauce, then basil (or anything else you're adding to personalize your pie).

Pizza

You'll Need:

Pizza Dough

Olive oil for brushing and drizzling

1½ cups fresh mozzarella, chopped

Normal packaged mozzarella is a fine substitute, but it's not as delicious.

1 **cup Tomato Sauce**

About 10 fresh basil leaves

- Preheat a grill using a two-zone fire (see page 40), one zone over high heat and the other over low. Close the lid so that the heat can effectively build up.

- Divide the dough into two equal balls. Working with one ball at a time on a well-floured work-space, use a rolling pin to stretch the dough into 10" circles.

- Have all of your toppings prepared and within arm's reach of your grill. Place one of the dough circles on a lightly floured pizza peel. Brush the top with oil and slide the dough directly onto the hot part of the grill. Cook for about 30 seconds, until the dough begins to brown and firm up, then use a pair of tongs to rotate

45 degrees and grill for another 30 seconds, creating diamond-shaped grill marks on the crust. Flip and place the raw side of the dough down on the cooler side of the grill. Working quickly, top with half of the mozzarella first, then half the sauce and basil leaves, and a drizzle of olive oil. Close the top and let the pizza grill for 2 to 3 minutes, until the cheese begins to melt. Use your tongs to carefully rotate the pizza 45 degrees and continue grilling for another minute or two, until the crust is lightly charred and crisp beneath and the cheese is fully melted. Repeat with the other pizza. Cut the pizzas into 6 slices each before serving.

Makes 4 servings

Pizza Dough

You'll Need:

1 **cup hot water**

1 **Tbsp sugar or honey**

½ **tsp salt**

1 **envelope instant yeast**

2½ **cups flour (we like King Arthur), plus more for kneading and rolling**

Any of the pizzas in the coming pages can be made healthier by using half whole-wheat and half all-purpose flour. That will boost both protein and fiber counts in all of your creations.

- Combine the water, sugar, and salt in a large bowl and sprinkle with the yeast. Allow to sit for 10 minutes while the water activates the yeast. Stir in the flour, using a wooden spoon to incorporate. When the dough is no longer sticky, place on a cutting board, cover with more flour, and knead for 5 minutes, folding the dough over on itself and using the heel of your hand to push it into the cutting board. Return the dough to the bowl, cover with plastic wrap, and let the dough rise at room temperature for at least 90 minutes. Makes enough dough for two 10" pizzas. The dough will keep, covered, in the refrigerator for up to 2 days.

Tomato Sauce

You'll Need:

1 **can (28 oz) whole peeled tomatoes**

Whole, peeled tomatoes are best because they are minimally processed and allow you to dictate the texture of your sauce.

1 **Tbsp olive oil**

½ **tsp salt**

- Discard the excess tomato juice in the can. Use your hands to thoroughly crush the tomatoes (careful, they're loaded with juice!) into a puree. Stir in the olive oil and salt. Makes about 2 cups sauce; keeps in the refrigerator for up to 1 week.

America's WORST Pizza

While it's our goal to teach you how to make the perfect pizza at home, remember there are hundreds of seriously imperfect pies lurking behind every delivery dude and deep-dish dispensary. These five offenders represent just a glimpse of what you're up against when you venture out into the pernicious world of mass-produced pizzas.

Uno Chicago Grill Chicago Classic Deep Dish Pizza (Individual)

2,310 calories,
165 g fat (54 g saturated)
4,650 mg sodium

Think of a deep dish pizza as a bread bowl filled with flab-inducing grease. We've chastised Uno for this "individual" pie before, but the chain refuses to lighten it up. Add one of these to your weekly diet and you'll gain nearly 8 pounds in 3 months.

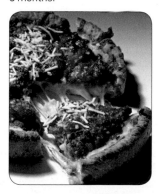

Domino's Deep Dish ExtravaganZZa Feast (2 slices, 14" pie)

840 calories
44 g fat
(16 g saturated)
2,280 mg sodium

Despite the fun name, this pie is a nutritional downer that derives nearly half its calories from fat. Blame the extra cheese and the fact that Domino's crowns it with four different meats. You know what's not fun? Jogging for an hour and a half to burn off your dinner.

Pizza Hut Stuffed Crust Meat Lover's Pizza (2 slices, 14" pie)

960 calories
52 g fat
(22 g saturated)
2,760 mg sodium

If this book proves anything, it's that we have no qualms about meat. But with this pie, Pizza Hut goes too far. They've piled this crust with pepperoni, ham, beef, bacon, and sausage. And they finish the pie—and your diet—by piping gobs of molten cheese into the crust. Urp. Hope you brought your Rolaids.

California Pizza Kitchen Tostada Pizza with Grilled Steak (½ pie)

840 calories
16 g saturated fat
1,649 mg sodium

This is the melting pot of pizza pies, drawing culinary influence from Italy, Mexico, and the dressing aisle of your local Piggly Wiggly. That's right, CPK has topped an Italian dish with Tex-Mex tortilla chips and fat-heavy ranch dressing. The innovation would be more laudable if it didn't come at such a staggering nutritional price.

DiGiorno Traditional Crust Four Cheese (1 pie)

710 calories
30 g fat
(11 g saturated,
3.5 g trans)
1,190 mg sodium

No, it's not delivery, but it's just as bad. Not only is DiGiorno's pie heavy with sodium and calories, but it also delivers nearly twice the maximum amount of trans fats that you should take in over the entire course of your day. Very few of DiGiorno's pizzas are fit for consumption.

Meatball Pizzas
with Olives & Caramelized Onion

Great cooking is all about balance, and that goes especially for pizza. A pepperoni, sausage, and bacon pie, for example, doesn't quite get you there; it's all fat and salt. This pie, our version of a slimmed-down supreme pizza, is sweet, salty, and savory in equal measure—an addictive equilibrium.

You'll Need:

- 1 **Tbsp olive oil, plus more for brushing**
- 2 **medium onions, thinly sliced**

Salt

Pizza Dough (page 110)

- 1½ **cups chopped fresh mozzarella**
- 1 **cup Tomato Sauce (page 110), heated**
- 8 **leftover Grilled Meatballs (from recipe on page 258), or store-bought meatballs, sliced**
- ¼ **cup Kalamata olives, chopped**

Homemade dough is always best, but for this and all the pizza recipes, fresh, store-bought dough will work just fine.

How to Make It:

- Heat the olive oil in a large saucepan over low heat. Add the onions and a pinch of salt and cover. Cook, stirring occasionally so that the onions don't stick, for about 15 minutes, until very soft and lightly browned.

- Preheat a grill using a two-zone fire (see "Go High and Low," page 40), one zone high and the other low. Close the lid so that the heat can effectively build up. While the grill heats, divide the dough into two equal balls. Using a well-floured work surface and a rolling pin, stretch the dough into 12" circles.

- Place one of the dough circles on a lightly floured pizza peel. Brush the top with oil and slide the dough directly onto the hot part of the grill. Cook for about 30 seconds, until the dough begins to brown, then use a pair of tongs to rotate it 45 degrees. Cook for another 30 seconds, creating diamond-shaped grill marks on the crust. Flip the dough and place, raw side down, on the cooler side of the grill. Working quickly, top first with half the mozzarella, then half the sauce, meatballs, olives, and onions. Close the grill top and let the pizza cook for 2 to 3 minutes, until the cheese begins to melt. Use your tongs to carefully rotate the pizza 45 degrees and continue cooking for another minute or two, until the crust is crisp beneath and the cheese is fully melted. Repeat with the other pizza.

Makes 4 servings

Per Serving:
$3.12

540 calories
18 g fat (6 g saturated)
900 mg sodium

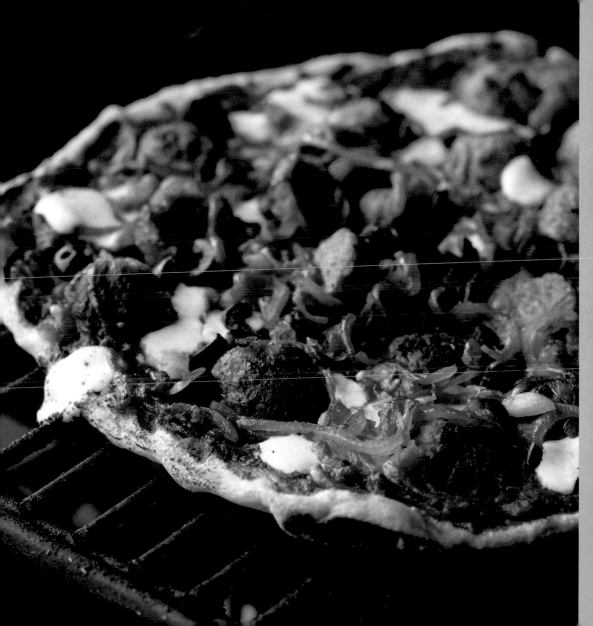

Artichoke Pesto Pizzas

Pizza done properly, with a fine balance of cheese, sauce, and toppings, can make for a surprisingly healthy meal. This is our favorite vegetarian pie of all time, equal parts nutritional powerhouse and deeply delicious comfort food.

You'll Need:

- ½ Tbsp olive oil, plus more for brushing
- 4 oz cremini mushrooms, stemmed and sliced
- 1 clove garlic, minced
- Salt and black pepper to taste
- Pizza Dough (page 110)
- ½ cup soft goat cheese
- ½ cup marinated artichoke hearts
- ¼ cup oil-packed sundried tomatoes
- ¼ cup prepared pesto
- 1 cup Tomato Sauce (page 110)

How to Make It:

- Heat the olive oil in a sauté pan over medium-high heat. Add the mushrooms and garlic and sauté for about 5 minutes, until the mushrooms are caramelized and soft. Season with salt and pepper.

- Preheat a grill using a two-zone fire (see "Go High and Low," page 40), one zone high and the other low. Close the lid so that the heat can effectively build up. While the grill heats up, divide the dough into two equal balls. Using a well-floured work surface and a rolling pin, stretch the dough into 12" circles.

- Place one of the dough circles on a lightly floured pizza peel. Brush the top with oil and slide the dough directly onto the hot part of the grill. Cook for about 30 seconds, until the dough begins to brown, then use a pair of tongs to rotate it 45 degrees. Cook for another 30 seconds, creating diamond-shaped grill marks on the crust. Flip the dough and place, raw side down, on the cooler side of the grill. Working quickly, top first with half of the cheese, then half the artichokes, sundried tomatoes, mushrooms, pesto, and pizza sauce. Close the top and cook for 2 to 3 minutes, until the cheese begins to melt. Use your tongs to carefully rotate the pizza 45 degrees and continue cooking for another minute or two, until the crust is crisp and the cheese is fully melted. Repeat with the other pizza.

Makes 4 servings

Per Serving:	510 calories
$1.94	16 g fat (6 g saturated)
	910 mg sodium

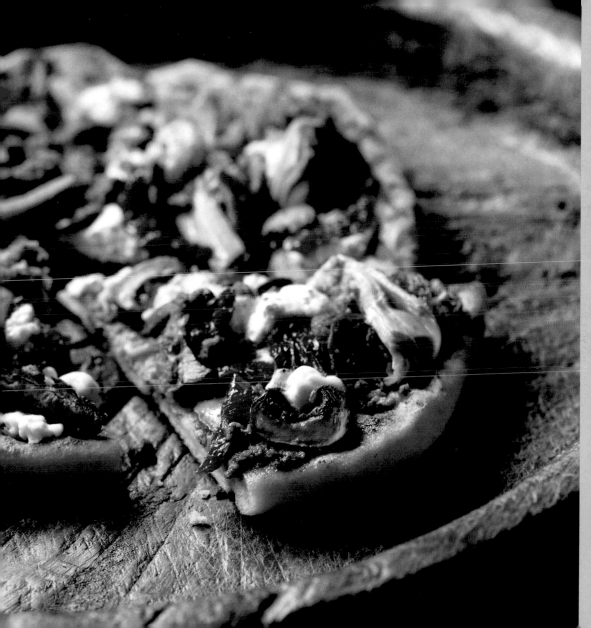

Sausage & Pepper Pizzas

We've spilled quite a bit of ink over the years warning readers about the hazards of sausage pizza at places like Pizza Hut. At home, though, you can have your sausage and eat it too, just as long as it's chicken or turkey sausage.

You'll Need:

2 links uncooked chicken sausage

2 medium bell peppers (green, red, or yellow), stemmed, cored, and quartered

1 large red onion, sliced into ¼"-thick rings and skewered with toothpicks

2 jalapeño peppers (optional)

Pizza Dough (page 110)

Olive oil for brushing

1½ cups diced fresh mozzarella

1 cup Tomato Sauce (page 110)

You can also use cooked chicken sausage from companies like Al Fresco. Just slice and lay them on top of the pizza.

How to Make It:

● Preheat a grill using a two-zone fire (see "Go High and Low," page 40), one zone high and the other low. Place the sausages, peppers, onions, and jalapeños (if using) over the hottest section of the fire. Grill, turning, for about 10 minutes, until the sausage is cooked all the way through, the onions are soft and browned, and the skin on the peppers is blistered. Slice both the sausage and the bell peppers into bite-size pieces and thinly slice the jalapeños.

● Divide the dough into two equal balls. Using a well-floured work surface and a rolling pin, stretch the dough into 12" circles.

● Place one of the dough circles on a lightly floured pizza peel. Brush the top with oil and slide the dough directly onto the hot part of the grill. Cook for about 30 seconds, until the dough begins to brown, then use a pair of tongs to rotate it 45 degrees. Cook for another 30 seconds, creating diamond-shaped grill marks on the crust. Flip the dough and place, raw side down, on the cooler side of the grill. Working quickly, top first with half the mozzarella, then half the sauce, sausages, onions, and peppers. Close the grill top and let the pizza cook for 2 to 3 minutes, until the cheese begins to melt. Use your tongs to rotate the pizza 45 degrees and continue cooking until the crust is lightly charred and the cheese is fully melted. Repeat with the other pizza.

Makes 4 servings

Per Serving:
$2.87

550 calories
15 g fat (8 g saturated)
950 mg sodium

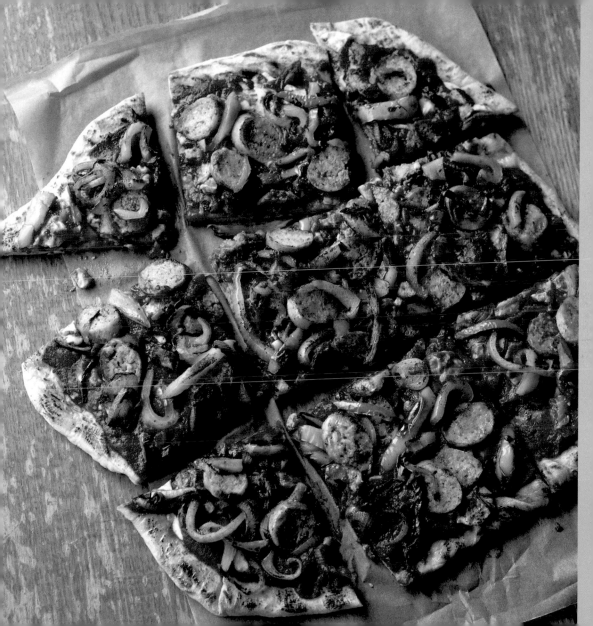

Kale & Bacon Pizzas

We've seen pizza topped with oysters, quail eggs, hot dogs, and dozens of other previously unthinkable pizza components. If there's anything America has taught the world about pizza, it's that anything goes, as long as it tastes good. Crispy kale, smoky bacon, and piquant provolone definitely qualify.

You'll Need:

Pizza Dough (page 110)

Olive oil for brushing

1½ cups shredded provolone, fontina, or smoked mozzarella

1 cup Tomato Sauce (page 110)

4 strips bacon, cooked until lightly crisp and broken into ½" pieces

Crack Kale (page 335), chopped into bite-size pieces

Feel free to replace grilled kale with sautéed spinach or broccoli rabe.

How to Make It:

● Preheat a grill using a two-zone fire, one zone high and the other low. Close the lid so that the heat can effectively build up.

● Divide the dough into two equal balls. Using a well-floured work surface and a rolling pin, stretch the dough into 12" circles.

● Place one of the dough circles on a lightly floured pizza peel. Brush the top with oil and slide the dough directly onto the hot part of the grill. Cook for about 30 seconds, until the dough begins to brown, then use a pair of tongs to rotate it 45 degrees. Cook for another 30 seconds, creating diamond-shaped grill marks on the crust. Flip the dough and place, raw side down, on the cooler side of the grill. Working quickly, top first with half the cheese, then half the sauce, bacon, and kale. Close the grill top and let the pizza cook for 2 to 3 minutes, until the cheese begins to melt. Use your tongs to rotate the pizza 45 degrees and continue cooking until the crust is lightly charred and crisp beneath and the cheese is fully melted. Repeat with the other pizza.

Makes 4 servings

SAVVY SHORTCUT ↑

Homemade dough is an incomparable component of a first-rate pizza. Rather than turning to the store-bought stuff, double or triple the dough recipe (page 110) and freeze the leftovers. It's simple: After the dough comes together, divide it into tennis ball-size portions, drizzle with a bit of olive oil, and wrap tightly in plastic. Place the balls in the refrigerator to defrost the night before.

Per Serving: $2.17	470 calories 12 g fat (4.5 g saturated) 800 mg sodium

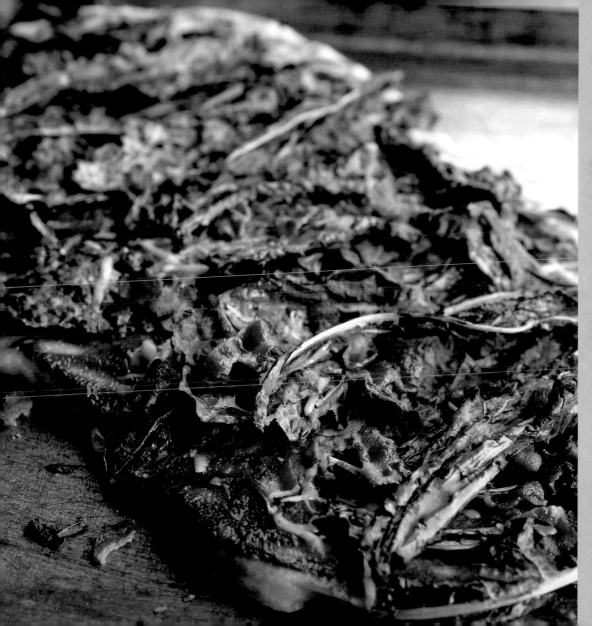

Pasta Primavera

Pasta primavera is one of the most misunderstood dishes in the restaurant universe. It appears on menus, beckoning health-conscious eaters with the promise of a cornucopia of vegetables. What the menu fails to mention is that the average bowl of restaurant pasta primavera contains nearly 1,000 calories, mostly from quick-burning pasta carbs and the oily cream sauce that traditionally dresses the dish. Our version is the real deal, made with more vegetables than pasta and dressed with a drizzle of olive oil and fresh basil.

You'll Need:

- 2 medium zucchini, sliced horizontally into ¼"-thick planks
- 2 medium yellow squash, sliced horizontally into ¼"-thick planks
- 12 asparagus spears, woody ends removed
- 1 red bell pepper, seeded, stemmed, and quartered
- 1 medium red onion, sliced into ¼" rings and skewered with toothpicks
- 2 Tbsp olive oil, plus more for coating the vegetables
- Salt and black pepper to taste
- 12 oz whole-wheat penne
- 20 cherry tomatoes, halved
- ½ cup grated Parmesan
- 1 cup chopped fresh basil

How to Make It:

- Preheat a grill over medium heat. Coat the zucchini, squash, asparagus, bell pepper, and onion with olive oil and season with salt and pepper. Grill the vegetables for 8 to 12 minutes (depending on the thickness of the vegetable), until tender and lightly charred on both sides.

- Bring a large pot of water to boil. Season with salt, add the penne, and cook until just al dente. Drain.

- Chop the grilled vegetables into bite-size pieces. In a large bowl, combine the vegetables and pasta with the 2 tablespoons olive oil, tomatoes, Parmesan, and basil.

Makes 4 servings

Any pasta shape will work just fine here, but the key is that the pasta has some fiber. Ronzoni Smart Taste is our favorite of the fiber-packed brands.

Per Serving:
$3.45

510 calories
13 g fat (3 g saturated)
600 mg sodium

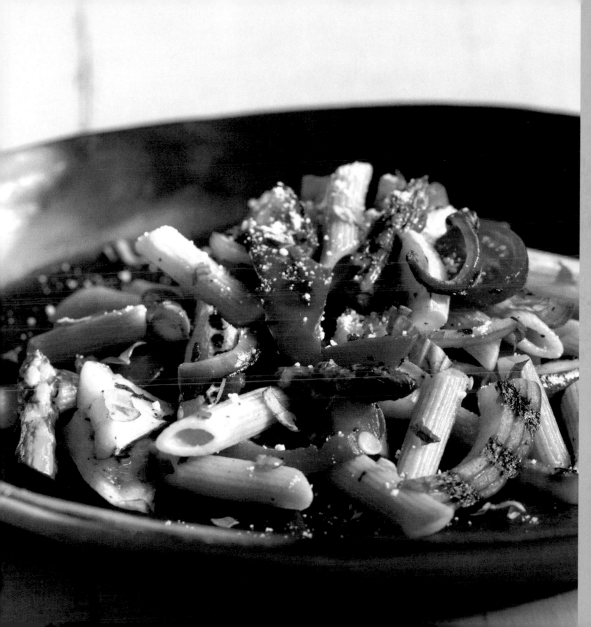

Sausage & Peppers
with Orecchiette

This ain't your grandma's bowl of noodles, that's for sure. No, this dish is a break from the standard stovetop creations, one that relies entirely on the power of the flame to create a robust sauce that dresses little ear-shaped shells. It might not be Italian, technically, but like the best Italian food it's based on a few simple ingredients, carefully prepared and thoughtfully combined. The results speak for themselves. (Note to campers, tailgaters, and people with electricity issues: You can even boil the pasta on the grill.)

You'll Need:

- 1 **bunch broccoli rabe, bottom 2" of stems removed**
- 2 **Tbsp olive oil**

Salt and black pepper to taste

- 2 **bell peppers, stemmed, seeded, and quartered**
- 2 **links hot Italian sausage**
- 10 **oz orecchiette pasta**

Grated Parmesan for serving

How to Make It:

- Preheat a grill over medium heat. Toss the broccoli rabe with 1 tablespoon of the olive oil, plus salt and pepper. Place the broccoli rabe, peppers, and sausages on the grill. Cook the peppers, turning, for about 10 minutes, until the flesh softens and the skin picks up a bit of char. Cook the broccoli rabe, turning once, for 12 to 15 minutes, until the stems are soft and tender and the florets begin to crisp up. Cook the sausages, turning, for about 15 minutes, until the skin is blistered and the meat is cooked through.

- Cook the pasta according to package instructions. Before draining, dip a coffee mug into the cooking water and reserve a few ounces for tossing with the pasta. While the pasta cooks, chop the peppers and broccoli rabe into bite-size pieces. Slice the sausages into thin rounds.

- Toss the vegetables and sausage with the drained pasta, the remaining 1 tablespoon olive oil, plus a splash of the pasta cooking water so that the pasta is moist. Serve with Parmesan over the top.

Makes 4 servings

Per Serving:
$2.23

520 calories
22 g fat (6 g saturated)
670 mg sodium

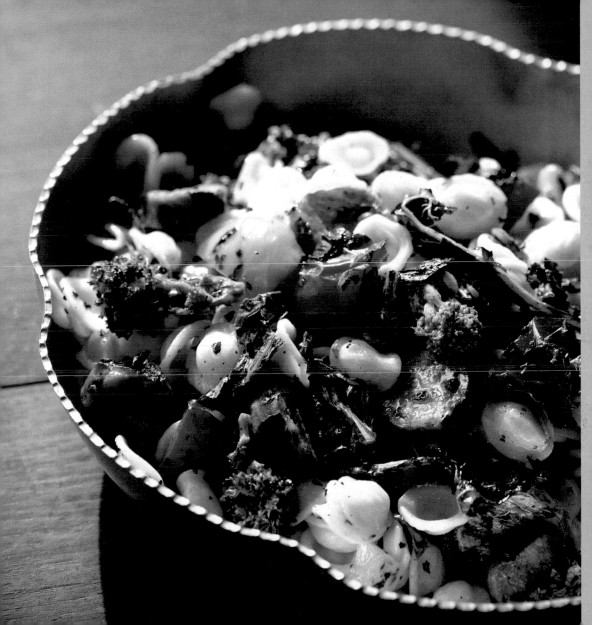

POULTRY

CHAPTER **5**

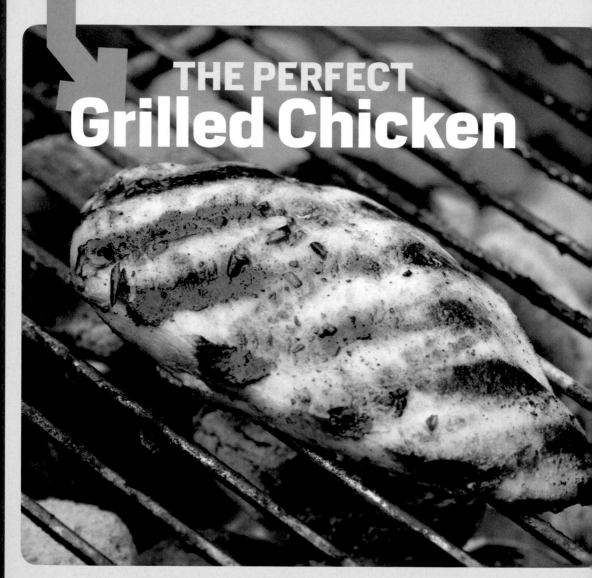

THE PERFECT
Grilled Chicken

The chicken breast is the Mitt Romney of the grill world: It neither excites nor offends anyone with its steady, predictable performance. But with a few minor adjustments, it can become something worthy of loving, even craving. Consider this your master recipe for chicken, whether you're planning to enjoy it in a sandwich, in a salad, or as is, right off the grill.

Buy high-quality chicken.

The reason "it tastes like chicken" became such a popular phrase is because most chicken tastes like nothing at all. Beyond the flavor issue, there's also a health issue at play here (for you and the bird): Most chicken is pumped full of so many drugs it's more science experiment than supermarket staple. Look for antibiotic-free and preferably free-range chickens; you'll pay extra, but you'll taste the difference.

Season in advance.

Every ingredient in the marinade here serves a specific purpose: Garlic, rosemary, and black pepper bring lively, but not over-whelming, flavor. Olive oil and a touch of sugar both help facilitate browning on the surface of the meat—an absolute must for a perfect piece of chicken. The acids in the lemon juice tenderize the meat. But most important, as always, is the salt—salting early will help season the entire chicken, not just the surface.

Cook carefully.

With little to no fat to help insulate it from overcooking, chicken breasts dry out quickly, mercilessly. Cook over a medium-high flame until both sides are nicely charred and the meat feels firm, but still gently yielding, like a tennis ball.

You'll Need:

- 4 **boneless, skinless chicken breasts**
- ¼ **cup olive oil**
- **Juice of 1 lemon**
- 2 **cloves garlic, minced**
- 1 **tsp chopped fresh rosemary, or 1 tsp dried rosemary**
- 1 **tsp sugar**
- 1½ **tsp salt**
- ½ **tsp black pepper**

- If the chicken breasts are uneven—thick in some parts, thin in others—cover with plastic and gently pound until they're a uniform ½" thick. Combine the olive oil, lemon juice, garlic, rosemary, sugar, salt, and pepper in a shallow bowl. Add the chicken breasts, turn to coat, and cover. Refrigerate and marinate for 30 minutes.

- Preheat a grill or grill pan over medium-high heat. When hot, remove the chicken from the marinade, pat thoroughly dry, and place on the grill. Cook for 2 minutes, then rotate 45 degrees and continue grilling for another 2 minutes, until the breasts have nice diamond-shaped grill marks. Flip and continue grilling for another 3 to 4 minutes, just until the meat is firm but yielding, like a tennis ball, and an instant-read thermometer inserted in the thickest part of the chicken registers 160°F. Makes 4 servings.

Ways to Cook a
CHICKEN BREAST

Chicken breast is the ultimate canvas, a lean, mild cut of meat that takes well to spice rubs and sauces. With a bit of international inspiration, we've created simple combinations that will turn a weekday staple into something spectacular. With this chart, you can take a spin around the globe without ever leaving your backyard.

	Season with	Sauce with	Serve with
Spanish	Smoked paprika	Romesco (page 50)	Grilled potatoes
Italian	Rosemary, garlic, and lemon	Pesto (page 49) or store bought	Grilled tomatoes
Indian	Curry powder	Mango chutney (page 200) or store bought	Sautéed spinach
Mexican	Chili powder	Grilled Corn Guacamole (page 266)	Black beans
Greek	Oregano, garlic, and olive oil	Tzatziki (page 48)	Warm pita
Argentinean	Cumin	Chimichurri (page 47)	Grilled asparagus
Southwestern	Magic Blackening Rub (page 51)	Mango Salsa (page 47)	Grilled zucchini

Meat Cheat Sheet
Chicken

Sometimes it feels as though the meat case—with its dizzying array of cuts and prices—should come with an instruction manual. To help simplify the process in the next two chapters, we've broken down chicken, beef, and pork by cut, providing you with the nutritional and cost information you need to make the best purchases possible.

Bone-in, skin-on wings (4 oz)
252 calories
21 g protein
18 g fat (5 g saturated)
Grill it right: Direct heat, medium
Average cost per lb: $2.22

Bone-in, skin-on breast (4 oz)
195 calories
24 g protein
10.5 g fat (3 g saturated)
Grill it right: Direct heat, medium
Average cost per lb: $2.56

Boneless, skinless thigh (4 oz)
135 calories
22 g protein
5 g fat (1 g saturated)
Grill it right: Indirect heat, medium
Average cost per lb: $2.92

Boneless, skinless breast (4 oz)
129 calories
24 g protein
3 g fat (0.5 g saturated)
Grill it right: Direct heat, medium-high
Average cost per lb: $3.29

Bone-in, skin-on thigh (4 oz)
248 calories
18.5 g protein
19 g fat (5 g saturated)
Grill it right: Indirect heat, medium
Average cost per lb: $1.66

Bone-in, skin-on drumsticks (4 oz)
180 calories
20 g protein
10.5 g fat (3 g saturated)
Grill it right: Indirect heat, medium
Average cost per lb: $2.16

* Prices for this and the other two Meat Cheat Sheets reflect the average cost obtained from a survey of butcher shops around the country. They may be higher or lower in your local market, depending on where you live.

The SPICE Route

These six exotic spice blends do wonders for food served around the world. They can do the same in your backyard.

ZA'ATAR

This all-purpose blend is used throughout the Middle East, usually as a condiment for sprinkling on breads and meats at the table. Sesame seeds add crunch and nuttiness, while sumac, a purple-hued Syrian spice, brings a pleasant acidic tang.

Grill This! Lamb chops and chicken drumsticks are prime candidates for a pre- or post-grilling sprinkle of za'atar. Or mix a spoonful with olive oil and use as a dip for toasted pita or a dressing for grilled eggplant, tomatoes, or zucchini.

HERBES DE PROVENCE

Long before spice companies started overcharging for their mediocre blends, cooks in southern France were using this floral mix of fennel, thyme, lavender, tarragon, and bay to season everything from a steak to homemade tomato sauce. This will end up being one of the most useful members of your entire spice rack.

Grill This! Rub all over a whole chicken before cooking it beer-can style, or toss with a mix of vegetables like squash, zucchini, and asparagus prior to grilling.

OLD BAY

This classic Chesapeake Bay spice blend was created by a German immigrant in 1939 as a crab companion, but these days its reach extends well beyond crustaceans. It packs a cabinet worth of seasonings, from ground mustard to cinnamon to mace.

Grill This! Toss medium unpeeled shrimp with a generous amount of Old Bay, then grill for an amazing peel-and-eat snack, or use it to convert wedges of grilled potatoes into Old Bay steak fries.

CHINESE FIVE-SPICE POWDER

This Eastern blend is made predominantly from warm cookie spices like cloves and cinnamon, which makes for a perfect yin-yang combination when rubbed on savory grilled meats. Look for a version with lip-tingling Szechuan peppercorns, which gives the blend some extra firepower.

Grill This! Rub it onto a steak, lamb chop, or duck breast, then serve with a dipping sauce of soy sauce, sesame oil, and a squirt of chili sauce.

SHICHIMI TOGARASHI

You don't have to be able to pronounce it to reap the rewards. This potent blend varies from one batch to the next, but expect sesame seeds, orange peel, dried seaweed, and a few different kinds of chiles.

Grill This! Japanese cooks use it to sprinkle on top of grilled chicken skewers, vegetables, and sliced steaks. You'd be wise to do the same.

GARAM MASALA

Nearly every constituent in this Indian spice blend falls well beyond the realm of the average American spice cabinet, but this heady mixture of star anise, cardamom, kalonji, and other exotic ingredients will feel right at home in your kitchen.

Grill This! Marinate chicken breasts or pork chops for an hour before cooking, or season shrimp, scallops, or vegetables just before grilling.

Power up your pantry:
Your local supermarket may not carry most of these spice blends, but online spice merchants Penzeys.com and Kalustyans.com do—along with hundreds of other exotic seasonings.

131

Classic Barbecue Chicken

There are just two factors that separate good barbecue chicken from bad barbecue chicken: technique and sauce. Barbecue chicken needs to be seasoned early (giving the chicken time to absorb the spices) and cooked over a low flame for even browning. As for sauces, we tested dozens of different recipes until finally settling on this homemade version, a perfect balance of sweet, salty, spicy flavors that will make your chicken sing.

You'll Need:

4 chicken legs, thighs and drumsticks separated

1 tablespoon All-Purpose Barbecue Rub (page 50)

Classic Barbecue Sauce (page 45)

How to Make It:

● Season the chicken all over with the rub. Do this at least 1 hour before cooking or up to 8 hours ahead, keeping the chicken refrigerated the whole time.

● Preheat a grill over medium-low heat. Pour ½ cup of the barbecue sauce into a small bowl for basting the chicken, reserving the rest to serve at the table. Place the chicken on the grill, skin side down. Grill for about 5 minutes, until the skin begins to lightly brown and the fat begins to render (which may create flare-ups on your grill; if need be, move the chicken to the cooler parts on the grill's perimeter).

● Turn the chicken and baste with the sauce, cooking for another 5 minutes. Continue turning and basting for 15 to 20 minutes total, until the chicken skin is deeply browned, the meat is firm to the touch and beginning to pull away from the bone, and an instant-read thermometer inserted into the thickest part of the meat registers 160°F. Pass the reserved sauce at the table.

Makes 4 servings

Per Serving:
$1.12

480 calories
26 g fat (9 g saturated)
580 mg sodium

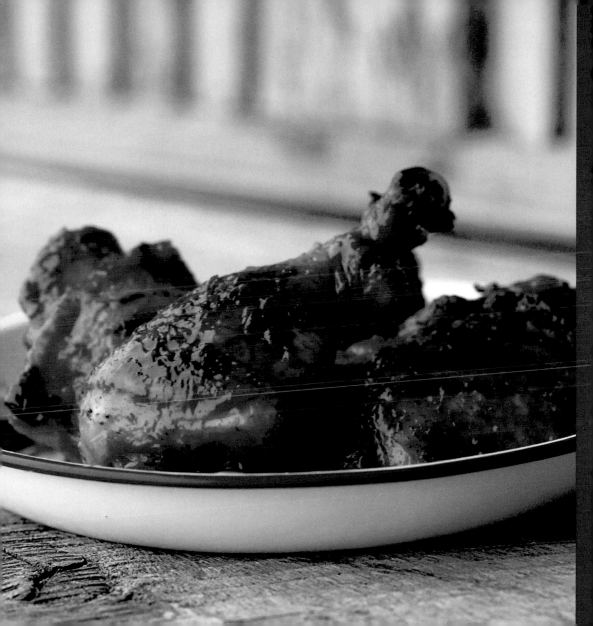

Chicken Yakitori

It's a sight beautiful enough to make a grown man weep: Long, narrow streets jam-packed with tiny restaurants serving nothing but grilled chicken parts and ice-cold beer. You'll find more than a few yakitori alleys throughout Tokyo, and you'll know them by the thick cloud of charcoal smoke that hangs over the street. This is the closest you'll get to Japan without a plane ticket.

You'll Need:

- ½ cup soy sauce
- ½ cup sake
- ½ cup mirin
- 2 cloves garlic, crushed and peeled
- 1" piece fresh ginger
- 1 bunch scallions
- 1 lb boneless, skinless chicken thighs, cut into ½" pieces
- Metal skewers, or wooden skewers soaked in water for 30 minutes
- Salt and black pepper to taste

How to Make It:

- Combine the soy sauce, sake, mirin, garlic, and ginger in a small saucepan over medium-low heat. Simmer until the sauce is reduced by three-fourths, about 15 minutes. Discard the garlic and ginger. Pour half the sauce into a small bowl and reserve for brushing on the chicken after it's cooked.

- Preheat a grill or grill pan over high heat. Remove the greens from the scallions and save for another use (or for garnish, if you like). Cut off and discard the bottoms, then chop the white parts into ½" pieces. Alternately thread the chicken and scallion pieces onto the skewers. Season with pepper and a light sprinkle of salt (the yakitori sauce packs plenty of sodium).

- Brush the chicken skewers all over with the sauce from the saucepan. Grill for 8 minutes, turning occasionally, until the chicken and scallions are lightly charred and the meat is firm to the touch and cooked through. Brush the skewers with the reserved sauce before serving. Serve with a scoop of steamed rice, if you like.

Makes 4 servings

Mirin is a sweetened rice wine that plays a huge role in Japanese sauces and marinades. You can find it in the Asian section of larger supermarkets, or you can substitute ½ cup sake plus 1 tablespoon honey.

Per Serving:
$1.45

260 calories
4.5 g fat (1 g saturated)
780 mg sodium

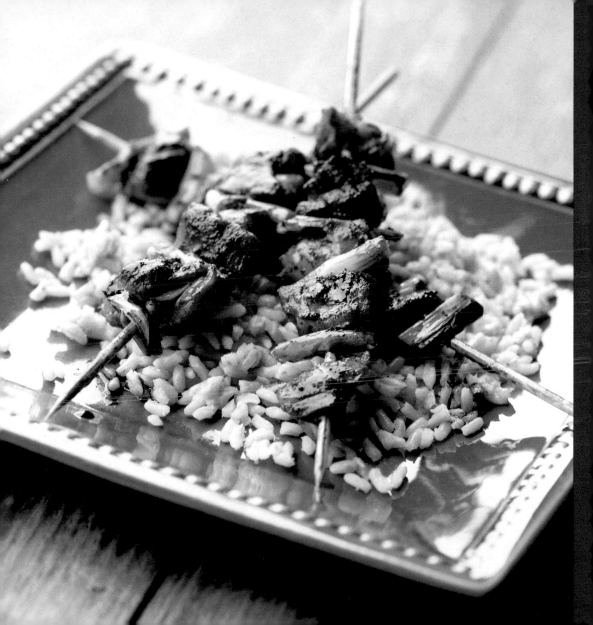

Prosciutto Pesto Chicken

Wrapping meats in other meats may seem like an overly indulgent way of tackling the issue of a weeknight dinner, but consider this: A slice of prosciutto has just 50 calories, many of which melt away under the intensity of an open flame. What you're left with is a crisp, intensely savory sheath that holds in place soft, melting goat cheese laced with the bright herbal notes of pesto. Try these tasty chicken thighs with a side of sautéed spinach and roasted potatoes, or stack them on toasted wheat buns for a heroic handheld meal.

You'll Need:

- 4 boneless, skinless chicken thighs (4 oz each)

Salt and black pepper to taste

- ½ cup fresh goat cheese, softened at room temperature for 30 minutes

- 2 Tbsp pesto (page 49 or store-bought)

- 4 thin slices prosciutto

How to Make It:

- Preheat a grill or grill pan over medium heat. Season the chicken all over with salt and pepper. Mix together the goat cheese and pesto until thoroughly incorporated. Slather the mixture down the center of each chicken thigh, then wrap with the prosciutto. The prosciutto should fit fairly tightly around the chicken, but as it cooks and the fat renders, it will tighten up even more.

- Grill the thighs for about 4 minutes per side, until the chicken is firm and cooked through and the prosciutto is browned and crisp around the edges.

Makes 4 servings

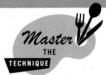

Master THE **TECHNIQUE**

Prosciutto wrapping

Chicken is just one of many grilled edibles made more delicious by the addition of a thin layer of prosciutto stretched across its surface. Other favorites include fillets of firm white fish like halibut or cod, scallops, shrimp, asparagus spears, and fresh figs. All follow the same technique: Wrap the meat, fish, fruit, or vegetable in just enough prosciutto to form a single secure layer and grill over medium heat until the prosciutto is crisp.

Per Serving:
$1.83

230 calories
14 g fat (6 g saturated)
600 mg sodium

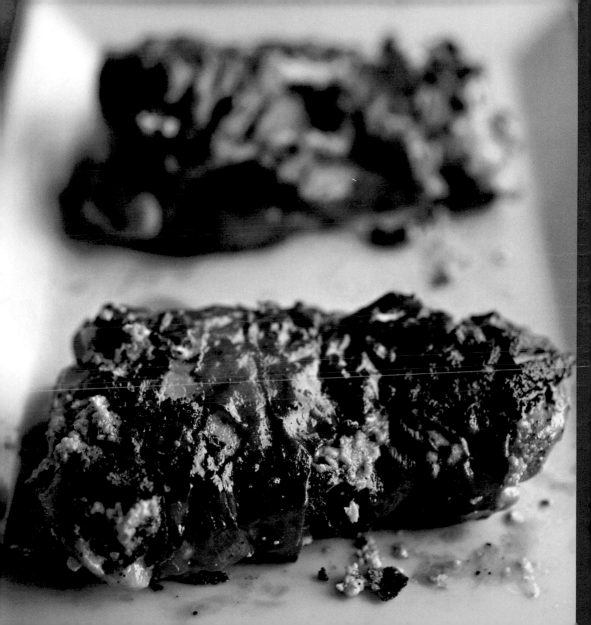

Hoisin-Lime Duck Breasts

For most people, duck is restaurant food, only to be enjoyed at white-linen fine-dining palaces or out-of-the-way Chinese spots. That's unfortunate, since it's not only intensely enjoyable, but also surprisingly lean and prime for the open flame. Its rich flavor is best when tempered with sweetness and acidity, both of which you'll find in our Asian-inspired glaze. Be sure to score the duck, as it will allow the fat underneath the skin to render out, leaving you with a crispy crust and soft, supple meat.

You'll Need:

¼ cup hoisin sauce

Juice of 2 limes

1 Tbsp reduced-sodium soy sauce

1 tsp toasted sesame oil

4 duck breasts (about 5 oz each)

Black pepper to taste

1 tsp Chinese five-spice powder

How to Make It:

- Preheat a grill or grill pan over medium heat. Combine the hoisin, lime juice, soy sauce, and sesame oil in a mixing bowl. Set aside half the sauce for serving.

- Score the duck: Make 3 diagonal cuts through the skin, then rotate 90 degrees and make 3 more cuts, creating diamonds in the skin. Season with pepper.

- Grill the breasts, skin side down, for 5 minutes, until the fat begins to render and a crust forms. Flip and baste with the hoisin mixture. Continue cooking and basting for 3 to 5 minutes, until the duck is firm but gently yielding to the touch and an instant-read thermometer inserted into the thickest part of the duck registers 135°F. Let the duck rest for 5 minutes before slicing. Serve with the reserved sauce.

Makes 4 servings

Per Serving:

$2.65

230 calories
8 g fat (2 g saturated)
470 mg sodium

SECRET WEAPON

Hoisin

Made from sweet potatoes, vinegar, garlic, and red chiles, among other ingredients, hoisin has become an indispensible part of our grill pantry; try it once and it's likely to get as much use in your kitchen as that bottle of Heinz. Brush this sweet-salty condiment on salmon or beef before grilling, combine with soy sauce and sriracha and use as a marinade for chicken drumsticks or wings, or swipe on burgers and chicken sandwiches for a low-calorie mayo replacement.

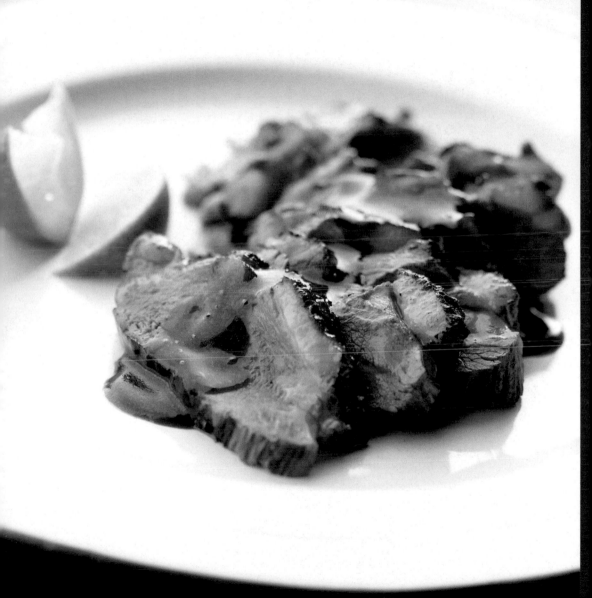

Beer-Can Chicken
Peruvian Style

El Pollo Rico, an unassuming Peruvian chicken spot on a tiny Arlington, VA, side street, serves America's greatest chicken, hauntingly delicious birds licked by the open flame of the restaurant's massive rotisserie setup. With a can of beer standing in for the spit and a fiery dipping sauce served on the side, we pay tribute to El Pollo Rico and their indecently juicy birds.

You'll Need:

1 **whole chicken (3½–4 pounds)**

½ **Tbsp ground cumin**

1 **tsp chili powder**

Juice of 2 limes

3 **cloves garlic, chopped**

1 **can (12 oz) beer**

Green Sauce (page 48)

Short of a rotisserie spit, there is no better way to grill a chicken than over a half-full can of beer. The steam from the beer produces an incredibly moist, tender bird.

How to Make It:

- Place the chicken in a large, sealable plastic bag. Add the cumin, chili powder, lime juice, and garlic. Seal, shake, and place in the refrigerator to marinate for at least 1 hour (but no more than 4 hours).

- Preheat a grill over medium-low heat. Open the beer and take a few spirited sips (or pour half of it down the drain, but why waste?). With the drumsticks facing down, carefully slide the chicken cavity over the beer can until it fits snugly. The chicken and beer should be able to stand freely on their own.

- Place the chicken on the grill grate and carefully close the lid. Cook for 35 to 45 minutes, depending on the size of the chicken. The chicken is done when the juices from the legs run clear (or until a thermometer inserted into the deepest part of a thigh reads 160°F). Check on the chicken occasionally; if the chicken fat is causing flare-ups, move the chicken to the coolest part of the grill. Allow the chicken to rest for 10 minutes before carving. Serve with the green sauce.

Make 4 servings

Per Serving:
$2.68

460 calories
26 g fat (7 g saturated)
680 mg sodium

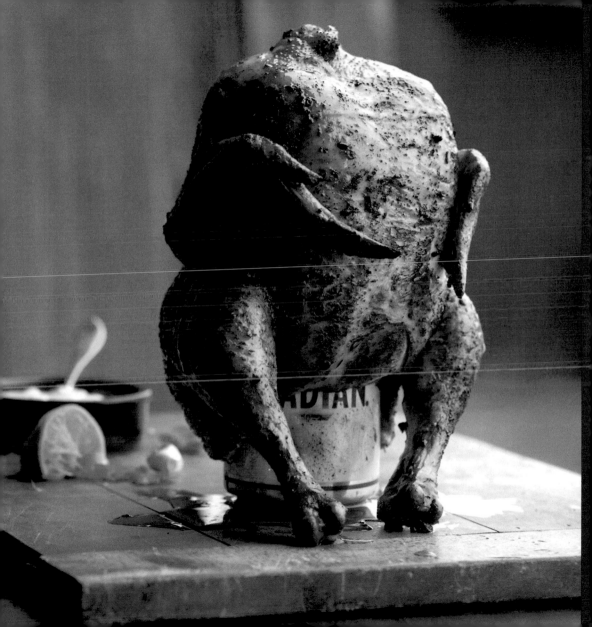

Balsamic Chicken Breasts

The best thing that can be said about a chicken breast—apart from the fact that it's a lean, powerful source of protein—is that it takes well to outside flavors. This balsamic barbecue sauce is pretty amazing stuff: Six ingredients that everyone has in their pantry come together to make a complex, deeply satisfying sauce that elevates the prosaic chicken breast to delicious new heights. It tastes every bit as good when painted onto pork chops, duck breasts, or flank steak.

You'll Need:

1 cup ketchup

1 cup balsamic vinegar

1 Tbsp brown sugar

1 Tbsp Dijon mustard

1 Tbsp Worcestershire sauce

1 clove garlic, minced

4 small chicken breasts (about 6 oz each)

Salt and black pepper to taste

How to Make It:

- Bring the ketchup, balsamic, brown sugar, mustard, Worcestershire, and garlic to a simmer in a saucepan set over medium heat. Simmer for about 5 minutes, until the liquid has reduced by half and the sauce is thick like a bottled barbecue sauce. Allow the sauce to cool, then set aside half of the sauce to serve with the chicken.

- Preheat a grill over medium heat. Season the chicken with salt and pepper. Paint the chicken all over with a thin layer of sauce from the saucepan and place on the grill. Cook for 2 minutes, turn the breasts 45 degrees, and cook for another 2 minutes, until nice diamond-shaped grill marks have developed. Flip, brush one more time with the sauce, and grill for another 3 minutes, until the chicken is firm to the touch and an instant-read thermometer inserted into the thickest part of the chicken registers 160°F. Brush the chicken with the reserved barbecue sauce before serving.

Makes 4 servings

Per Serving: $1.97	270 calories 4.5 g fat (1 g saturated) 610 mg sodium

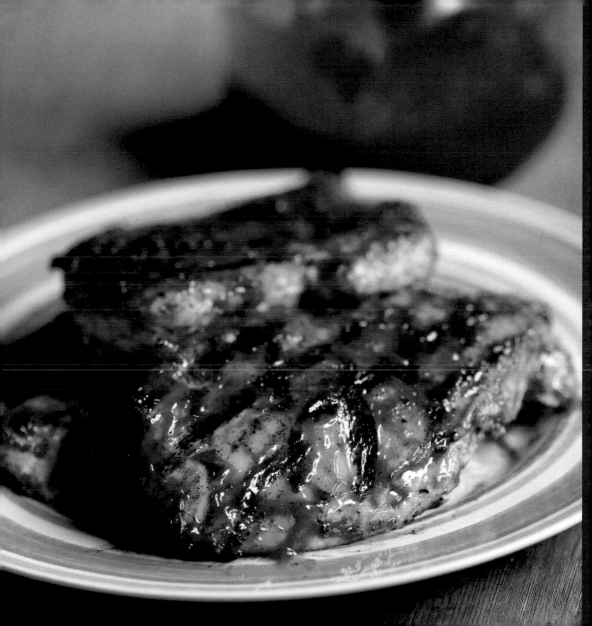

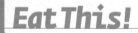

Chimi Skewers

Argentina lays claim to one of the world's greatest grill cultures, thanks in large part to the cattle-wrangling gauchos of Patagonia. Massive *asados,* epic feats of grilling often involving whole animals, are a common catalyst for social gatherings in this magical part of the world. While these spreads usually involve a staggering variety of smoked and grilled meats and fish, the one common thread tying them all together is chimichurri, the garlicky herb sauce that is paired with everything from thick-cut steaks to piles of crispy french fries. Here, we use it to top skewers of grilled chorizo and chicken, but it works just as well with fish, pork, and beef.

You'll Need:

- 1 lb boneless, skinless chicken breasts, cut into ¾" chunks
- 2 links chorizo, cut into ¾" chunks
- 1 medium onion, coarsely chopped
- 1 red or green bell pepper, cored and coarsely chopped
- ½ Tbsp olive oil
- Salt and black pepper to taste
- 8 metal skewers, or wooden skewers soaked in water for 30 minutes
- Chimichurri (page 47)

How to Make It:

- Preheat a grill or grill pan over medium heat. Combine the chicken, chorizo, onion, red pepper, and olive oil in a large mixing bowl. Season with salt and black pepper and toss. Alternating among chicken, chorizo, and vegetables, thread the ingredients onto the skewers.

- Grill the skewers, turning occasionally, for 3 to 4 minutes per side, until the meat and vegetables are nicely colored and the chicken and chorizo are firm to the touch and cooked through. Serve with the chimichurri drizzled over the skewers.

Makes 4 servings

Al Fresco makes an excellent lean chicken chorizo that would be perfect for these skewers.

Per Serving:

$2.24

300 calories
15 g fat (5 g saturated)
500 mg sodium

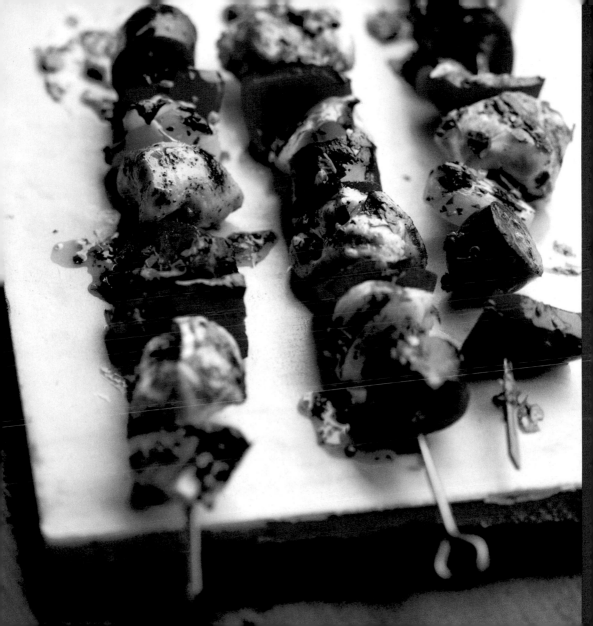

Eat This!

Smoked Turkey Breast

This recipe is a strong argument for eating fresh-cooked turkey more than once a year. Hot off the grill, it's excellent with all the traditional Thanksgiving fixings, but even better as leftovers. Cook this on Sunday and you'll be eating the best turkey sandwiches of your life all week long.

You'll Need:

- ¼ cup salt
- ¼ cup sugar
- 16 cups water
- 1 boneless turkey breast (3–4 lb)
- Black pepper to taste
- 2 cups wood chips (mesquite, oak, or apple), soaked in warm water for 30 minutes
- ¼ cup Dijon mustard
- ¼ cup maple syrup
- 2 Tbsp apple cider vinegar
- 2 Tbsp canola oil, plus more for coating the turkey

Turkey breasts are often sold in mesh netting, ready for cooking. If not, roll the breast and secure it with twine on both ends and in the middle.

How to Make It:

- Heat the salt, sugar, and water in a large pot set over medium heat until the sugar and salt dissolve. Allow to fully cool, then place the turkey in the brine. Refrigerate for at least 4 hours (or up to 12 hours). If the pot doesn't fit in the fridge, add a few big scoops of ice to the brine every few hours.

- Preheat a grill over low heat. Remove the turkey from the brine, pat dry, and lightly coat with oil. Season with pepper. Place the chips in a wood-chip box and place the basket directly over the flame. Place the turkey on the grill and close the lid. Grill, turning occasionally, for about 30 minutes, until the turkey is lightly browned on all sides.

- Combine the mustard, maple syrup, vinegar, and the 2 tablespoons canola oil. Grill the turkey for another 15 minutes, using a brush to continuously glaze the turkey with the sauce. The turkey is done when an instant-read thermometer inserted into the thickest part registers 155°F. Wait 15 minutes before slicing.

Makes 8 servings

Per Serving: **$1.63**

270 calories
5 g fat (0.5 g saturated)
620 mg sodium

LEFTOVER LOVE

As great as this turkey is on its own, it's even better dressed up and stacked between two pieces of bread. Here are three different ways to do it well:

- On a toasted English muffin with tomatoes, pepper-Jack cheese, and guacamole
- On sourdough with avocado and cranberry-spiked cream cheese
- On toasted rye with melted Swiss, sauerkraut, and Thousand Island dressing

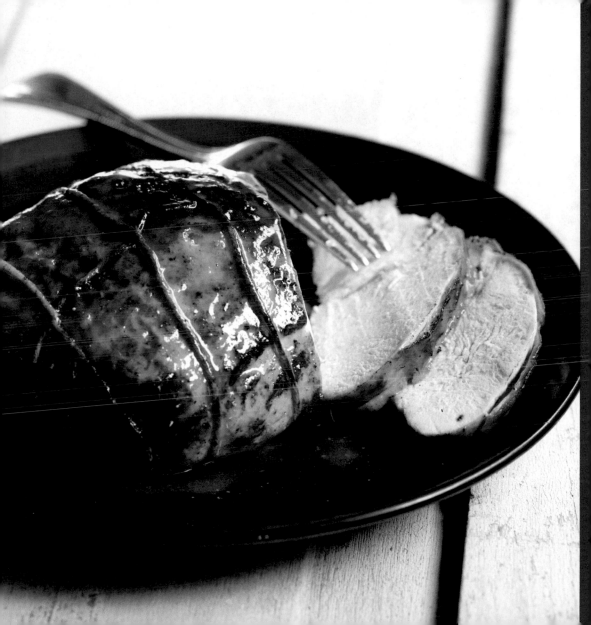

Korean-Style Drumsticks

Koreans are chicken geniuses, able to perform dazzling acts of alchemy with the humble bird. Unfortunately, most of those acts involve the use of a deep fryer, which is both inconvenient and ultimately deleterious for the home cook. Instead, we've taken some of their classic flavors and adapted them for the grill, using drumsticks to ensure the same type of juicy, succulent chicken you'd get from a deep fryer. This sweet, spicy glaze would work just as well on grilled chicken breasts or pork chops.

You'll Need:

- 3 cloves garlic, minced
- 1 Tbsp minced fresh ginger
- ¼ cup honey
- 2 Tbsp sesame oil
- 2 Tbsp chili garlic sauce (sambal oelek is best, but sriracha will do)
- 2 Tbsp rice wine vinegar
- 8 chicken drumsticks

Salt and black pepper to taste

How to Make It:

- In a mixing bowl, whisk together the garlic, ginger, honey, sesame oil, chili sauce, and vinegar. Season the chicken all over with salt and pepper. Place the chicken in a sealable plastic bag and pour in half of the marinade, reserving the other half. Seal the bag and refrigerate for at least 1 hour (but not more than 8 hours).

- Preheat a grill over medium heat. Remove the chicken from the marinade and grill, turning occasionally, for about 15 minutes, until the skin is nicely caramelized and the meat feels firm to the touch and is cooked through. If the rendered chicken fat causes flare ups, turn down the heat or move the chicken to a cooler side. Toss the cooked chicken with the reserved marinade and serve.

Makes 4 servings

Per Serving:
$1.07

300 calories
16 g fat (4 g saturated)
490 mg sodium

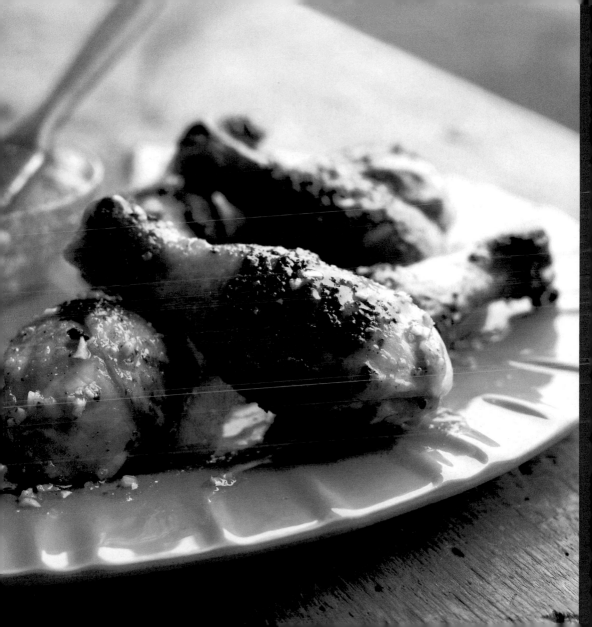

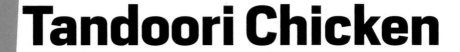

Tandoori Chicken

The Indians know better than anyone the potential for yogurt beyond the breakfast table. It acts as a sauce, a binder, and, perhaps most effectively, an excellent marinade base, where its natural acids help break down tough muscle tissue. Yogurt is at the heart of one of India's most famous dishes, tandoori chicken, where it's combined with a host of aromatic spices to transform an otherwise boring cut of meat. These skewers are killer on their own, but perhaps even better with a bit of Mango Chutney (page 200) drizzled over the top.

You'll Need:

- ¾ cup plain Greek yogurt
- 2 cloves garlic, minced
- 1 Tbsp minced fresh ginger
- ½ tsp cumin
- ½ tsp ground coriander
- ¼ tsp turmeric
- ⅛ tsp cayenne pepper
- 1 lb boneless, skinless chicken breasts, cut into ¾" cubes
- 4 metal skewers, or wooden skewers soaked in water for 30 minutes

How to Make It:

- In a large mixing bowl, combine the yogurt, garlic, ginger, cumin, coriander, turmeric, and cayenne and mix thoroughly. Submerge the chicken in the marinade, cover with plastic, and refrigerate for at least 2 hours (but no more than 8 hours).

- Preheat a grill or grill pan over high heat. Thread the chicken onto the skewers. Cook the skewers, rotating 90 degrees every few minutes, for about 8 to 10 minutes, until the chicken is firm to the touch and nicely browned all over.

Makes 4 servings

Per Serving:
$1.45

160 calories
4 g fat (1 g saturated)
370 mg sodium

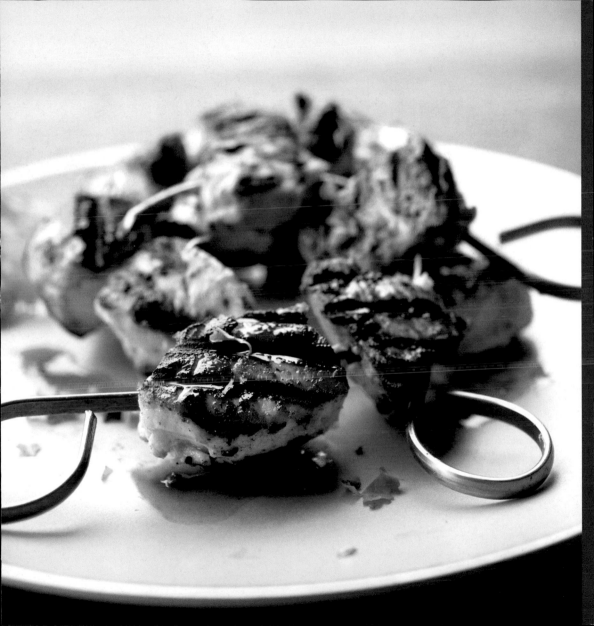

Fried Chicken
with Honey and Hot Sauce

We're using the term "fried" very liberally here, as this chicken contains not a single drop of oil. But the spirit of the dish is the same: chicken soaked in buttermilk, dredged in bread crumbs, and grilled until crisp and juicy. It might not replace Grandma's fried chicken in your world of comfort foods, but dipped into a mix of honey and hot sauce, it will wiggle its way into your heart nonetheless.

You'll Need:

1 **lb boneless, skinless chicken thighs**

1 **cup buttermilk**

6 **tablespoons hot sauce (we like Frank's RedHot)**

2 **cups panko bread crumbs**

1 **Tbsp butter, melted**

Salt and black pepper to taste

4 **Tbsp honey**

Panko is a light, flat Japanese bread crumb that produces crispier crusts than standard bread crumbs.

Chicken breasts work fine here, too, but they should first be pounded until they're uniformly ½" thick

How to Make It:

● Combine the chicken, buttermilk, and 2 tablespoons of the hot sauce in a sealable plastic bag. Seal and marinate in the refrigerator for up to 4 hours.

● Preheat a grill or grill pan over medium-low heat. Combine the bread crumbs and butter, plus a few pinches of salt and pepper, in a shallow baking dish. Working with a few pieces at a time, remove the chicken from the buttermilk and roll it in the bread crumbs, using your hands to gently press the crumbs into the flesh.

● Grill the chicken (if using a regular grill, keep the lid closed for about 4 minutes, until the bread crumbs begin to color and turn crisp). Flip and continue cooking for another 3 to 4 minutes, until golden and cooked through and an instant-read thermometer inserted into the thickest part of the chicken registers 160°F.

● Place 1 tablespoon of honey in each of four ramekins. Top with 1 tablespoon of hot sauce and serve alongside the chicken thighs.

Makes 4 servings

Per Serving:
$1.73

360 calories
8 g fat (3 g saturated)
630 mg sodium

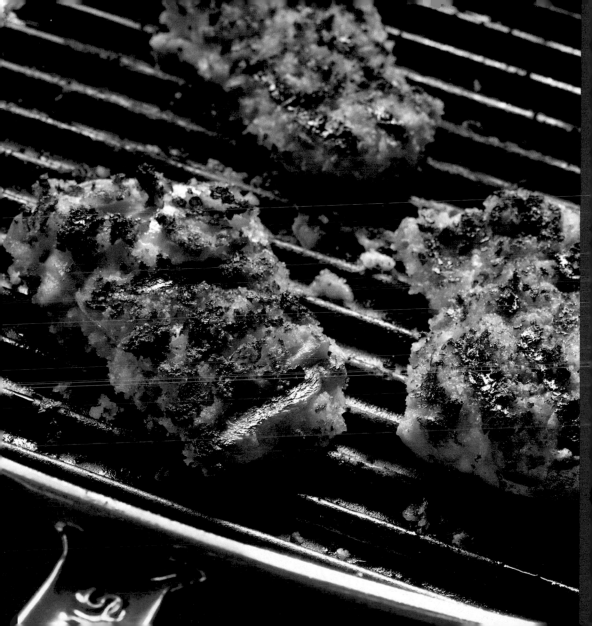

Asian Chicken Meatballs

Most of the world has its own spin on the meatball, and you'd be wise to embrace a few in your kitchen. These meatballs are inspired by street-corner grills in Vietnam and Thailand, where ginger, garlic, and chiles reign supreme. Wrap them in lettuce leaves for a lean, boldly-flavored Asian-style burrito.

You'll Need:

- 1 lb ground chicken or pork
- 1 small red onion, minced
- 2 cloves garlic, minced
- 1 Tbsp minced fresh ginger
- 1 Tbsp minced lemongrass (optional)
- 1 jalapeño pepper, minced
- 2 tsp sugar
- 1 tsp salt
- 4–8 wooden skewers, soaked in water for 20 minutes
- Boston lettuce, steamed rice, pickled cucumbers and onions (see Master the Technique to the right), hoisin, and/or sriracha for serving

How to Make It:

- Preheat a clean, lightly oiled grill or grill pan over medium heat. In a large mixing bowl, combine the ground meat with the onion, garlic, ginger, lemongrass if desired, jalapeño, sugar, and salt, stirring gently to evenly distribute all the ingredients. Roll the mixture into golf ball–size orbs, then carefully thread 3 or 4 onto each skewer.

- When your grill is hot, add the meatball skewers and grill for 4 to 5 minutes per side, until a light char has developed on the outside and the meatballs are cooked through. When done, they should feel firm, but springy to the touch.

- Use the lettuce and rice to make little Asian-style wraps with the meatballs, topping with cucumbers and your choice of sauces.

Makes 4 servings

Per Serving:	
$2.11	230 calories 12 g fat (3.5 g saturated) 670 mg sodium

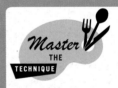

Master **THE** TECHNIQUE

Quick Pickling

A quick soak in seasoned vinegar can turn a raw vegetable into something special, perfect for topping grilled creations or eaten on its own as a snack. Combine ½ cup rice wine vinegar or white vinegar with ½ cup water and ½ tablespoon each salt and sugar. This basic solution can be used for onions, cucumbers, jalapeños, and pretty much any cooked vegetable you can imagine. Let them soak for at least 15 minutes before eating.

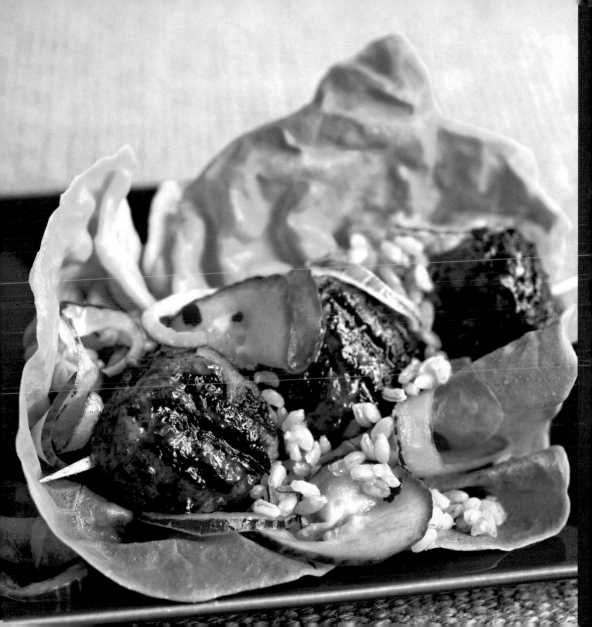

Moroccan Turkey Legs

These days it's easy to spot turkey legs at state fairs, carnivals, and ballparks across the country: They're those massive hunks of flesh that look more like caveman clubs than a grab-and-go snack. But the carnies and ballpark vendors are definitely on to something: The hearty cut of turkey makes for good eats hot off the grill—a far cry from the dry turkey most people are used to.

You'll Need:

¼ cup salt

¼ cup sugar

16 cups water

4 turkey drumsticks (about 1 lb each)

1 Tbsp Moroccan Spice Rub (page 51)

¼ cup honey

¼ cup red wine vinegar

2 Tbsp olive oil, plus more for coating the turkey legs

2 cloves garlic, minced

Buy the smallest turkey legs you can find. If your market only sells large legs, count on one leg for two people.

How to Make It:

● Heat the salt, sugar, and water in a large pot over medium heat just long enough to dissolve the salt and sugar. Allow to fully cool, then place the turkey legs in the brine. Refrigerate for 4 to 6 hours (or up to 12 hours). (If the pot doesn't fit in the fridge, add a few big scoops of ice to the brine every few hours.)

● Preheat a grill over low heat. Remove the turkey legs from the brine and pat dry with paper towels. Drizzle the legs with enough oil to lightly coat, then season them all over with the Moroccan Spice Rub.

● Grill the legs with the lid closed, turning occasionally, for about 45 minutes, until the skin is lightly browned all over and the meat begins to pull away from the bone. Stir together the honey, vinegar, the 2 tablespoons olive oil, and garlic. Use a brush to glaze the legs with the mixture, and grill for another 15 to 20 minutes, until the turkey has developed a dark crust all over (if using a gas grill, you can turn the fire up a notch to facilitate the browning) and an instant-read thermometer inserted into the thickest part of the turkey registers 155°F.

Makes 4 servings

Per Serving:
$3.39

380 calories
18 g fat (4.5 g saturated)
900 mg sodium

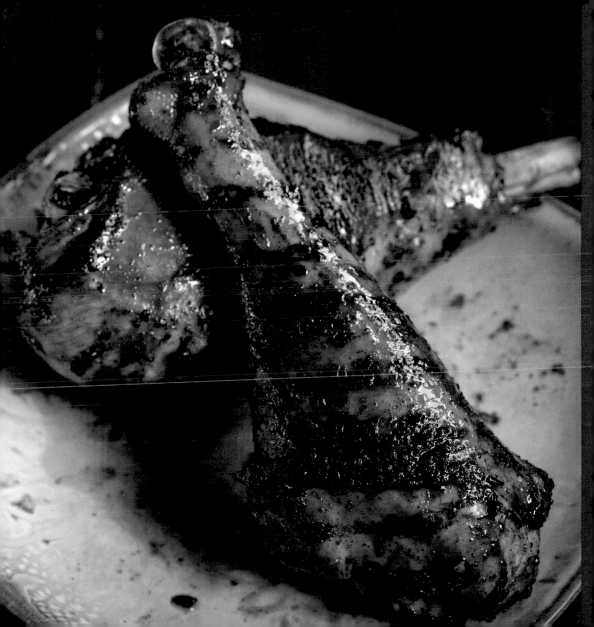

Eat This!

Chicken Under a Brick

Brick chicken, or *pollo al mattone* as the Tuscans call it, has been a favorite in central Italy for many years; taste it once and you'll see why. The concept is simple: By exposing as much of the chicken as possible to the hot grate, and by weighing it down with something heavy like a foil-wrapped brick, you encourage even cooking and deep crisping of the skin.

You'll Need:

- ¼ cup white or red wine vinegar
- ¼ cup olive oil
- 2 Tbsp Dijon mustard
- 1 Tbsp honey
- 1 tsp black pepper
- 1 tsp chili powder
- 1 tsp smoked paprika
- ½ tsp garlic powder
- ½ tsp cumin
- ½ tsp allspice
- 1 tsp red pepper flakes
- ¾ tsp salt
- 1 whole chicken (about 3 lb), backbone removed
- 2 lemons (optional)

How to Make It:

- Whisk together the vinegar, olive oil, mustard, honey, and ¾ tsp of the black pepper in a bowl. Reserve.

- One hour before cooking, combine the chili powder, paprika, garlic powder, cumin, allspice, red pepper flakes, salt, and remaining ¼ teaspoon black pepper in a bowl, and season the chicken all over with the mixture.

- Preheat a grill over medium-low heat. Grill the chicken, back side down, with the lid closed for 15 minutes, until the bones have begun to brown. Flip, top with a heavy object (preferably a brick wrapped in foil) and close the top. Grill for about 20 minutes longer, until the skin is lightly charred and crispy and an instant-read thermometer inserted into the thickest part of the breast registers 160°F. If the fire flares up, move the chicken to a cooler part of the grill and continue cooking. Serve the chicken with the sauce and grilled lemon halves, if you like.

Makes 4 servings

Per Serving:
$2.83

470 calories
28 g fat (8 g saturated)
780 mg sodium

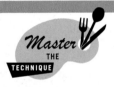

Master THE TECHNIQUE

Breaking down a chicken

Any butcher worth his salt will remove the chicken backbone with a few cleaver whacks, but doing it yourself at home is easy: Take a pair of kitchen scissors (or, failing that, a sharp, heavy knife) and cut your way through the chicken back immediately to the right of the spine. Repeat on the left side until the entire spine can be separated from the back. Toss the spine (or save for chicken stock), open the bird and flatten it out, and proceed with the recipe.

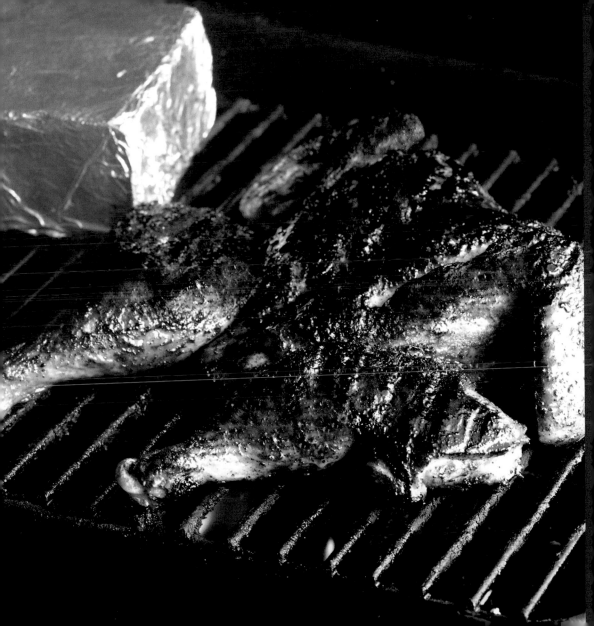

Paella

When it comes to making authentic paella at home, there's no better place to start than with the grill. That's because the traditional paella of central Spain has always been cooked over an open fire, which perfumes the rice with smoke and assures that the large paella pan cooks the dish evenly.

You'll Need:

- 1 Tbsp olive oil
- 1 small yellow onion, minced
- 1 large tomato, diced
- 2 cloves garlic, minced
- 1 link Spanish-style chorizo, diced
- 4 bone-in chicken thighs

Salt and black pepper to taste

- 1 cup bomba, Arborio, or other short-grain rice
- 3 cups low-sodium chicken broth

Pinch of saffron

- 8 medium shell-on shrimp
- 8 mussels, scrubbed under water and debearded

How to Make It:

- Preheat a grill over high heat. Place a large stainless steel sauté pan directly on the grate and close the lid to allow the heat to build up. When the pan is hot, add the olive oil, onion, tomato, garlic, and chorizo and sauté for about 10 minutes, until the vegetables are very soft and caramelized and the chorizo is lightly browned. Remove to a plate and reserve.

- Season the chicken thighs with salt and pepper and place in the pan, skin side down. Cook for about 5 minutes, until the skin is deeply browned, then flip. Return the vegetables and chorizo to the pan, along with the rice, chicken broth, and saffron. Simmer the paella, undisturbed, for 15 minutes, until most of the liquid has been absorbed by the rice (if the liquid isn't simmering, close the lid to speed the process). Arrange the shrimp and mussels around the paella, close the lid, and cook for about 5 minutes, until the shrimp are pink and firm, and the mussels have opened. If you like an extra crispy crust on the bottom of the paella (called *socarrat* in Spain, it's the most important part of paella), leave the pan on the hottest part of the grill for an extra minute or two before serving.

Makes 4 servings

Per Serving:	510 calories
$2.91	21 g fat (5 g saturated)
	980 mg sodium

SECRET WEAPON

Paellera

To make a great paella, you can't crowd the rice. Doing so will result in a wet, unevenly cooked paella rather than the dry, almost crunchy rice dish that paella is supposed to be. That's why Spaniards have always used paelleras, flat pans with ample surface area, to give the rice a chance to absorb every last drop of flavorful liquid. Pick one up (along with the chorizo and other great Spanish products) at Tienda.com. If you don't feel like investing in a paella pan, use the largest, shallowest oven-safe sauté pan you have.

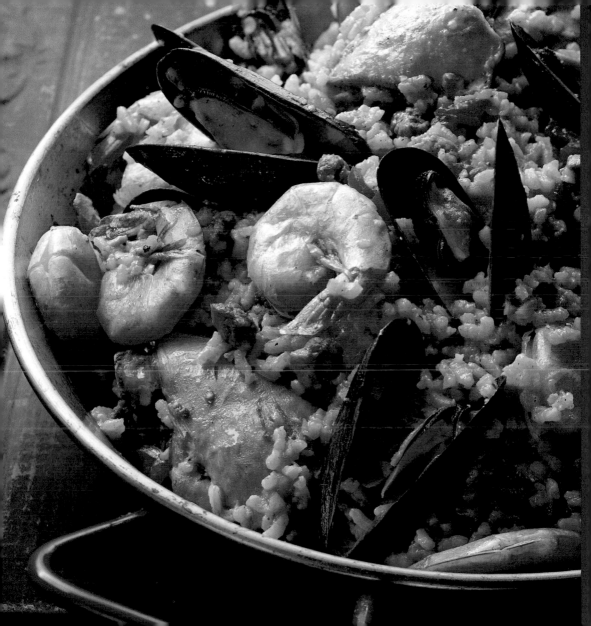

RED MEAT

CHAPTER **6**

Meat Cheat Sheet
Beef

We've all been there before: You stand at the meat case and a sprawling diversity of cuts spreads out before you. Unless you grew up in a butcher shop, it's tough to know where to start. There's a time and a place for nearly every cut of cow, but when it comes to everyday grilling, look for lean, affordable beef that can be cooked over direct heat. Take a close look at the chart breakdown and a few favorites stand out: flank steak, skirt steak, and oft-overlooked round provide a great balance of price, protein, and calories, while sirloin emerges as the best of the common steak cuts.

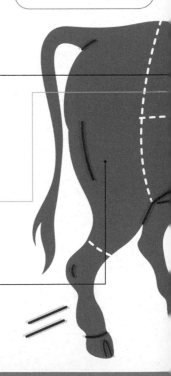

Tenderloin (4 oz)*
280 calories

22 g protein

20.5 g fat
(8 g saturated)

Grill it right: Direct heat, medium

Average cost per lb: $15.16

Sirloin (4 oz)
228 calories

23 g protein

14.5 g fat
(6 g saturated)

Grill it right:
Direct heat, high

Average cost per lb: $7.05

Porterhouse/ T-bone (4 oz)
280 calories

21 g protein

21 g fat (8 g saturated)

Grill it right: Direct heat, medium-high

Average cost per lb: $10.49

Round (4 oz)
188 calories

25 g protein

9 g fat
(3.5 g saturated)

Grill it right: Direct heat, medium-high

Average cost per lb: $5.49

* Fillet (aka filet mignon) comes from the tapered end of the tenderloin. As such, its cost and its nutritional numbers are essentially the same.

Rib-eye/ prime rib (4 oz)

277 calories

21.5 g protein

21 g fat (9 g saturated)

Grill it right: Indirect heat, medium

Average cost per lb: $10.66

Short ribs (4 oz)

266.5 calories

20 g protein

21 g fat (9 g saturated)

Grill it right: Marinate first; indirect heat, low

Average cost per lb: $3.92

Shoulder roast (4 oz)

140 calories

24 g protein

5 g fat (2 g saturated)

Grill it right: Direct heat, medium-high

Average cost per lb: $5.08

Hanger steak (4 oz)

174 calories

24 g protein

8 g fat (3 g saturated)

Grill it right: Direct heat, medium-high

Average cost per lb: $13.32

Brisket (4 oz)

285 calories

21 g protein

22 g fat (8.5 g saturated)

Grill it right: Indirect heat, medium-low

Average cost per lb: $4.66

Flank steak (4 oz)

176 calories

24 g protein

8 g fat (3.5 g saturated)

Grill it right: Direct heat, medium-high

Average cost per lb: $7.66

Skirt steak (4 oz)

212 calories

23 g protein

13 g fat (5 g saturated)

Grill it right: Direct heat, medium-high

Average cost per lb: $6.32

Pork

No animal produces meat with a wider range of nutritional numbers than the humble hog. A serving of pork tenderloin has just 7 more calories than a serving of boneless, skinless chicken breast, while a piece of pork belly the size of a deck of cards packs more than a day's worth of saturated fat. As a general rule, the cuts from the perimeter of the pig are lightest on your wallet, while the center cuts are lightest on your waistline. Your best strategy? Grab any loin cut you can get your hands on.

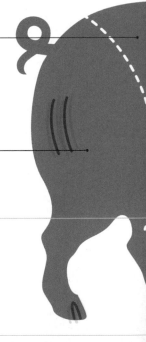

Chops (4 oz)
239 calories

22.5 g protein

16 g fat
(5.5 g saturated)

Grill it right: Direct heat, medium-high

Average cost per lb: $4.83

Tenderloin (4 oz)
136 calories

23.5 g protein

4 g fat
(1 g saturated)

Grill it right: Direct heat, medium-high

Average cost per lb: $3.89

Ham, fresh, uncured (4 oz)
278 calories

20 g protein

21.5 g fat
(7.5 g saturated)

Grill it right: Indirect heat, medium

Average cost per lb: $2.49

Pork belly/fresh bacon (4 oz)
587 calories

10.5 g protein

60 g fat
(22 g saturated)

Grill it right: Indirect heat, medium

Average cost per lb: $3.82

Spareribs/Kansas City ribs (4 oz)
314 calories

17.5 g protein

26.5 g fat
(8.5 g saturated)

Grill it right: Indirect heat, low

Average cost per lb: $2.65

Loin roast (4 oz)
188 calories

24 g protein

9.5 g fat
(2 g saturated)

Grill it right: Direct heat,
medium-high

Average cost per lb: $5.16

Rib roast (4 oz)
211 calories

23 g protein

12.5 g fat
(3 g saturated)

Grill it right: Indirect heat,
medium

Average cost per lb: $5.09

Shoulder roast/
Boston butt (4 oz)
211 calories

20 g protein

14 g fat
(5 g saturated)

Grill it right: Indirect heat, low

Average cost per lb: $2.79

Baby back ribs
(4 oz)
254 calories

22 g protein

18.5 g fat
(6.5 g saturated)

Grill it right:
Indirect heat, low

Average cost per lb: $5.16

Sirloin/roast
(4 oz)
191 calories

23 g protein

10 g fat
(2 g saturated)

Grill it right: Indirect heat,
medium

Average cost per lb: $2.89

THE PERFECT
Grilled Steak

There's a big difference between good steak and great steak. A good steak requires a decent cut of meat and a general idea of what you're doing on the grill; a great steak needs careful provisioning, true finesse, and a bit of patience—but all are within your grasp. Follow these steps to ensure that you never eat a merely good steak again.

Take the chill off the meat.

Allowing the steak to rest at room temperature before grilling helps erase the discrepancy between the warm surface of the meat and the cold center, making for more even cooking. A thick steak needs at least 40 minutes at room temperature; a thinner steak needs about 20 minutes to warm up.

Create a crust.

A steak without a well-developed crust can never be a truly great steak. Meat browns through a process called the Maillard reaction (a process similar to caramelization in vegetables) that is largely responsible for beef tasting, well, beefy. To ensure your steak has a deep, almost-crunchy crust, you need a steak with no excess water on its surface (which will cause it to steam rather than brown) and a very hot grill.

Flip the steak three times.

A hot grill facilitates browning, but you also want even cooking, minimizing that unappetizing gray area between the crust and the pink center of your steak. To do this, ignore the advice of the TV chefs who implore you to flip your meat only once. By flipping your steak more often, the heat of the grill is better distributed throughout the meat, which not only ensures more even cooking, but also encourages faster cooking. Aim for at least three flips in total, one every 2 minutes or so, depending on the thickness of your steak.

Be patient.

We can't say this strongly enough: Cut into your steak hot off the grill and you're compromising your dinner. The juices inside a hot steak are looking for an exit plan and an overeager knife and fork will provide the perfect escape route. By waiting 5 to 10 minutes for the internal temp of the steak to cool, you ensure yourself a juicier steak, from the first bite to the last.

You'll Need:

4 sirloin or strip steaks (about 6 oz each)

Olive oil for coating the steaks

Kosher salt and fresh cracked black pepper

- Preheat a grill or grill pan over high heat. Just before cooking, coat the steaks with a light layer of olive oil and season both sides aggressively with salt and black pepper.

- Place the steaks on the grill and cook for 2 minutes, until light grill marks have developed, then flip. Grill for another 2 minutes and flip again. Flip one more time, grilling for 8 to 10 minutes in total, until the steak is firm but very yielding to the touch. (For medium-rare, an instant-read thermometer inserted into the center of the steak should register between 130 and 135°F). Allow the steak to rest for at least 5 minutes before eating. Makes 4 servings.

These rules apply to any kind of steak you like to cook. Some of our favorites come from Nimanranch. com and Snakeriverfarms.com.

THE PERFECT
Grilled Pork Chop

In 1987, the National Pork Board created the slogan "The Other White Meat," meant to tout pork's healthfulness and versatility, but mostly what it achieved was to remind people that pork can be dry and boring. But with our simple steps, you can restore pork to its rightful place as both a lean protein and incredibly delicious hunk of red meat.

Choose wisely.

Major domestic hog producers have steadily bred the flavor out of pork over the years, hence the comparisons to chicken and turkey. Fortunately, excellent small-scale pig farmers are selling high-quality meat that actually tastes like pork at local farmers' markets and grocers like Whole Foods. If you can't find someone locally, order a few chops online from nimanranch.com—they're life changing.

Stick to the bone.

Bones impart both moisture and flavor to meat, which is why buying bone-in chops, steaks, and chicken is always a good idea when looking for full-on meat flavor.

Soak your chops.

Remember osmosis and diffusion from high school science? Well, these are some of the same concepts at work when you brine meat. By submerging a chop in a liquid seasoned with lots of salt and sugar, the end result is a more tender and moist piece of pork. If you don't have time to do a full brine, then salt each chop a few hours before cooking. The meat will absorb the salt, which helps break down tough proteins, leaving you with a more flavorful, tender chop.

Ease off the gas.

It's been beaten into our heads over the years that pork must be incinerated for it to be safe to eat, but according to the Centers for Disease Control and Prevention, trichinosis has been all but eliminated in domestic swine. Just to be safe, harmful bacteria is killed off at 145°F, while the meat begins to dry out around 160°F degrees, so aim for 150°F and you'll be amazed at how juicy a chop can be.

You'll Need:

½ **cup salt**

½ **cup sugar**

8 **cups water**

4 **thick bone-in pork chops (about 8 oz each)**

Olive oil for coating the chops

1 **tsp fennel seeds, roughly chopped**

Consider the fennel seeds optional, but if Italian sausage has taught us anything, it's that fennel brings out the best in pork.

Black pepper to taste

- Combine the salt, sugar, and water in a large pot and heat just enough for the sugar and salt to dissolve. Cool thoroughly, then place the chops in the brine and refrigerate for at least 2 hours (but no more than 4 hours).

- Preheat a grill or grill pan over medium-high heat. Remove the chops from the brine and pat thoroughly dry. Coat the chops with a thin layer of olive oil, then season on both sides with the fennel and black pepper.

- When the grill is very hot, place the chops on the grate and grill for 2 to 3 minutes, until grill marks have formed. Rotate 45 degrees and continue grilling for another 2 minutes, until you have nice diamond-shaped grill marks. Flip and continue grilling for 4 to 5 minutes, until the chops feel firm but gently yielding to the touch and an instant-read thermometer inserted in the thickest part of a chop registers 150°F. Let the chops rest 5 minutes before serving. Makes 4 servings.

Marinade Matrix

Marinades serve many purposes: First, they infuse cuts of meat and fish with flavor and moisture. The acids in marinades also help break down tough muscle tissue, turning chewy cuts as tender as their more expensive counterparts. But marinades also have a serious health function: Research from the Food Science Institute of Kansas State University found that the polyphenols in marinades cut carcinogen levels in grilled foods by up to 88 percent. Time for a soak!

Four Quick Recipes

Build the base of your marinade with an acid, fill it out with another source of liquid, then punch up the flavor with aromatics and a secret weapon or two. It's a recipe for grilling greatness every time.

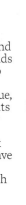

CHOOSE AN ACID

RED WINE

Balsamic is the sweetest of the vinegars and will cause your food to brown faster. The wine vinegars (red, white, rice) have less sugar and a more intense acidity.

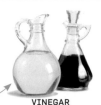
VINEGAR

CHOOSE A LIQUID

SOY SAUCE

WORCESTERSHIRE SAUCE

CHOOSE AROMATICS

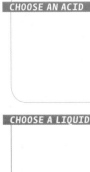
GARLIC

FRESH GINGER

CHOOSE A SECRET WEAPON ▶

Even better than the chipotle peppers themselves is the piquant, smoky sauce they come in. A few spoonfuls add a ton of flavor.

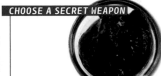
CHIPOTLE PEPPERS

Mirin is a sweet Japanese wine available in the international section of large supermarkets.

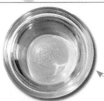
MIRIN

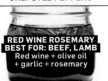
RED WINE ROSEMARY
BEST FOR: BEEF, LAMB
Red wine + olive oil + garlic + rosemary

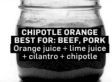
CHIPOTLE ORANGE
BEST FOR: BEEF, PORK
Orange juice + lime juice + cilantro + chipotle

ORANGE JUICE

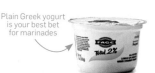

Plain Greek yogurt is your best bet for marinades

YOGURT

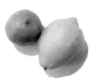

LEMON OR LIME JUICE

Marinade Basics

Rule 1

As a general rule, the less you spend on a cut of meat, the more likely it is that it will benefit from a marinade. That $20 fillet mignon? Don't bother. The $5 piece of flank steak? Time for a soak.

Combine with olive oil, lime juice, and honey for a bold beef, pork, and vegetable marinade.

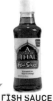

FISH SAUCE

Olive oil is great for Mediterranean-style marinades, sesame oil adds a touch of Asian flavor, and a neutral oil like canola or vegetable helps moisten proteins and keep them from getting dry without altering their inherent flavor.

OIL

Rule 2

Marinades by definition contain some type of acid, which is the critical ingredient that helps break down muscle tissue and make proteins more tender. If you're looking for flavor but not tenderness, you can skip the acid, but then it's not really a marinade.

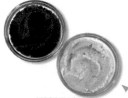

SLICED ONIONS

Stronger herbs like rosemary, thyme, oregano, and bay leaf work best.

FRESH HERBS

Rule 3

Marinade times should correspond to the size and intensity of the cut. A brisket or a pork shoulder can withstand an overnight marinade, but fish and shrimp should be marinated for no more than 30 minutes, otherwise the acid will begin to "cook" your food, turning your seafood into ceviche. Mid-range cuts like chicken breasts and pork chops are best if marinated between 1 and 4 hours.

White miso paste is sweeter and goes best with chicken and seafood, while red miso's intensity pairs nicely with beef and pork.

MISO PASTE

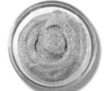

SPICY MUSTARD

SPICY YOGURT
BEST FOR: LAMB, CHICKEN, PORK
Yogurt + lemon juice
+ garlic + sriracha

SWEET MISO
BEST FOR: FISH, SCALLOPS, CHICKEN
Rice wine vinegar + canola oil
+ mirin + miso paste

Porterhouse
with Soy-Dijon Dipping Sauce

There is something magical about meat cooked on the bone, and it's not just the sheer primal joy of having a Flinstonian cut of meat before you. No, bones impart both flavor and moisture to meat, which is why T-bones and porterhouses are the undisputed kings in America's greatest steakhouses. Go for the thickest steak you can get your hands on, even if it means begging the butcher to saw one especially for you. This is caveman eating, with just a hint of sophistication.

You'll Need:

- 1 **small shallot, minced**
- 2 **Tbsp minced fresh ginger**
- 2 **Tbsp soy sauce**
- 2 **Tbsp Dijon mustard**
- 1 **Tbsp honey**
- Juice of 1 lime
- ¼ **cup canola oil**
- 1 **very large (18–20 oz) or 2 smaller (10–12 oz) T-bone or porterhouse steaks**
- Salt and black pepper to taste

How to Make It:

- Preheat a grill or grill pan over high heat. In a food processor, combine the shallot, ginger, soy sauce, mustard, honey, and lime juice. Pulse, slowly adding the oil to obtain a smooth, nicely emulsified sauce.

- Season the steak(s) all over with salt and pepper. Grill for 3 to 4 minutes, then rotate 45 degrees and continue grilling on the same side for another 2 to 3 minutes. Flip and repeat on the other side. Depending on how thick your steak is, it will take between 12 and 18 minutes total to hit medium-rare, when a thermometer inserted into the center of the steak (close to the bone) reads 135°F. Allow the steak to rest for 10 minutes before slicing into thick pieces. Serve with the soy-Dijon sauce.

Makes 4 servings

Per Serving:
$4.15

460 calories
35 g fat (10 g saturated)
910 mg sodium

SECRET WEAPON

Salt and pepper

Throw away your salt and pepper shakers immediately! Seasoning food with imprecise shaking is a recipe for disaster. Keep a small bowl of kosher salt on your countertop and season with your fingers; the large flakes make it easier to season your food with precision. Always use whole peppercorns ground in a pepper mill. Fresh cracked pepper is ten times more flavorful than the preground stuff These two small upgrades will make everything you cook taste better.

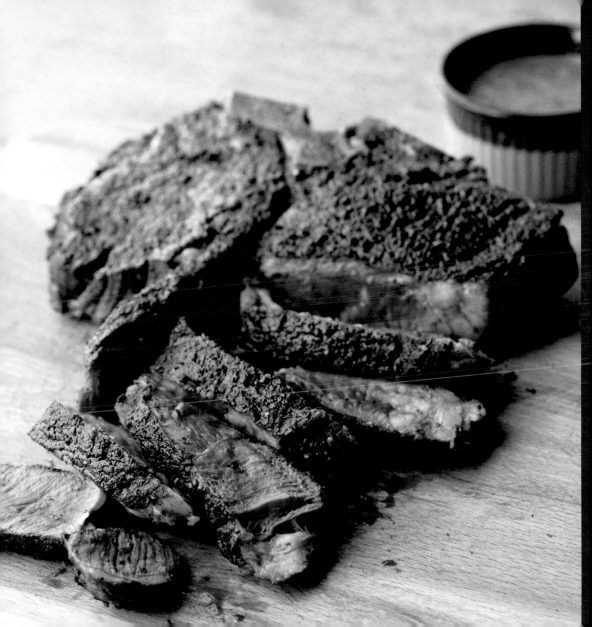

Lamb Kofta

Nobody on the planet has been grilling as long and consistently as the rich cultures of the Middle East, so when a popular dish emerges from these parts, savvy cooks should pay attention. Kofta, a mixture of ground meat and spices, is a ubiquitous staple found all across the region, albeit in many different guises. According to a study from 2005, Turkey alone lays claim to 291 different types of kofta. This one here, made from lamb spiced with cayenne pepper and cinnamon, is as good a place to start as any.

You'll Need:

- 1 lb ground lamb
- ¼ cup chopped fresh parsley
- ¼ cup minced onion
- 2 cloves garlic, minced
- ½ tsp cumin
- ⅛ tsp cinnamon
- ⅛ tsp cayenne pepper
- 1 tsp salt
- ½ tsp black pepper
- 4 metal skewers, or wooden skewers soaked in water for 30 minutes

Tzatziki (page 48)

How to Make It:

- Preheat a grill or grill pan over medium-high heat. In a large mixing bowl, combine the lamb, parsley, onion, garlic, cumin, cinnamon, cayenne, salt, and pepper. Gently mix to distribute the spices, then pack around the skewers to form two 3"-long oblong kebabs on each. (The colder the meat is, the more easily it will hold its shape on the skewers. To that end, it may be helpful to refrigerate the formed skewers for 15 or 20 minutes before grilling.)

- Grill the kebabs, turning them so that all sides pick up a nice char from the fire, for about 10 minutes, until the meat is cooked all the way through. Serve each skewer with a generous scoop of tzatziki on the side.

Makes 4 servings

If your market doesn't sell ground lamb, ask the butcher to grind a pound of lamb stew meat, usually cut from the lamb leg or shoulder. Or use ground chuck as a substitute.

Per Serving:
$2.30

290 calories
22 g fat (8 g saturated)
650 mg sodium

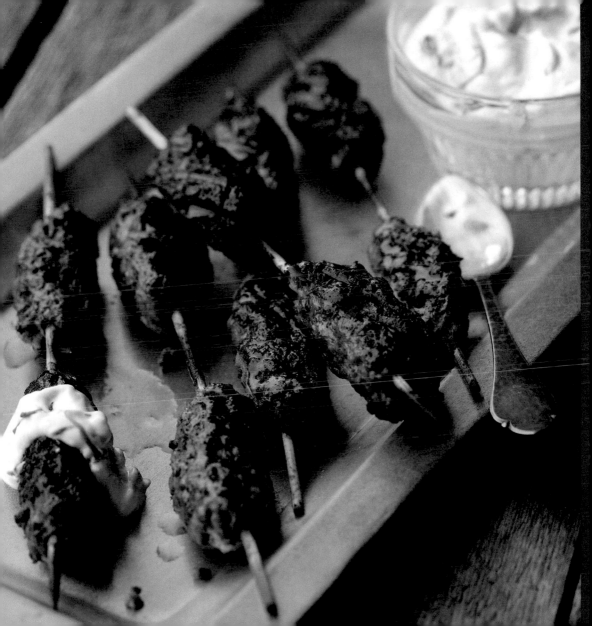

Stuffed Pork Chops

A pocket in a pork chop presents the cook with a world of opportunities. Savory, salty, sweet, spicy: All effects can be obtained with just a few carefully considered ingredients stuffed inside the chop. Do it right and there's no sauce or other bells and whistles required. It's restaurant-quality food (and by restaurant, we don't mean Applebee's or Outback, we mean the good ones), achieved for a few bucks a plate in the amount of time it takes you to load up the car and drive to the nearest lackluster chain. Who can argue with that?

You'll Need:

- **4 boneless pork chops** (about 6 oz each)
- **Salt and black pepper to taste**
- **½ cup dried cranberries**
- **½ cup fresh goat, feta, or blue cheese**
- **¼ cup walnuts, chopped**
- **1 tsp fennel seeds, roughly chopped**

Look for chops that are at least ¾" thick to make the stuffing easier.

How to Make It:

- Preheat a grill over medium heat. Use a paring knife to cut a pocket in the side of each chop, making it as deep and as long as you can without actually puncturing any other part of the meat. Use your fingers to carefully stretch out the pocket to create a bit of extra space. Season the chops all over with salt and pepper.

- Combine the cranberries, goat cheese, walnuts, and fennel seeds in a mixing bowl. Stuff the chops with the mixture until they're very full and secure with toothpicks. Place the chops on the grill, close the lid, and grill, turning once, for about 15 minutes, until browned and cooked all the way through.

Makes 4 servings

MEAL MULTIPLIER

Three more ways to successfully stuff a chop or a chicken breast:

- Apples, onions, chicken sausage, bread crumbs, fresh sage—all sautéed for 5 minutes in olive oil

- Wild rice, caramelized onions, crumbled bacon

- Sautéed broccoli florets, caramelized onions, and sharp Cheddar cheese

Per Serving:
$2.28

410 calories
19 g fat (8 g saturated)
460 mg sodium

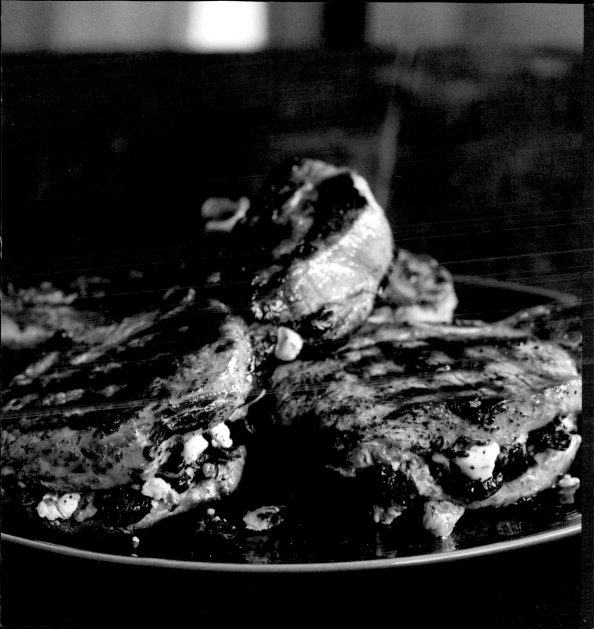

Grilled Steak Fajitas

On paper, fajitas look to be among the healthiest options at any Tex-Mex restaurant. The reality isn't so rosy; excess oil, cheese, and sour cream invariably saddle restaurant fajitas with more than 1,000 calories. Our version, done entirely on the grill, packs half the calories and twice the flavor.

You'll Need:

¼ cup vegetable or canola oil

Juice of 2 limes

1 Tbsp sugar

1 chipotle pepper in adobo

2 cloves garlic, crushed and peeled

1 tsp chili powder

¼ tsp cumin

1 lb skirt or flank steak

Salt and black pepper to taste

1 large sweet onion, sliced into ¼"-thick rings and skewered with toothpicks

2 large bell peppers (a mix of green and red is best), stemmed, seeded, and quartered

FOR SERVING

Guacamole (page 49)

Pico de Gallo (page 46)

Shredded Jack cheese

8 small flour or corn tortillas, warmed on the grill

There are few ingredients we love more than chipotle pepper. Its mixture of spice and smoke is a perfect addition to marinades and sauces.

How to Make It:

● Combine the oil, lime juice, sugar, chipotle, garlic, chili powder, and cumin in a food processor or blender. Puree until you have a smooth, uniform sauce. Combine with the skirt steak in a sealable plastic bag, seal, and marinate in the refrigerator for at least 1 hour (or up to 4 hours).

● Preheat a grill over high heat. Remove the steak from the marinade and pat dry with a paper towel. Season all over with salt and pepper and grill for 4 to 5 minutes per side, until a crust has formed, the meat is firm but yielding to the touch, and an instant-read thermometer inserted into the thickest part of the steak registers 135°F. While the steak cooks, grill the onions and peppers, turning, for 8 to 10 minutes, until soft and caramelized.

● After the steak has rested for at least 5 minutes, slice into thin pieces against the natural grain of the meat. Roughly chop the onions and peppers. Serve the steak and vegetables with the guacamole, pico de gallo, cheese, and warm tortillas.

Makes 4 servings

Per Serving:
$3.86

430 calories
16 g fat (7 g saturated)
810 mg sodium

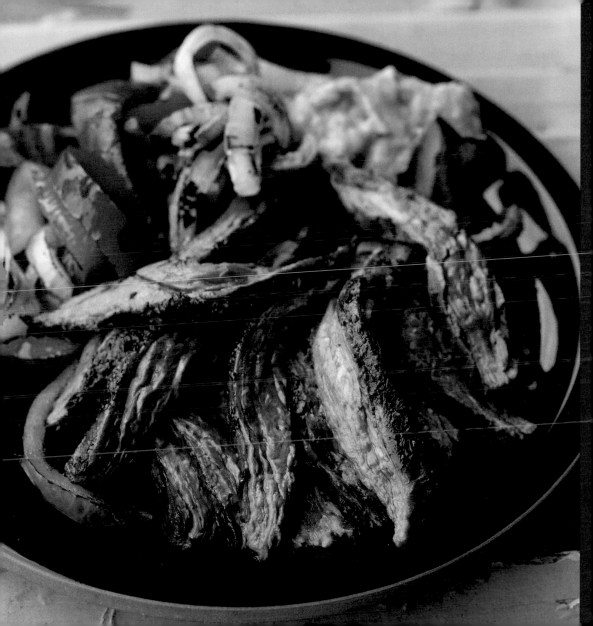

Classic Baby Back Ribs

In 2004, *Advertising Age* placed the "Baby Back Ribs" jingle from Chili's restaurant at the top of the list of the "10 songs most likely to get stuck in your head." The rib business exploded, and thousands of American waistlines followed suit, taking in 2,170 calories per rack (not to mention 6,510 milligrams of sodium). Ribs by their very nature are fatty, which is why we crave them, but there are two effective ways to tame the caloric intake: Cut back on the gloppy, candy-sweet sauce and dish out the final product in reasonable portions. We've done both here and still put out ribs with more appeal than those that have been stuck in all of our heads this past decade.

You'll Need:

- 2 **small racks baby back ribs**
- ¼ cup **All-Purpose BBQ Rub** (page 50)
- 2 cups **mesquite or hickory wood chips,** soaked in warm water for 30 minutes
- **Classic Barbecue Sauce** (page 45)

Serve the ribs with a few healthy sides (Barbecued Carrots and Cowboy Beans are perfect), which allow you to dish out smaller serving sizes and save everyone serious calories.

How to Make It:

- Preheat the oven to 250°F. Remove the thin membrane from the back of each rack of ribs (if not already removed by the butcher). Rub the ribs all over with the spice rub. Place in a large baking dish, cover tightly with aluminum foil, and bake for about 90 minutes, until the meat is tender and just beginning to pull away from the bone.

- Preheat a grill over medium heat. Place the mesquite or hickory chips in a wood-chip box and place the box directly over the flame. (If using charcoal, you can add the chips directly to the hot coals.) Brush the ribs with barbecue sauce and place on the grill. Cook, basting continuously with the sauce, for 15 to 20 minutes, until a deep, dark crust forms on the surface of the ribs.

Makes 6 servings

Per Serving: $2.93	370 calories 15 g fat (4.5 g saturated) 870 mg sodium

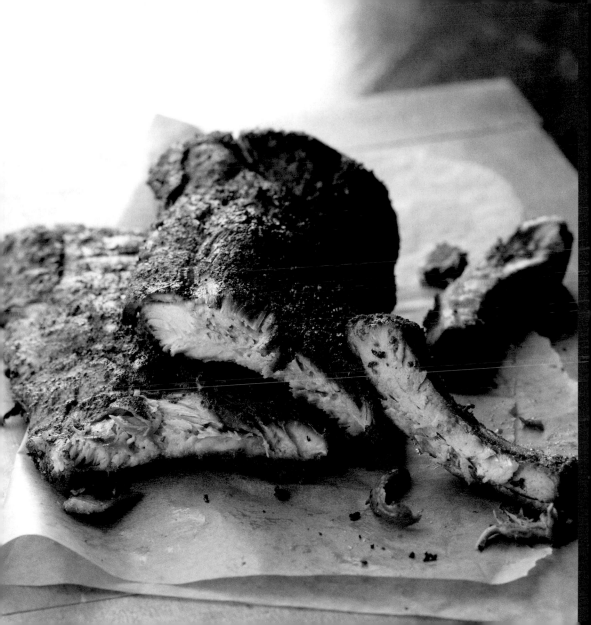

Balsamic Lamb Chops

Lamb chops can be pricey, but as a special occasion or an impressive appetizer for a group, they're pretty tough to top. They cook quickly on the grill, emerging juicy even if you go a minute or two too long. And because they're lean and tender, they carry less of the gamy taste many people associate with lamb. Lamb loves rosemary and garlic, which by itself would make this a perfectly good dish, but the sweetness of the balsamic drizzle really takes it over the top.

You'll Need:

- 2 Tbsp olive oil
- 2 cloves garlic, minced
- 1 Tbsp finely chopped fresh rosemary
- 1 lb lamb rib chops
- ½ cup balsamic vinegar
- Salt and black pepper to taste

Cut the cost in half by going with shoulder chops. They're not quite as pretty as the petite loin chops, but they're every bit as tasty.

How to Make It:

- Whisk together the olive oil, garlic, and three-fourths of the chopped rosemary. Place the lamb chops in a sealable plastic bag and pour the marinade over them. Seal the bag and refrigerate for up to 4 hours.

- Combine the remaining rosemary and the balsamic vinegar in a small saucepan set over medium heat. Cook until the vinegar reduces by about three-fourths (it should easily coat the back of a spoon), about 10 minutes.

- Preheat a grill over high heat. When very hot, season the lamb chops all over with salt and pepper and cook for 2 to 3 minutes per side, until firm but still yielding. Serve with the balsamic syrup drizzled over the chops.

Makes 4 servings

Per Serving: **$3.66**

280 calories
21 g fat (8 g saturated)
435 mg sodium

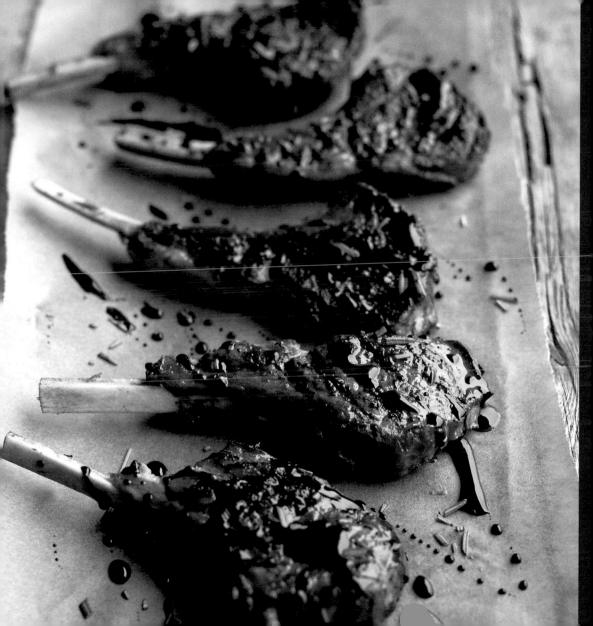

Carolina Pulled Pork (2 Ways)

The best barbecue in the world comes from the Carolinas, where whole hogs are smoked over hickory until the meat falls off the bone, then dressed in a vinegar-, ketchup-, or mustard-based sauce, depending on where you're eating. Which one is best? We'll let you decide for yourself.

You'll Need:

1 8–10-lb piece pork shoulder (preferably one with a generous crown of fat on top)

Salt and black pepper to taste

4 cups hickory wood chips, soaked in warm water for 30 minutes

NC Vinegar Sauce (page 46), SC Mustard Sauce (page 46), or Classic Barbecue Sauce (page 45)

Cole Slaw (page 337)

Potato rolls, warmed

How to Make It:

- A few hours before cooking, season the pork shoulder all over with salt and pepper and return to the refrigerator.

- Preheat a grill over low heat. You want to maintain a temperature between 200 and 300°F, which on a large gas grill means lighting just one or two burners on the lowest setting. Place a cup of the hickory chips in a wood-chip box and place the box beneath the grate, over the flame. (If using charcoal, you can add the chips directly to the hot coals.) Place the pork on the grill and close the lid. Grill for 3 to 4 hours, refreshing the wood chips occasionally and basting the meat with half of the NC Vinegar Sauce every 30 minutes or so. The exterior of the pork should be a deep amber color and the meat should pull away easily with a set of tongs.

- Let the pork rest for 15 to 20 minutes, then use tongs or forks to shred it into long strands. Alternatively, you can use two knives to chop it into fine pieces (the traditional way Eastern-style Carolina barbecue is served).

- Serve the barbecue with any or all of the sauces, along with slaw and buns on the side for making sandwiches.

Makes 12 to 16 servings (depending on the size of the shoulder)

The fat cap renders slowly while it cooks, basting your pork naturally without dramatically affecting the calorie count.

Per Serving:
$1.31

350 calories
16 g fat (5 g saturated)
650 mg sodium

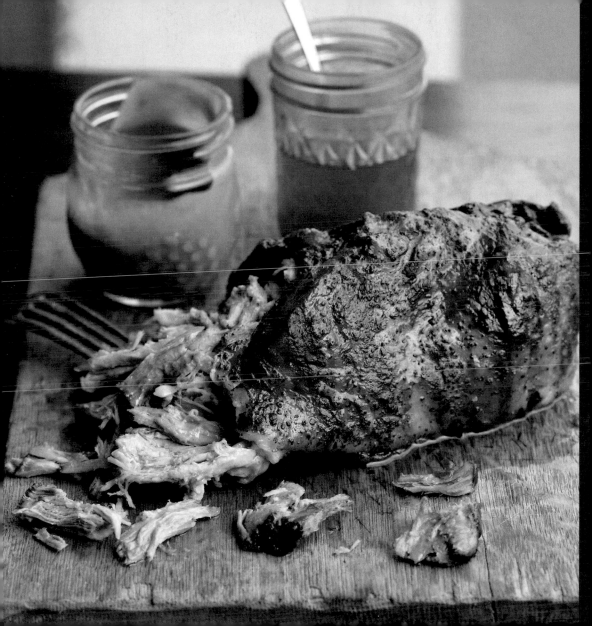

Grilled 'Carpaccio' with Arugula

Raw slices of beef have been a staple on fancy restaurant menus for decades now, allowing diners the privilege of paying $15 for what amounts to a couple ounces of meat and some token greenery. We propose you could do a better job at home for a third of the cost, especially with the help of a screaming-hot grill. A quick sear on all sides gives the carpaccio texture and depth of flavor while making it easier to eat for those squeamish about eating rare meat.

You'll Need:

- ¼ cup pine nuts
- 1 lb beef tenderloin (about 2 medium steaks)
- Salt and black pepper to taste
- 4 cups baby arugula
- 2 Tbsp olive oil (the best you have)
- Juice of 1 lemon
- Shaved Parmesan

How to Make It:

- Preheat a grill or grill pan over high heat. While the grill warms up, toast the pine nuts in a lightly oiled sauté pan set over medium heat until lightly browned, about 3 minutes.

- Season the tenderloins all over with salt and pepper and grill on the hottest part of the grill for no more than 2 to 3 minutes per side, until the outside of the meat is nicely browned but the inside is still rare. Rest the meat for 5 minutes before slicing into thin pieces.

- Toss the arugula with the toasted pine nuts, olive oil, and lemon juice and season with salt and pepper. Arrange the slices of beef in a wide circle on each of 4 plates and season with a pinch of salt. Place a pile of the arugula mixture in the center of each circle and garnish with the shaved Parmesan.

Makes 4 servings

Per Serving:
$4.96

320 calories
21 g fat (5 g saturated)
440 mg sodium

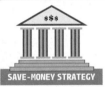

SAVE-MONEY STRATEGY

It's true that tenderloin makes for fine eating, especially in a dish as straightforward as this, but at $15 a pound or more, it's just not in the budget for most people. Truth is, many restaurants make their expensive carpaccio plates with cheaper cuts of beef, so there's no reason you can't do the same. Your best bets are eye of round or sirloin, both of which will cost you less than half of what you pay for tenderloin.

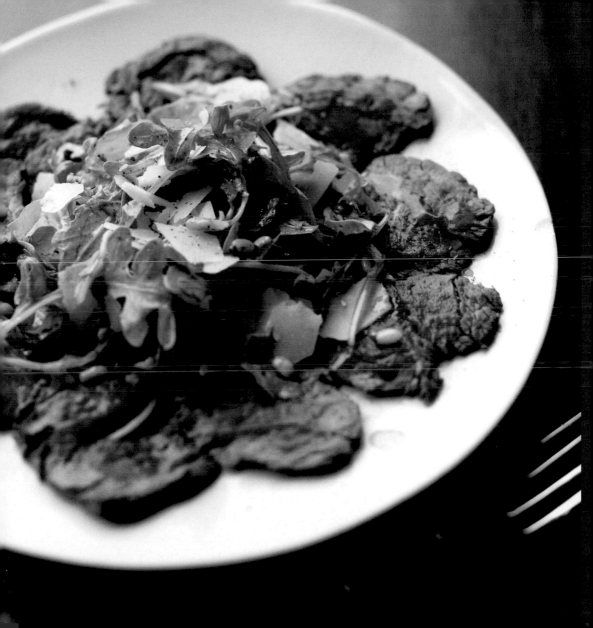

Tacos al Pastor

In Mexico, the *al pastor* taco is king. All throughout Mexico City you'll find late-night *taquerias* outfitted with giant spits of chile-rubbed pork turning over an open flame. Most wear a pineapple crown, the warm juices dripping down to commingle with the rendered pork fat. It's a glorious union of smoke and spice and sweet, one that we've done our best to recreate here.

You'll Need:

- 2 Tbsp white vinegar
- ½ Tbsp orange juice
- 1 onion, chopped
- 2 cloves garlic, chopped
- 2 Tbsp chipotle pepper in abodo
- ½ Tbsp guajillo chile powder
- Pinch cinnamon
- 1 lb pork loin, sliced into ½" rounds
- Salt and black pepper
- 1 avocado, peeled and pitted
- 1 cup Tomatillo Salsa (page 204) or store-bought salsa verde
- 2 thick slices pineapple
- 8 corn tortillas
- 1 handful cilantro, chopped
- Lime wedges

How to Make It:

- In a food processor or blender, combine the vinegar, orange juice, onion, garlic, chipotle pepper, guajillo, and cinnamon and pulse to a uniform puree. Season the slices of pork all over with salt and pepper, then combine with the marinade in a sealable plastic bag. Seal and refrigerate for at least 1 hour (or up to 4 hours).

- In a small mixing bowl, mash the avocado into a smoothish puree, then stir in the salsa to form a thick sauce. Reserve.

- Preheat a grill or grill pan over high heat. Remove the pork pieces from the marinade and grill for 2 to 3 minutes per side, until browned on the outside, firm to the touch, and cooked through. While the pork cooks, grill the slices of pineapple for 2 to 3 minutes per side, until light grill marks develop on the flesh.

- Warm the tortillas (on the grill or in a clean, damp towel in the microwave), then fill each with pork and pineapple and top with the avocado mixture and cilantro. Serve with lime wedges on the side.

Makes 4 servings

If you can't find guajillo chile powder, a standard chili powder can be substituted.

Per Serving: **$3.12**

370 calories
11 g fat (2 g saturated)
380 mg sodium

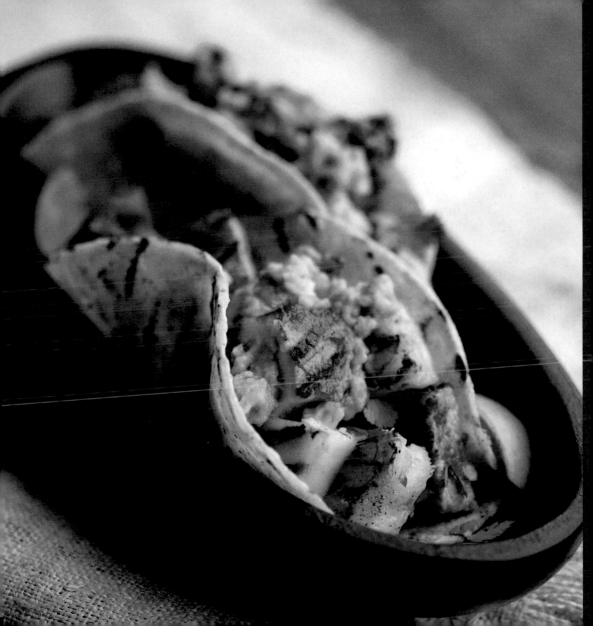

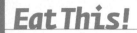

Santa Maria Tri-Tip
with Pico de Gallo

Tri-tip is a cut of meat taken from the bottom sirloin. It's an inexpensive and intensely beefy cut, and if cooked correctly and sliced across the natural grain of the meat, it can be perfectly tender and juicy too. Originally available primarily on the West Coast, supermarkets and independent butchers around the country are finally recognizing tri-tip's inherent awesomeness. This recipe is based on the specialty of Santa Maria, a farming town in central California with a long history of putting out soulful hunks of garlicky tri-tips.

You'll Need:

- 1 tri-tip steak (about 1½ lb)
- 1 Tbsp garlic powder
- Salt and black pepper to taste
- Mesquite or oak chips soaked in warm water for 30 minutes (optional)
- Pico de Gallo (page 46)
- Cowboy Beans (page 341)

How to Make It:

- Rub the tri-tip with the garlic, plus plenty of salt and pepper, using your fingers to gently press the spices into the meat. Let stand for 30 minutes at room temperature.

- Preheat a grill over medium-low heat. If using the wood chips, place them in a wood-chip box and place the box directly on the fire just before you start grilling. (If using charcoal, you can add the chips directly to the hot coals.) Grill the tri-tip, turning occasionally, for 20 to 25 minutes, until firm but yielding and a thermometer inserted into the thickest part of the meat registers 135°F. Rest for at least 10 minutes before slicing against the natural grain of the meat. Serve with the Pico de Gallo and Cowboy Beans.

Makes 4 servings

Santa Maria tri-tip is traditionally cooked over big hunks of red oak. Even a touch of smoke from a handful of chips will add to its authenticity.

Per Serving:
$2.36

280 calories
15 g fat (6 g saturated)
675 mg sodium

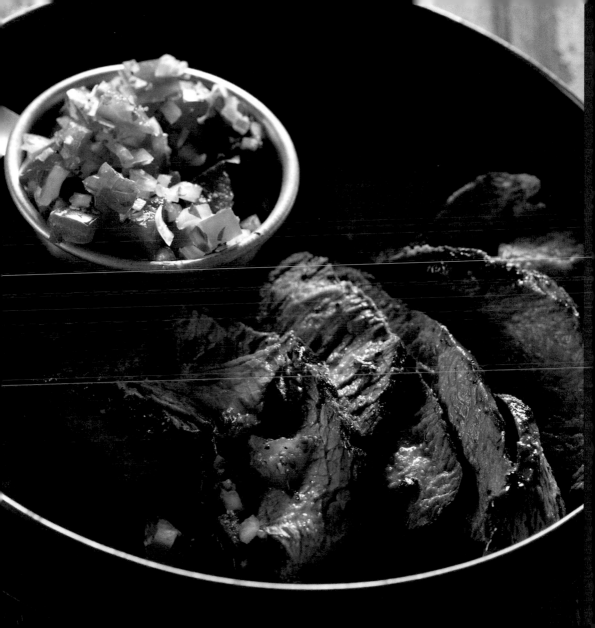

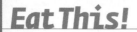

Chinese Spareribs

As much as we love baby back ribs for being obscenely tender, spareribs pack more protein and generally cost about half as much as the more popular baby backs. The trick to making them every bit as rib-stickingly delicious is a low, slow cook in the oven, which helps to break down the tough muscle tissue that holds the ribs together. Then a high-heat blast on the grill imparts that smoky outdoor flavor we crave from ribs and turns the sweet, sticky hoisin glaze into a lovely crust that contrasts nicely with the moist, tender meat inside.

You'll Need:

- 1 **rack St. Louis–style spareribs, cut into individual ribs**
- 1 **Tbsp Chinese five-spice powder**
- 1 **cup hoisin sauce**
- ½ **cup soy sauce**
- ¼ **cup honey**
- 2 **Tbsp rice wine vinegar**
- 2 **cloves garlic, minced**
- 1 **Tbsp minced fresh ginger**

Because spareribs are naturally such a fatty cut, this is the most caloric recipe in the book. Our suggestion? Serve just a few ribs per person and round out dinner with plenty of grilled vegetables.

How to Make It:

- Rub the ribs with the five-spice powder and place inside a sealable plastic bag. Combine the hoisin, soy sauce, honey, vinegar, garlic, and ginger in a bowl and whisk thoroughly. Pour half of the sauce over the ribs, seal the bag, and refrigerate the ribs overnight. Reserve the sauce remaining in the bowl.

- Preheat the oven to 300°F. Remove the ribs from the marinade and spread across a wire rack set in a baking dish. (If you don't have a rack, oil the baking dish and place the ribs directly in it.) Cover with aluminum foil. Bake for 1 hour, until the meat begins to pull away from the bone.

- Preheat a grill over high heat. Baste the ribs with some of the reserved marinade and grill for about 15 minutes, until the sauce caramelizes and the ribs pick up a nice char. Serve with the leftover sauce for slathering.

Makes 4 servings

Per Serving: **$1.97**

600 calories
35 g fat (11 g saturated)
1,010 mg sodium

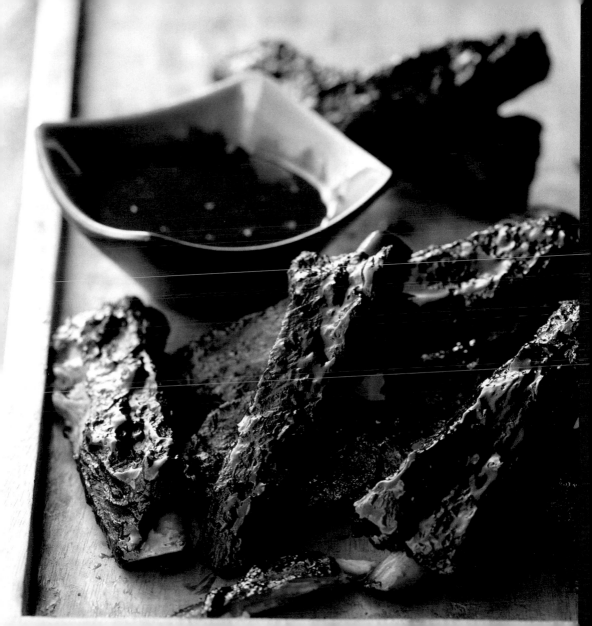

Strip Steaks
with Blue Cheese Butter

Beef and blue cheese are common menu partners for a reason: The subtle funk of blue cheese echoes and elevates the beefiness of a good steak, creating something much more than the sum of the two parts. If you don't have the time to form the butter and refrigerate, simply mix the ingredients in a bowl and serve each plate with a scoop slowly melting on top of the beef.

You'll Need:

- ¼ cup (½ stick) butter, softened at room temperature for 30 minutes
- 2 Tbsp crumbled blue cheese
- 1 Tbsp chopped fresh chives
- 1 shallot, minced
- 1 clove garlic, minced
- Black pepper and salt to taste
- 1 lb New York strip steak (about 2 medium steaks)
- 1 tsp smoked paprika

Normal paprika has almost no flavor at all, but Spanish-style smoked paprika is an explosive spice, perfect for steaks, chops, and chicken breasts.

How to Make It:

- Mix the butter, blue cheese, chives, shallot, garlic, and pepper together in a bowl. Spoon the butter into the center of a long piece of plastic wrap, fold the plastic around the butter, and twist the ends to create a log about an inch in diameter. Place in the refrigerator to firm up. Before cooking, remove the butter and slice into 4 thick coins.

- Preheat a grill or grill pan over high heat. Season the steaks with the paprika, salt, and pepper. Grill the steaks, flipping every two minutes, until nice grill marks have developed, the steaks are firm but still yielding to the touch (like a Nerf football), and an instant-read thermometer inserted into the thickest part of the steaks registers 135°F. Allow the steaks to rest for at least 5 minutes before slicing into thick pieces. Arrange on 4 plates and top with the butter.

Makes 4 servings

Per Serving: $2.92	300 calories 20 g fat (10 g saturated) 510 mg sodium

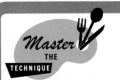

Master THE TECHNIQUE

Flavored butters

Spiking softened butter with assertive flavors is a great way to add an instant "sauce" to your dinner. And adding coins of compound butters (which keep for weeks in your fridge) to high-carb foods like baked potatoes actually works to mitigate blood-sugar spikes. Try any of these combinations on meat, fish, or vegetables.

- Reduced red wine, garlic, and rosemary
- Maple syrup and a slug of bourbon
- Minced sundried tomatoes and olives with goat cheese

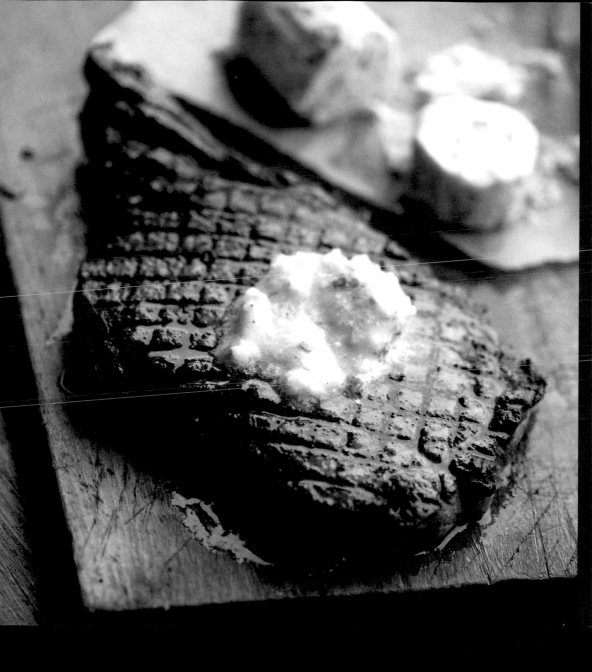

Steak-and-Potato Skewers
with Horseradish Steak Sauce

The classic steak-and-potato dinner can pack up to 1,200 calories on its own. This interpretation retains all the best parts of the steak dinner but puts it all on one skewer, shedding more than 700 calories in the process.

You'll Need:

16 **golf-ball size yellow or red potatoes**

Salt

2 **Tbsp prepared horseradish**

2 **Tbsp ketchup**

2 **Tbsp Dijon mustard**

2 **Tbsp brown sugar**

2 **Tbsp Worcestershire sauce**

1 **Tbsp honey**

1 **lb sirloin, cut into ¾" cubes**

Freshly cracked black pepper to taste

4 **metal skewers, or wooden skewers soaked in water for 30 minutes**

How to Make It:

- Place the potatoes in a pot, cover with water, season with salt, and set over high heat. Cook for about 15 minutes, until just tender. Drain.

- Preheat a grill over high heat. To make the sauce: Combine the horseradish, ketchup, mustard, brown sugar, Worcestershire, and honey in a mixing bowl. Set aside a few tablespoons of the sauce to serve with the grilled steak and potatoes.

- Season the sirloin with salt and lots of black pepper. Thread the skewers with chunks of sirloin and the potatoes. Grill the skewers, turning once and basting with the sauce, for about 5 minutes per side, until the steak is browned, slightly firm to the touch, and an instant-read thermometer inserted into the thickest part of the steak registers 135°F. Brush the reserved sauce on the steak and potatoes just before serving.

Makes 4 servings

If you can't find small potatoes, buy normal Yukon gold potatoes and cut them into ¾" pieces.

Per Serving:
$2.74

440 calories
15 g fat (6 g saturated)
710 mg sodium

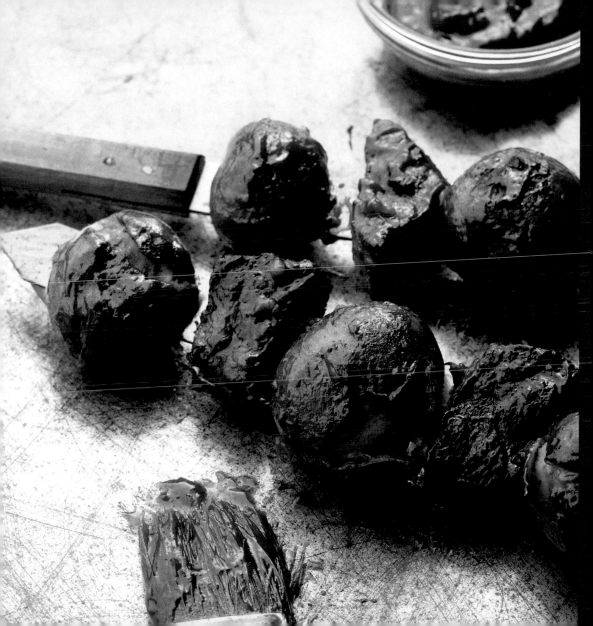

Curried Lamb Chops
with Mango Chutney

The average American consumes more than 60 pounds of beef a year. By comparison, that same average American consumes less than 1 pound of lamb a year. It's an astounding discrepancy, especially when you consider that lamb is widely available, easy to cook, and relatively lean. Here's a recipe we hope takes a bit of the pressure off the cows of this country.

You'll Need:

MANGO CHUTNEY

2 fresh mangos, peeled and diced

1 small red onion, diced

½ Tbsp minced fresh ginger

1 jalapeño pepper, minced

1 cup orange juice

2 Tbsp apple cider vinegar

2 Tbsp brown sugar

½ Tbsp curry powder

Salt and black pepper to taste

LAMB CHOPS

1½ lb lamb shoulder or loin chops

½ Tbsp curry powder

Salt and black pepper to taste

How to Make It:

- To make the mango chutney: Combine the mangos, onion, ginger, jalapeño, orange juice, vinegar, brown sugar, and curry powder in a saucepan set over medium heat. Simmer, stirring occasionally, for about 20 minutes, until the liquid has reduced into a thick syrup and the fruit and vegetables are very soft. Season with salt and pepper.

- To grill the lamb chops: Preheat a grill or grill pan over high heat. Season the lamb chops on both sides with the curry powder and salt and pepper. Grill for about 5 minutes per side, until nicely charred on the outside, firm but yielding to the touch, and an instant-read thermometer inserted into the thickest part of the lamb registers 135°F. Serve with the mango chutney.

Makes 4 servings

Shoulder lamb chops are cheaper, but also contain more fat than loin chops. The choice is yours.

Frozen mango also works great here. Defrost 2 cups, then chop into small pieces before cooking.

Per Serving:
$3.84

380 calories
10 g fat (3.5 g sat)
510 mg sodium

LEFTOVER LOVE

Mango chutney is one of those heroic condiments that seems to make most everything better—duck breast, bone-in pork chops, salmon steaks, even turkey sandwiches. Make up a double batch and keep it on hand for any time you're looking for a quick cure for the common dinner. Here's a favorite: Rub a chicken breast with chili powder and grill until cooked through. Serve over basmati rice with a side of sautéed spinach and a huge scoop of mango chutney.

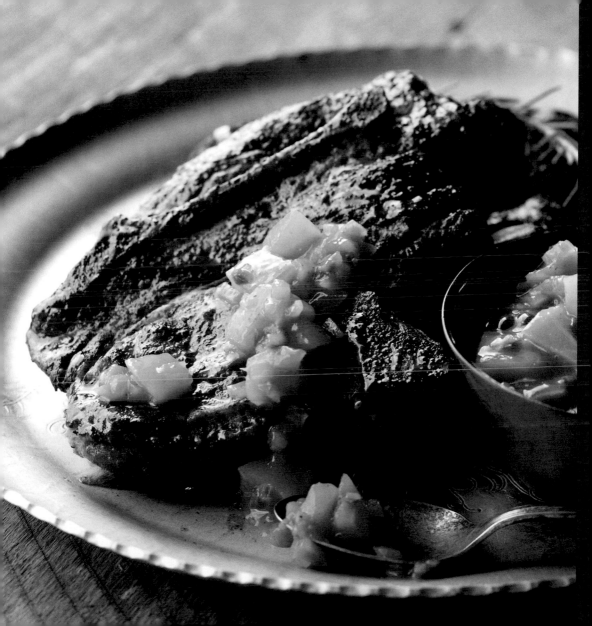

Stuffed Flank Steak

Stuffing meat is one of those great kitchen tricks that takes very little time or effort, but makes you look like a culinary genius. This is a simple three-step process: Pound the meat until flat, spread with the spinach-raisin mixture, then roll up and tie with a few pieces of butcher twine. To turn this into an Italian-style braciole, all you need is a few ladles of simmered tomato sauce.

You'll Need:

- 1 flank steak (1–1½ lb)
- 1 tsp olive oil
- 2 cloves garlic, thinly sliced
- ¼ cup pine nuts
- 1 bunch spinach, washed, bottom half of the stems removed
- ¼ cup raisins (preferably golden raisins)
- Pinch of nutmeg
- Salt and black pepper to taste
- 1 cup shredded provolone (or 3 thin deli slices)
- Butcher twine

How to Make It:

- Preheat a grill over medium heat. Place the steak on a cutting board, cover with a sheet of plastic wrap, and using a meat mallet or a heavy-bottomed pan, pound the meat until it's uniformly about ¼" thick.

- Heat the oil in a large sauté pan over medium heat. Sauté the garlic and pine nuts for a minute, until the garlic softens, then stir in the spinach and cook until it's fully wilted, about 5 minutes. Pour off any water in the bottom of the pan, then add the raisins, nutmeg, and salt and pepper.

- Season the steak on both sides with salt and pepper. Distribute the spinach mixture and provolone evenly over the meat. Roll the meat up tight, as if making a jelly roll (or rolling a sleeping bag). Use butcher twine to secure the meat on both ends and in the middle.

- Place the flank steak on the grill and close the lid. Grill until the bottom is nicely browned, about 5 minutes, then roll 90 degrees and continue grilling. Repeat the process until the steak is browned on all sides and cooked all the way through (an instant-read thermometer inserted into the thickest part should read 135°F). Wait 10 minutes before slicing.

Makes 4 servings

Per Serving:

$3.35

430 calories
23 g fat (9 g saturated)
610 mg sodium

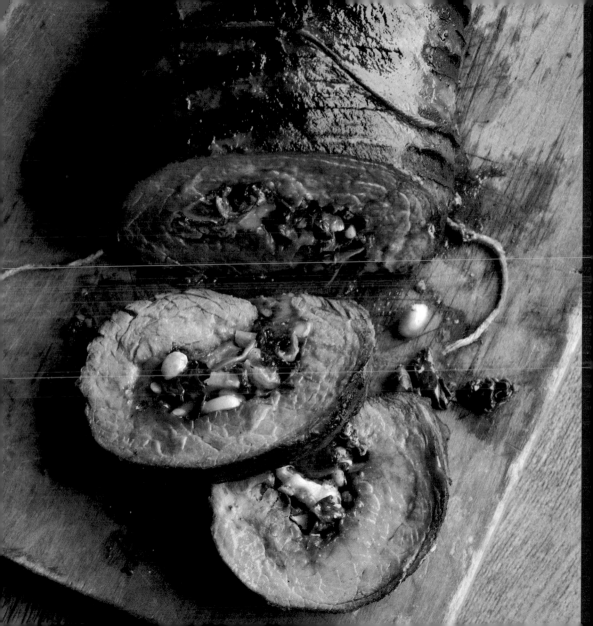

Pork Tenderloin
with Grilled Tomatillo Salsa

Pork tenderloin offers everything you should be looking for in a cut of meat: It's inexpensive (about $5 a pound), lean (with about the same amount of fat found in a chicken breast), and packs more flavor than any other protein in its calorie range. It also takes well to bold flavors and a huge variety of treatments, from spice rubs to sauces, both of which are in use here.

You'll Need:

- 1 **pork tenderloin (1–1½ lb)**
- 1 **Tbsp Southwestern Rub (page 51)**
- **Salt to taste**

TOMATILLO SALSA

- 1 **lb tomatillos, husks removed**
- 1 **small yellow onion, halved**
- 1 **jalapeño pepper**
- ½ **cup cilantro leaves**
- **Juice of 1 lime**
- 2 **cloves garlic, chopped**
- 8 **corn tortillas, heated on the grill**

How to Make It:

- Season the pork with the spice rub and salt, cover, and refrigerate for at least 1 hour (or up to 8 hours).

- Preheat a grill over medium heat. When hot, grill the pork, turning occasionally, for 12 to 15 minutes, until nicely browned on all sides, firm but gently yielding to the touch, and an instant-read thermometer inserted into the thickest part of the pork registers 150°F. While the pork cooks, grill the tomatillos, onion, and jalapeño, turning, for about 10 minutes, until soft and lightly blistered from the heat.

- While the pork rests, combine the tomatillos, onion, jalapeño, cilantro, lime juice, and garlic in a blender. Pulse until smooth. Season with salt.

- Slice the pork and serve with the tomatillo salsa and tortillas.

Makes 4 servings

MEAL MULTIPLIER

Pork tenderloin is a perfect canvas for a grill master to paint with spices and sauces. Here are a few ideas to get the creative juices flowing:

- Rub with curry powder and serve with Mango Chutney (page 200)
- Brush with a mixture of Dijon, bourbon, and maple syrup during and after grilling and serve with grilled peaches
- Marinate in fish sauce, garlic, and honey and serve with a generous scoop of Peanut Sauce (page 48)

Per Serving:
$2.37

320 calories
6 g fat (1.5 g saturated)
550 mg sodium

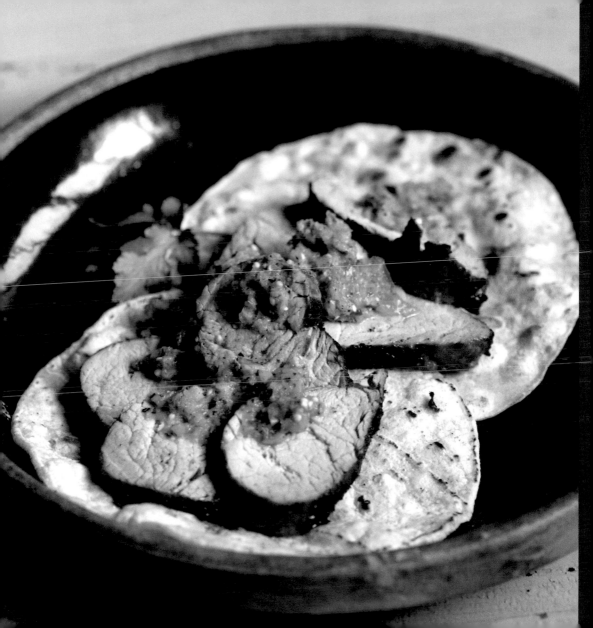

Smoked Brisket
with Chimichurri

Brisket offers tough love for the home cook, but when it's done right, few things are better. Great brisket demands slow, steady cooking in a moist environment, which is achieved easily enough with a bit of help from Mr. Beer. By placing a pan of beer next to the huge hunk of beef, you create a constant source of moisture that bastes the brisket as it cooks. Save this recipe for a down weekend. Though it cooks for a long time, it requires absolutely nothing from you, so just take it easy and let the grill do the work.

You'll Need:

2 **cups wood chips (preferably oak), soaked in warm water for 30 minutes**

1 **center-cut beef brisket (3–4 lb)**

2 **Tbsp Southwestern Rub (page 51)**

1 **can beer**

Chimichurri (page 47)

How to Make It:

- Preheat a grill over low heat. You want to maintain a temperature between 200 and 300°F, which on a large gas grill means lighting just one or two burners on the lowest setting. On a charcoal grill, this means banking all of the charcoal to one side, leaving a generous space for indirect cooking. (For more on two-zone fires, see "Go High and Low," page 40). Place the 2 cups of hickory chips (or as many as will fit) in a wood-chip box and place the box beneath the grate, directly over the flame. (If using charcoal, you can add the chips directly to the hot coals.)

- Season the brisket all over with the rub and place on the coolest part of the grill. Pour the beer into a flame-proof baking dish and place beside the brisket. Close the lid and grill, turning, over low heat for 3 to 4 hours, until the brisket is very tender and an instant-read thermometer inserted into the thickest part of the meat registers 180°F. Let rest for at least 15 minutes before slicing. Serve with the chimichurri.

Makes about 8 servings (depending on the size of the brisket)

Per Serving:
$2.38

360 calories
20 g fat (6 g saturated)
790 mg sodium

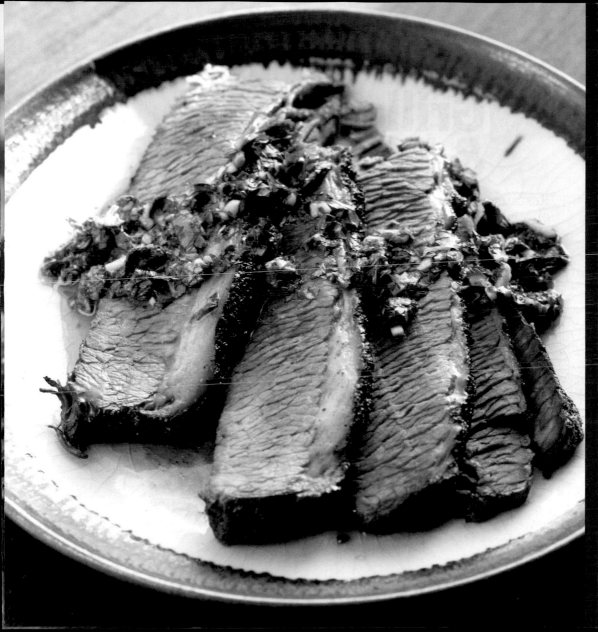

Leg of Lamb
with Gremolata

Few cuts of meat are better suited for the grill than a leg of lamb. The mix of lean meat studded with small, soft deposits of fat means you get juicy results off the grill without a glut of calories. Gremolata, the classic Mediterranean-style mix of garlic, parsley, and lemon, can be sprinkled on pretty much anything—chicken legs, flank steak, pork tenderloin—to great effect, but it works especially well when bringing lamb to life.

You'll Need:

¼ cup olive oil

4 cloves garlic, peeled

2 Tbsp chopped fresh rosemary

1 boneless leg of lamb (2–3 lb)

Salt and black pepper to taste

Butcher twine

GREMOLATA

Zest of 2 lemons

4 cloves garlic, finely minced

1 cup finely minced parsley

To make the gremolata, simply mix together the three ingredients in a bowl.

How to Make It:

- Combine the olive oil, garlic, and rosemary in a food processor and pulse. Place the lamb in a shallow dish, season with salt and pepper, and spread the garlic mixture all over. Cover and marinate in the refrigerator for at least 1 hour (or up to 4 hours).

- Preheat a grill over medium-low heat. Remove the lamb from the marinade, roll tight like a jelly roll, and tie at both ends and in the middle with the twine.

- Place the lamb on the grill and close the lid. Grill, turning occasionally, for about 25 minutes, until the outside is deeply browned and an instant-read thermometer inserted into the thickest part of the meat registers 130°F.

- Allow the lamb to rest for 10 minutes before slicing. Serve with a bit of gremolata sprinkled on top.

Makes about 6 servings (depending on the size of the lamb)

Per Serving:
$3.34
340 calories
19 g fat (5 g saturated)
660 mg sodium

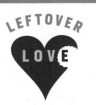

LEFTOVER LOVE

These are precious leftovers to have on hand. Make the most of them with one of these next-day treatments:

- Stuff into a toasted pita with tomato and onion, then top with Greek yogurt spiked with garlic and lemon

- Cradle in warm tortillas with salsa and guacamole

- Stack on focaccia (or a crusty roll), then top with caramelized onions, olives, roasted red peppers, and a few crumbles of feta

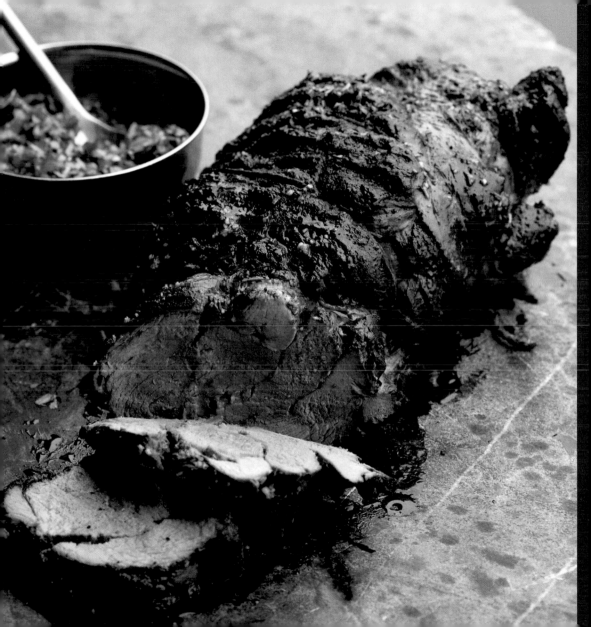

GRILL
THIS
NOT
THAT!

FISH & SEAFOOD

CHAPTER **7**

THE PERFECT
Grilled Fish

Even the most confident spatula-wielders tend to seize up in terror at the prospect of grilling fish. It's too expensive, they say, too delicate, too easy to mess up. Our response? Fish is at its finest hot off the grill, which means it's time to conquer any fears and hesitations and learn how to do it right every time. This is your blueprint.

Shop at a market with a real fish counter.

Too many American supermarkets have traded in a dedicated fishmonger for a section of shrink-wrapped plastic trays of fish. More than any other purchase you make in the market, fish is one that demands some basic inquiries, which requires human contact. You'll find it at places like Whole Foods, though it can be pricey. An even better source? Asian markets, where high turnover, low prices, and expert fishmongers make buying fresh fish simple and inexpensive.

Choose freshness over fish type.

The first question you ask your fish guy should always be: "What's fresh today?" No fish dish can be rescued if it starts with lousy fish, so make sure you source the fillet carefully. More important than getting the exact fish in the recipe is getting a piece of fish that's as fresh as possible, so substitute freely with any of the recipes in this chapter.

Scrape the grate.

You want clean grill grates for everything you cook, but nowhere is it more essential than when you cook fish. Use a grill brush, or failing that, a large piece of crumpled aluminum foil, to scrape away any lingering adherents from the grate, then thoroughly oil the grill (and the fish) before you cook.

Leave it alone.

Fish will stick to the grate every time if you try to flip it too early. Place the more attractive side of the fillet down on the grill (always start with the side you want to see when you sit down to eat) and leave it untouched for 3 to 4 minutes. Once grill marks develop, the flesh will release naturally from the grate. Flip and continue cooking for another minute or two.

You'll Need:

Olive oil for coating the grate and fish

4 **fillets firm white fish like halibut, mahi-mahi, or sea bass (about 6 oz each)**

Salt and freshly ground pepper to taste

White pepper is almost always better with fish, not just because it looks better, but because it has a gentler heat than black pepper.

- Preheat a grill or grill pan over medium heat. As the grill is warming up, drizzle a bit of oil onto a paper towel and use it to wipe down the grate.

- Coat the fish with a light layer of oil and season on both sides with salt and pepper. When the grill is hot, place the fish on the grate with the pretty side facing down (this is the side you want to see when you serve the fish). Grill without touching for 3 to 4 minutes, until nice grill marks have developed and the flesh releases easily from the grate. Flip and continue grilling for another 2 to 3 minutes, until the thickest part of the fillet flakes with gentle pressure from your finger and an instant-read thermometer inserted in the thickest part of the fish registers 140°F. Makes 4 servings.

Grill This!
The Packet Matrix

The French call it *en papillote;* for the Italians it's en *cartoccio;* but for us, it's simply a meal in a bag. It might not sound as fancy in English, but it makes for an extraordinary way to eat dinner. And regardless of how refined your grill skills are, the method is almost impossible to screw up because the food steams inside the enclosed packet, making for moist, flavorful results. It's the grilling equivalent of the one-pot meal, with even less cleanup.

Four Quick Recipes

Place a piece of fish or chicken on a sheet of foil, drizzle with a bit of flavorful liquid, top with a few vegetables, and seal the deal. The ratio of effort to deliciousness is unmatched anywhere in the culinary galaxy.

CHOOSE A PROTEIN

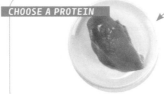

This technique works best with fish and other types of seafood because they're naturally so tender. When it comes to meat, chicken is best.

CHICKEN BREAST

SCALLOPS

CHOOSE A LIQUID

When cooking with wine, no need to break out the big expensive guns, but if you wouldn't drink it, you shouldn't cook with it.

WHITE WINE

REDUCED-FAT COCONUT MILK

CHOOSE VEGETABLES

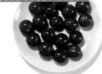

Potatoes work best when sliced and parboiled for 10 minutes.

CHERRY TOMATOES

SLICED POTATOES

SLICED ONION OR FENNEL

CHOOSE AROMATICS

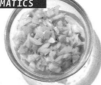

Parsley, basil, tarragon, thyme, and oregano are all excellent herb choices.

MINCED GARLIC

FRESH HERBS

CATFISH CURRY
Catfish + coconut milk + broccoli + red curry paste + ginger

DIJON CHICKEN
Chicken breast + white wine + cherry tomatoes + potatoes + Dijon + garlic

SALMON

Peeled shrimp cook very fast inside the packet. Be ready to pull them off the grill in about 5 minutes.

SHRIMP

MUSSELS

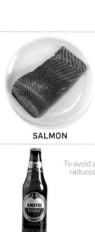

BEER

To avoid a salt overload, opt for reduced-sodium soy sauce.

SOY SAUCE

OLIVE OIL

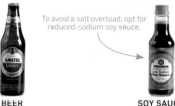

Want a vegetarian meal? Skip the protein entirely and load up on the vegetables. The combo of mushrooms, broccoli, and butternut squash is an excellent way to start.

BROCCOLI FLORETS OR ASPARAGUS

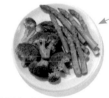

Sliced white or cremini mushrooms or shiitake caps work best.

MUSHROOMS

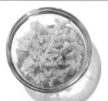

MINCED FRESH GINGER

CHILES

Squeeze in the juice, grate in the rind, or top the protein with thin slices of the citrus.

LEMON OR LIME

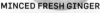

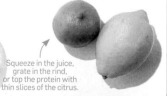

DRUNKEN MUSSELS
Mussels + dark beer + fennel + fresh parsley + Dijon + garlic + butter

SOY-GINGER SALMON
Salmon + soy sauce + asparagus + mushrooms + ginger + garlic

Packet Basics

Rule 1
Everything you place in the packet needs to cook in the same amount of time. A big hunk of carrot or potato will still be raw by the time a catfish fillet is cooked through. When using denser vegetables, slice them thin so they cook fast.

Rule 2
Create a sturdy, fully enclosed packet. Fold a two-foot piece of heavy-duty foil in half. Place all of the ingredients on the bottom third of the foil, then fold the opposite end of the sheet over to completely cover the food. Roll up the edges of the foil tightly.

Rule 3
Cooking time is essential. A medium chicken breast cooked over medium heat takes about 12 minutes; a thin fish like catfish cooks in about half that time. It's better to err on the side of overcooking. Because of the abundance of moisture trapped inside the packet, you can afford to cook the protein an extra minute without losing much in terms of flavor or texture.

217

Grill This!
The Sauce Matrix

Why work so hard to grill something correctly only to cover it in a tide of sugary, salty goop? That's what you get more often than not when you invite a bottled sauce into your backyard. As long as you have a decently stocked pantry, an incredible homemade sauce is never more than a few minutes away. Balance the flavors by choosing one product from each category and you'll have something that will improve your next meal without tarnishing the health benefits of grilling.

Four Quick Recipes

A properly made sauce is the kind of game-changing flourish that makes culinary geniuses out of everyday cooks. Use these creations before, during, and after cooking for amazing results.

CHOOSE SOMETHING SWEET

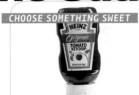

KETCHUP

HONEY

BROWN SUGAR

CHOOSE SOMETHING SALTY

SOY SAUCE

Fish sauce is at the heart of Southeast Asian cuisine. It adds an addictive salty-sweet punch to sauces for everything from catfish to steak.

FISH SAUCE

CHOOSE SOMETHING SOUR

BALSAMIC VINEGAR

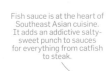

RED OR WHITE WINE VINEGAR

APPLE CIDER VINEGAR

CHOOSE SOMETHING SPICY

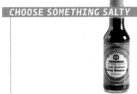

Sriracha is king of the chili sauces, but chili-garlic and sweet chili sauces are also great.

ASIAN CHILI SAUCE

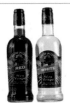

Tabasco and Frank's Red Hot are our favorite sources of heat and vinegar tang.

HOT SAUCE

GRATED HORSERADISH

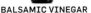

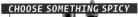

HOISIN LIME
BEST FOR: SALMON, DUCK, BEEF
Hoisin + soy sauce + lime juice + sriracha

MAPLE DIJON
BEST FOR: PORK CHOPS, CHICKEN
Maple syrup + Worcestershire + white wine vinegar + Dijon

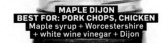

218

MOLASSES

MAPLE SYRUP

HOISIN

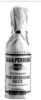

WORCESTERSHIRE

MISO PASTE

PEANUT BUTTER

LEMON OR LIME JUICE

ORANGE JUICE

DIJON MUSTARD

You're not after the peppers themselves, but rather a spoonful or two of the spicy sauce they come packed in.

CHIPOTLE PEPPERS

CAYENNE PEPPER

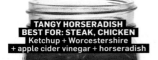

TANGY HORSERADISH
BEST FOR: STEAK, CHICKEN
Ketchup + Worcestershire
+ apple cider vinegar + horseradish

SPICY PEANUT
BEST FOR: CHICKEN AND PORK SKEWERS,
AS A DIPPING SAUCE FOR GRILLED SHRIMP
Honey + peanut butter + fish sauce
+ lime juice + sriracha

Sauce Basics

Rule 1

Balance is everything. Make a sauce with ketchup, honey, brown sugar, and maple syrup and you'll bury your taste buds in a tide of sweetness. As a general principle, try to make your sauces with nearly equal amounts (by volume) of sweet, salty, and sour ingredients, then adjust the heat level to your liking.

Rule 2

Thickness counts. Make your sauce too thin and it will slide off the food rather than cling to it; make it too thick and it will dominate whatever dish it touches. The consistency of bottled barbecue sauce is ultimately what you're aiming for.

Rule 3

Know when to sauce. Thinner cuts of meat can be spread with sauce before cooking, but if you sauce items like thick steaks or whole chickens too early, the sugars will burn long before the meat is fully cooked. A good rule of thumb: If it takes more than 10 minutes to cook, don't sauce the food before it goes on the grill.

Grilled Whole Fish

We tend to like our meat and fish to resemble anything but the animals they come from. We're accustomed to packaged chicken breasts, neatly trimmed steaks, and ivory fillets of fish. Fair enough, but when it comes to seafood, that means missing out on one of the best ways to eat fish—and easily the most common form of fish consumption beyond the borders of the United States. Since the bones help impart moisture and the skin protects the flesh from the intensity of direct heat, fish cooked whole emerges effortlessly moist and tender. All it needs is a squeeze of lemon and a drizzle of olive oil.

You'll Need:

4 **whole sea bass (1–1½ lb each)**

Olive oil, for coating and drizzling

Salt and black pepper to taste

Fresh thyme sprigs (optional)

2 **lemons, halved**

Asian markets are the best places to buy whole fish. If you can't find fish this small, buy larger fish, about 2 pounds each, and divide between two people.

How to Make It:

- Preheat a grill over medium heat. Coat the fish with olive oil and season all over with salt and pepper. Place the thyme, if using, inside the fish cavities.

- Place the fish on the grill, close the lid, and grill for 6 to 7 minutes, until the skin is browned and easily pulls away from the grill. Flip and repeat, grilling for 5 to 7 minutes longer, until the flesh at the thickest part flakes with gentle pressure from your finger and an instant-read thermometer inserted into the thickest part of the fish registers 140°F. While the fish cooks, place the lemons on the grill, cut side down, and grill for about 5 minutes, until deeply caramelized and juicy.

- Serve the fish with the grilled lemons and an extra drizzle of olive oil.

Makes 4 servings

Per Serving: $7.35	210 calories 10 g fat (1.5 g saturated) 295 mg sodium

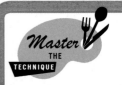

Master THE **TECHNIQUE**

Filleting fish

You can serve these lovely whole fish as is, or you can quickly fillet these after cooking. Run a long, thin knife along the spine of the fish, from head to tail, to loosen the meat from the bones. Gently slide a spatula underneath the fillet, starting at the tail and moving it up toward the head. The fillet should slide effortlessly off the spine and onto the spatula. It's so easy that servers at fancy restaurants often do it with a spoon.

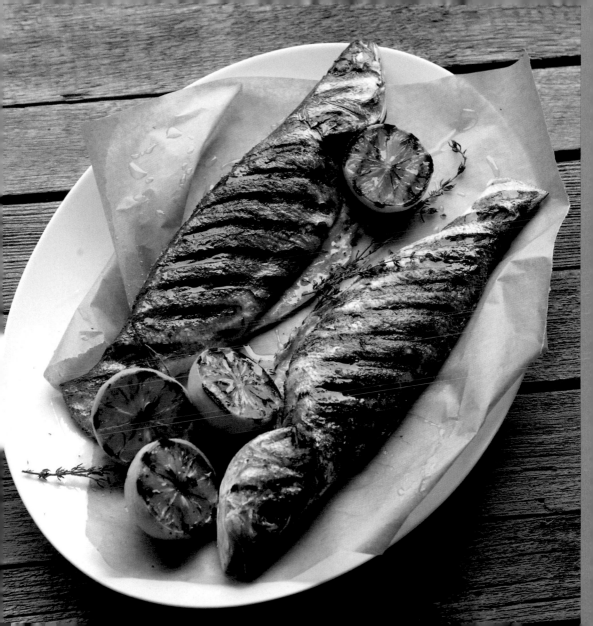

Cedar Plank Salmon

The tradition of cooking salmon over cedar comes from the Pacific Northwest, where Native Americans have been using large planks over fire pits for hundreds of years. For the home cook equipped with a few store-bought slats of cedar, it's an easy way to suffuse salmon with toasty, smoky flavor without calories and without the fear of the fish drying out. Whatever you do, don't throw the plank out. You paid serious cash for that little piece of wood and you should be sure to reuse it.

You'll Need:

- 2 Tbsp grainy mustard
- 2 Tbsp light brown sugar
- ½ Tbsp fresh thyme leaves (or 1 tsp dried thyme)
- 1 large salmon fillet (1–1½ lb)
- 1 large cedar plank, soaked in water for 30 minutes
- Salt and black pepper to taste

No planks? No problem. This is a simple, satisfying way to prepare salmon directly on the grill or in a 300°F oven.

How to Make It:

- Preheat a grill over medium-low heat. Combine the mustard, brown sugar, and thyme in a bowl. Place the salmon, skin side down, on top of the cedar plank, season with salt and pepper, and spread the mustard mixture on the top.

- Place the plank directly on the grill grate and close the lid. Grill for about 20 minutes, until the center of the fillet flakes with gentle pressure from the finger and an instant-read thermometer inserted into the thickest part of the salmon registers 135°F.

Makes 4 servings

$$(\text{\ff} + \text{I})^2$$

MEAL MULTIPLIER

Salmon is the most famous of the planked proteins, but the plank is no one-trick pony. Save the slats of cedar and use them to add a dimension of smoke to any of the following dishes:

- Burgers topped with sautéed mushrooms, Swiss, and steak sauce
- Chicken breasts brushed with Classic Barbecue Sauce (page 45)
- Pork chops glazed with a mixture of honey, bourbon, and spicy mustard

Per Serving:
$2.91

240 calories
9 g fat (1.5 g saturated)
470 mg sodium

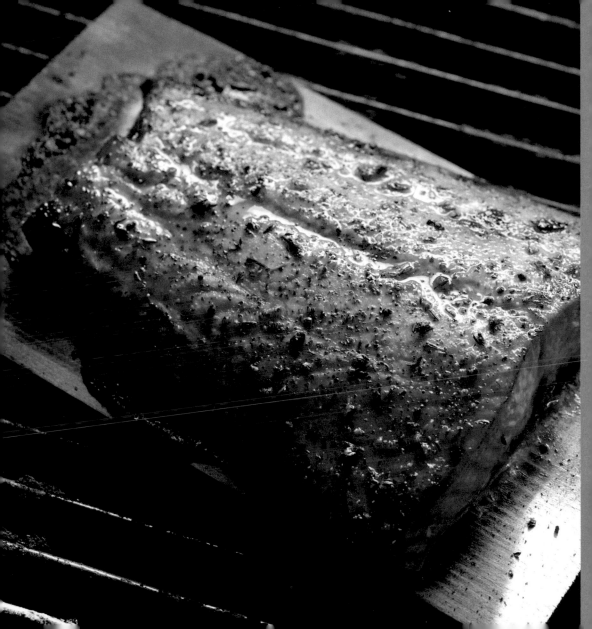

Scallops
with Orange-Soy Glaze

Scallops rarely make an appearance in the average American kitchen. Perhaps that stems from the days when supermarket seafood sections were awash in shrimp, mussels, and lobsters, but finding a scallop required a scuba mask and an oxygen tank. But now that scallops are a steady staple of the American food supply, they should be regular guests in your backyard. They are lean, meaty, take well to big flavors, and, best of all, impossible to screw up.

You'll Need:

- 1 cup orange juice
- 1 Tbsp soy sauce
- 2 Tbsp butter
- 1 lb large sea scallops, tough muscles removed
- Salt and black pepper
- 1 Tbsp minced fresh chives or scallions

Make sure there is no milky liquid accumulated beneath the scallops in the fish case, a sign that the scallops have likely been dyed or pumped full of additives.

How to Make It:

- Combine the orange juice and soy sauce in a small saucepan over medium heat. Simmer until the liquid is reduced by three-fourths (it should easily cling to the back of a spoon). Remove from the heat and stir in the butter.

- Preheat a grill or grill pan over high heat. Season the scallops with a bit of salt and pepper. Pour about 1 tablespoon glaze into a small bowl and use to brush both sides of the scallops with a light film. Grill the scallops on one side for 2 to 3 minutes, until a nice char has developed. Flip and grill for 1 more minute, until just firm to the touch. Brush with the glaze in the saucepan and top with the chives.

Makes 4 servings

Per Serving:
$3.60

180 calories
7 g fat (3.5 g saturated)
550 mg sodium

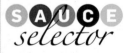

SAUCE *selector*

Scallops' creamy texture and neutral flavor make them a perfect canvas for improvised sauces and toppings. Feel free to swap out the orange-soy glaze for one of these tasty stand-ins:

- Equal parts Dijon mustard, white wine vinegar, honey, and crumbled bacon
- Tomatillo Salsa (page 204)
- Smoky Aioli (page 242)
- Chimichurri (page 47)

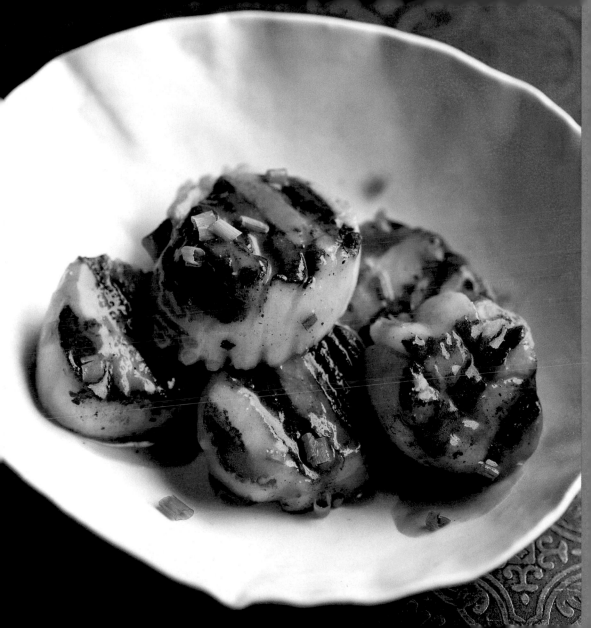

Snapper à la Veracruz

Veracruz is a coastal city in southern Mexico with a rich culinary history, one largely revolving around heaps of insanely fresh seafood. The most famous dish involves roasting a whole snapper, then topping it with a tomato sauce spiked with salty notes from capers and olives. This streamlined approach puts all the same great flavors inside a single package, quickening the cooking time (and the cleanup), but still giving you a dish elegant enough to serve on a serious occasion.

You'll Need:

- 1 pint cherry tomatoes
- 1 handful fresh parsley or cilantro, roughly chopped
- ¼ cup chopped green olives
- 2 Tbsp capers, rinsed
- Juice of 1 lime
- ¼ cup olive oil
- Chopped fresh or pickled jalapeño peppers (optional)
- 4 snapper (or other firm white fish like cod or halibut) fillets (4–6 oz each)
- Salt to taste

How to Make It:

- Preheat a grill over medium-low heat. Combine the cherry tomatoes, parsley, olives, capers, lime juice, olive oil, and jalapeños (if using) in a mixing bowl.

- Lay out one 2' sheet of aluminum foil on the kitchen counter and fold in half lengthwise. Season one snapper fillet with salt and place toward the right edge of the folded sheet. Top with one-fourth of the olive-tomato mixture. Fold the foil over so that it covers the fish completely, then carefully roll the corners tightly to create a fully sealed package. Repeat to make 4 packets.

- Place the packets directly on the grill grate and close the top (with the top closed, the grill temperature should max out around 450°F). Cook for 8 to 10 minutes, depending on the thickness of the fillets and the heat of the grill. Slash open the packets just before eating. The fish is done when it flakes with gentle pressure from your fingertip.

Makes 4 servings

Per Serving:	290 calories
$4.28	12 g fat (2 g saturated)
	370 mg sodium

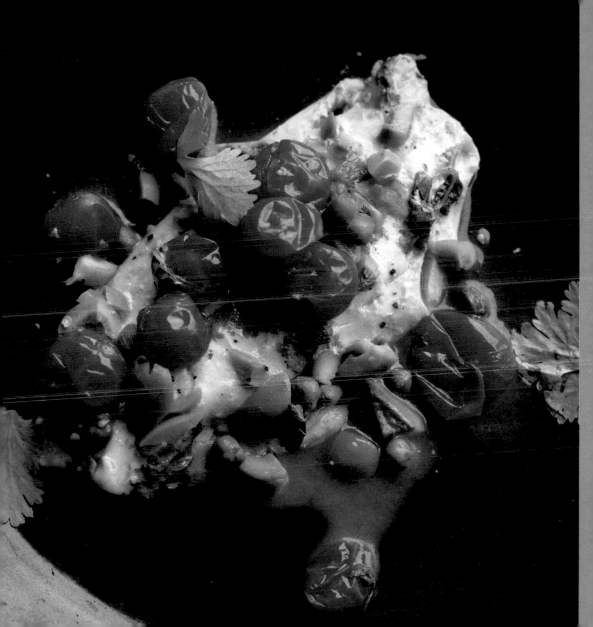

Grilled Halibut Skewers with Charmoula

Charmoula is one of those magical herb sauces, like pesto and chimichurri, that works wonders on almost any food that touches the grill: chicken legs, pork tenderloin, zucchini, asparagus. More than anything, though, charmoula is fit for fish. The cilantro- and spice-charged sauce is uniquely capable of elevating tender chunks of firm white fish (like halibut, cod, and swordfish) into near-sacred territory.

You'll Need:

- 1 cup fresh parsley leaves
- 1 cup fresh cilantro leaves
- 2 cloves garlic, peeled
- Juice of ½ lemon
- ½ cup olive oil
- 1 tsp paprika (preferably smoked paprika)
- ½ tsp ground cumin
- ½ tsp cayenne pepper
- Salt and black pepper to taste
- 1 lb halibut, cut into 1" pieces
- Metal skewers, or wooden skewers soaked in water for 30 minutes

How to Make It:

- Combine the parsley, cilantro, garlic, lemon juice, olive oil, paprika, cumin, and cayenne, plus a few pinches of salt and pepper, in a food processor or blender. Puree until you have a smooth, uniform sauce.

- Preheat a grill or grill pan over medium heat. Thread the halibut chunks onto the skewers and season with salt and pepper. Spoon enough of the charmoula over the skewers to cover the fish; let sit for 10 minutes.

- Grill the halibut, turning once, for 3 to 4 minutes per side, until the fish is lightly charred and flakes with gentle pressure from your finger. Serve with more charmoula spooned over the top.

Makes 4 servings

Per Serving:
$4.47

280 calories
22 g fat (2 g saturated)
510 mg sodium

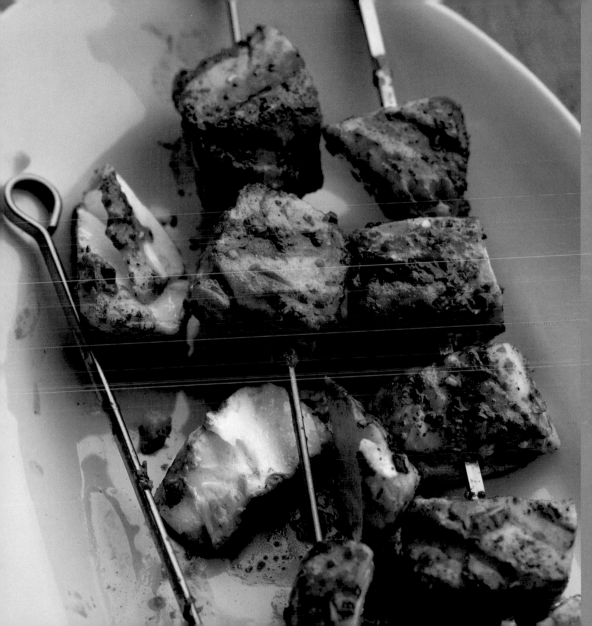

Tequila-Jalapeño Shrimp

Shrimp need help. With nary a speck of fat to insulate them from the heat of the flame, they go from perfectly cooked to dry and lifeless in a matter of seconds. That's where our boozy, jalapeño-laced marinade comes into play: Not only does it impart huge amounts of spicy flavor to a normally neutral protein, it also helps keep the shrimp as juicy as possible while they cook. Still, the shrimp require careful monitoring on the grill: When they've turned pink and their tails begin to curl, they're done. These spicy shellfish are best served alongside a scoop of black beans and a few warm tortillas.

You'll Need:

Juice of 1 lime

2 Tbsp tequila

1 Tbsp vegetable oil

½ medium onion, chopped

Handful of cilantro

2 jalapeño peppers, chopped

1 clove garlic

Salt and black pepper

1 lb medium shrimp, peeled and deveined

Metal skewers, or wooden skewers soaked in water for 30 minutes

How to Make It:

- Preheat a grill or grill pan over high heat. Combine the lime juice, tequila, oil, onion, cilantro, jalapeños, garlic, and a few pinches of salt and pepper in a food processor. Pulse until the mix has the consistency of a pesto.

- Thread the shrimp onto the skewers. Slather the shrimp with enough marinade to fully cover; let marinate for 15 minutes.

- Grill the shrimp for 1 to 2 minutes per side, until pink and firm.

Makes 4 servings

Per Serving:
$2.98

170 calories
5 g fat (0.5 g saturated)
410 mg sodium

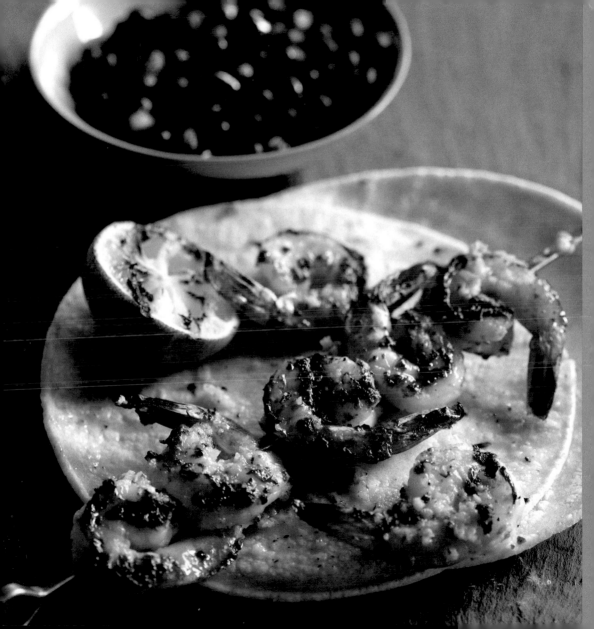

Grilled Mussels
with Garlic Butter

Compared with other shellfish stars like shrimp, clams, and oysters, mussels get little love from cooks. It's tough to imagine why: Not only are mussels considerably cheaper than their more popular counterparts, they also cook in a matter of minutes and are nearly impossible to mess up. And, surprisingly enough, they're perfect grill food. Contained within a foil packet with white wine, garlic, and butter, they're steamed into a state of sauce-absorbing submission. Use the side of grilled bread to soak up all that luscious liquid.

You'll Need:

- 4 (2'-long) pieces aluminum foil
- 1 lb mussels, scrubbed under water and debearded •⎯
- 4 cloves garlic, minced
- 2 Tbsp butter, cut into small pieces
- ½ cup chopped fresh parsley
- ½ cup white wine
- 4 thick slices sourdough or country-style bread, grilled for a few minutes

How to Make It:

- Preheat a grill over medium-low heat. Fold the sheets of foil in half crosswise. Place an equal amount of mussels in the center of each sheet, then divide the garlic, butter, and parsley among the four piles. For each packet, bring the ends of the foil up over the mussels to create a tent, then fold the foil together to create a tightly sealed package. Just before making the final seal, pour a few tablespoons of white wine into each packet.

- Place the packets directly on the grill grate, fold side facing up, and grill for 10 minutes, until the mussels have all opened. Serve with wedges of grilled bread for dipping.

Makes 4 servings

⎯ *Debearding just means removing any of the long "hairs" that sometimes come attached to mussel shells.*

Per Serving:	
$2.83	260 calories 10 g fat (4 g saturated) 530 mg sodium

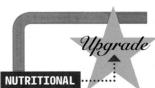

Upgrade

NUTRITIONAL

Mussel power

When it comes to nutrition, mussels are no wimps. Three ounces of cooked mussels packs in more than a day's worth of selenium and three days' worth of manganese, a mineral best known for strengthening bones and stabilizing blood sugar levels. Mussels also really flex in the B12 department, boasting three full days' worth of the vitamin, which is essential in keeping your cells (i.e., your body and everything that it does) functioning properly.

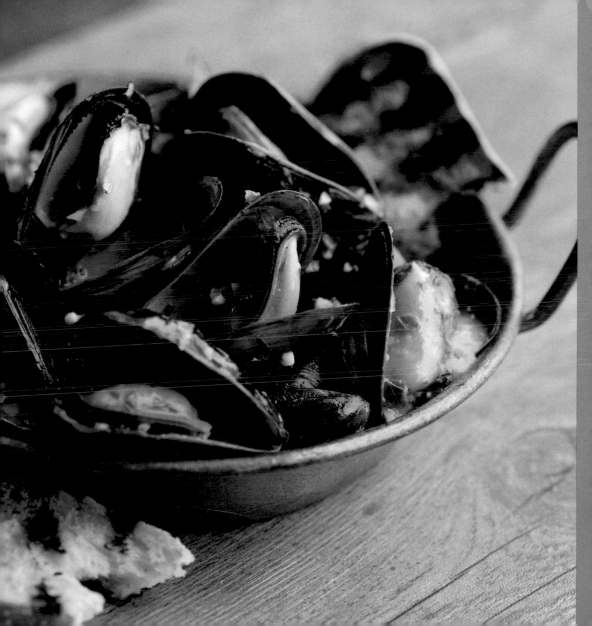

Mahi-Mahi
with Fennel-Orange Salsa

Mahi is perhaps the most grill-friendly fish of all: Not only does its meaty flesh stand up beautifully to the heat, but its skin is perfect for crisping over the open flame. Most people are accustomed to peeling off the skin, either before cooking or after, but with the right fish (sea bass, salmon, snapper), the skin is not only the healthiest part of the fillet, but also the most delicious, contrasting a deep, almost nutty flavor and a satisfying crunch with the flaky meat of the fish. To do it right, you want to grill the fish 75 percent of the way on the skin, then flip and finish it off quickly on the flesh side.

You'll Need:

2 **medium oranges (preferably blood oranges, if available), peeled**

1 **bulb fennel, cored and thinly sliced**

½ **small red onion, very thinly sliced**

½ **Tbsp minced fresh ginger**

2 **Tbsp olive oil, plus more coating the fish**

1 **Tbsp reduced-sodium soy sauce**

Salt and black pepper to taste

4 **mahi-mahi fillets (4–6 oz each)**

How to Make It:

- Preheat a grill over high heat. To make the salsa, use a paring knife to cut out the individual segments of the oranges, leaving the tough membranes behind. Combine the orange segments with the fennel, onion, ginger, olive oil, and soy sauce in a mixing bowl. Stir in a handful of chopped fennel fronds (the leafy tops of the fennel bulb) and season with pepper.

- Coat the fish with olive oil and season on all sides with salt and pepper. Place skin side down on the grill and cook for 5 to 6 minutes, until the skin is crispy and easily pulls away from the grill. Flip and cook for about 2 minutes longer, until the flesh is nicely browned and flakes with gentle pressure from your finger and an instant-read thermometer inserted into the thickest part of the fish registers 140°F. Serve the fish with the crispy skin facing up and the salsa on the side.

Makes 4 servings

Per Serving: **$4.11**

230 calories
8 g fat (1 g saturated)
290 mg sodium

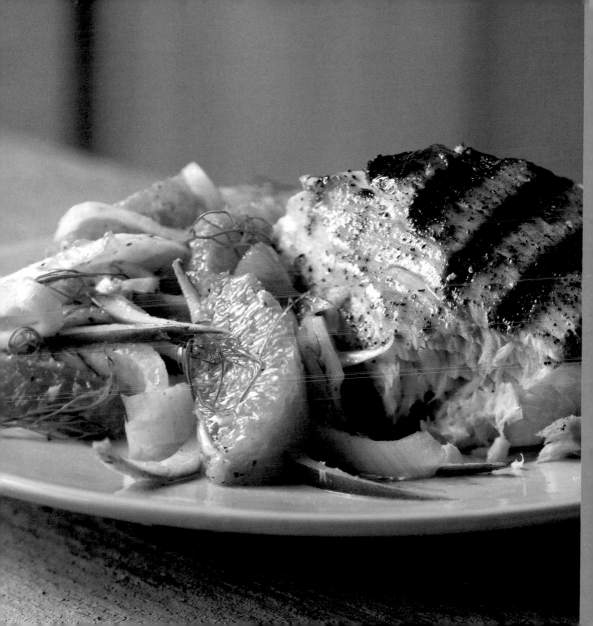

Grilled Lobster Tails with Chipotle-Lime Butter

It's not an exaggeration to say that 95 percent of all lobsters consumed are boiled. Both for convenience and for tradition, boiling has always been the preferred cooking method, but that doesn't make it the only way, or even the best way. The clean, sweet flavor of lobster is especially excellent when grilled over a hot flame and braced with a bit of fat (olive oil or butter) and a few drops of acidity (lemon, lime, vinegar). While grilling isn't the most convenient way to cook whole lobsters, it works perfectly for the individual lobster tails that are sold frozen in larger supermarkets everywhere.

You'll Need:

- ¼ cup (½ stick) butter, softened at room temperature
- ½ cup chopped cilantro
- Zest of 1 lime
- 1 Tbsp chipotle pepper puree
- 1 clove garlic, minced
- 4 lobster tails (about 7 oz each; if frozen, thawed)
- Olive oil for drizzling
- Salt and black pepper to taste

How to Make It:

- Preheat a grill over medium heat. Combine the butter, cilantro, lime zest, chipotle, and garlic in a small mixing bowl. Squeeze in a few drops of lime juice and stir to combine.

- Drizzle the lobster tails with olive oil and season with salt and pepper. Place flesh side down on the grill and cook for 5 minutes, until the meat is lightly browned. Flip and continue grilling for about 5 minutes, until the meat pulls away from the shell. Immediately serve each tail with a generous scoop of the compound butter over the top.

Makes 4 servings

Per Serving:
$9.23

220 calories
15 g fat (8 g saturated)
420 mg sodium

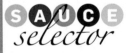

SAUCE selector

Grilled lobster tails are perfectly delicious with nothing more than a bit of butter, but it never hurts to dress them up a bit. Here are a few suggestions:

- Juice of 1 lemon, ¼ cup olive oil, 2 cloves minced garlic, and 1 cup fresh herbs like parsley and basil
- 1 cup chopped scallions, 2 tablespoons minced ginger, ¼ cup canola oil, and the juice on 1 lime
- Chimichurri (page 47)

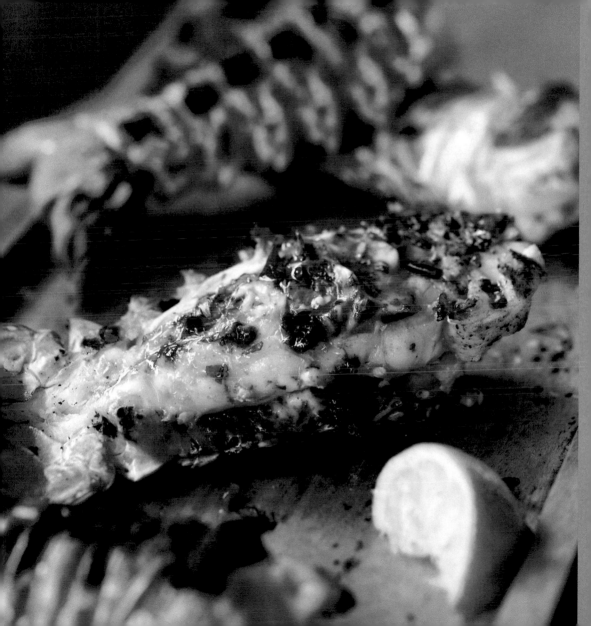

Grilled Fish Tacos

The famous fish tacos of Baja California are born of a simple formula: warm tortilla, fried fish fillet, mayonnaise-based sauce. Delicious for a bite or two, but by the time the fried crust is reduced to a mushy paste under the cover of the mayo, you have to wonder what you're wasting all of those calories on. That's why we prefer the fish in our tacos grilled: Smoky, tender, and the perfect vessel for bold condiments, it won't ever cross your mind how healthy this meal really is.

You'll Need:

Juice of 4 limes

¼ cup canola oil

1 tsp chili powder

1 lb fresh white fish (tilapia, catfish, snapper, halibut, etc.)

Salt and black pepper to taste

½ cup reduced-fat sour cream

½ cup chopped cilantro

8 corn tortillas

Pico de Gallo (page 46)

Hot sauce to taste

Any hot sauce will do, but the smokiness of Tabasco Chipotle really ties this dish together beautifully.

How to Make It:

● Preheat a grill or grill pan over medium-high heat. Combine half of the lime juice, the oil, and chili powder in a sealable plastic bag. Season the fish with salt and pepper and place in the marinade for no more than 20 minutes (any longer and the citric acid from the lime juice will begin to "cook" the fish). In a small mixing bowl, combine the remaining lime juice with the sour cream and cilantro.

● Grill the fish for 3 to 4 minutes, until the flesh begins to brown and easily pulls away from the grill. Flip and continue grilling for 3 to 4 minutes longer, until the fish flakes with gentle pressure from your finger and an instant-read thermometer inserted into the thickest part of the fish registers 140°F. Grill the tortillas until lightly toasted.

● Divide the fish among the tortillas and top with the lime sour cream, pico de gallo, and hot sauce.

Makes 4 servings

Per Serving:	
$2.89	320 calories 13 g fat (2 g saturated) 490 mg sodium

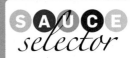

SAUCE *selector*

When it comes to dressing up a fish taco, there are many paths to success. Our tacos here combine lime-spiked sour cream with pico de gallo, but any of these other condiments would make a delicious alternative:

● Mango Salsa (page 47)
● Tomatillo Salsa (page 204)
● Grilled-Corn Guacamole (page 266)
● Asian Slaw (page 340)

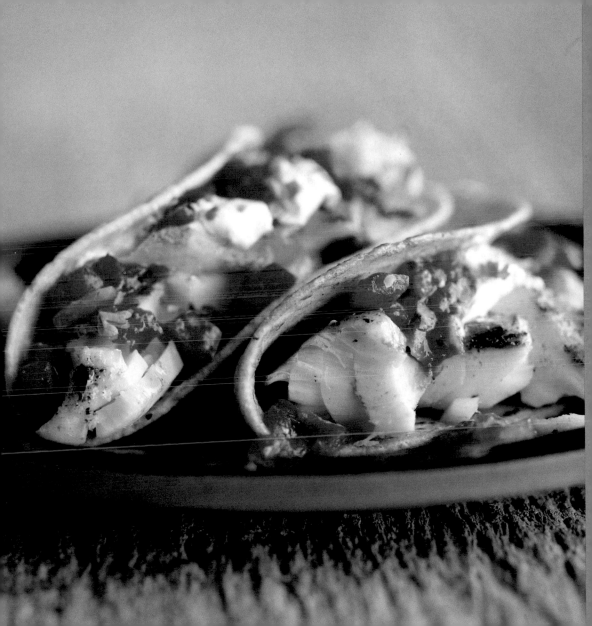

Salmon
with Ginger Soy Butter

It's well known that salmon is one of the world's healthiest foods, dense with protein and flush with a tide of heart-protecting, cancer-fighting omega-3 fatty acids. And yet, it's not uncommon to find restaurant salmon dishes packing 800 calories or more. Even with a generous mound of this incredible compound butter, our salmon doesn't break the 400-calorie barrier.

You'll Need:

2 Tbsp unsalted butter, softened

½ Tbsp minced chives

½ Tbsp grated fresh ginger

Juice of 1 lemon

½ Tbsp low-sodium soy sauce

4 salmon fillets (4–6 oz each)

Salt and black pepper to taste

1 Tbsp olive oil

The best way to peel ginger? With a spoon. That's right; the edge of a spoon easily scrapes away ginger's thin skin without wasting any of the fragrant flesh inside.

How to Make It:

- Mix the butter, chives, ginger, lemon juice, and soy sauce. Set aside.

- Preheat a grill or grill pan over medium heat. Season the salmon with salt and pepper and rub with the oil. Wipe the grill grates clean and rub with a paper towel dipped in oil. Add the salmon skin side down and cook for 4 to 5 minutes, until the skin is lightly charred and crisp.

- Flip the fish and cook for another 2 to 3 minutes on the flesh side, until the flesh flakes with gentle pressure from your finger but is still slightly translucent in the middle. (We believe salmon is best served medium, but if you want yours completely cooked, leave it on for another 2 minutes.)

- Serve the salmon with a generous spoonful of the flavored butter, which should begin to melt on contact.

Makes 4 servings

Per Serving:	
$2.46	390 calories 26 g fat (7 g saturated) 710 mg sodium

MEAL MULTIPLIER

Salmon's rich flavor stands up to more aggressive spices and sauces than white fish. Try one of these potent spice rubs to bring out the best in this versatile superfood:

- Pastrami Salmon: Rubbed with equal parts ground ginger, allspice, onion powder, garlic powder, paprika, and ground mustard

- Moroccan Salmon: Rubbed with the Moroccan Spice Blend (page 51)

- Thai Salmon: Rubbed with red curry paste and served with Peanut Sauce (page 48)

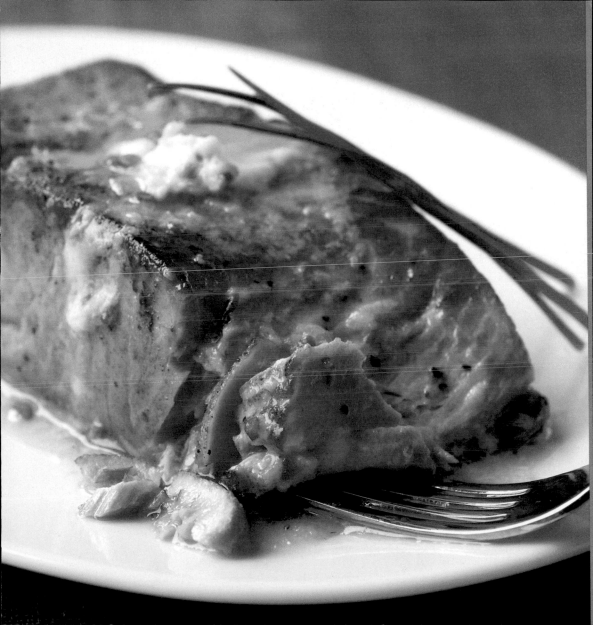

Grilled Swordfish
with Smoky Aioli

Sometimes the only thing dividing good food from great food is a simple embellishment: a quick spice rub, a light dressing, an improvised sauce. The only rule we stick to is that the embellishment, whatever it may be, doesn't overpower the dish. A red wine sauce on a fish fillet? Too much. But a smoky, garlic-spiked mayonnaise on a meaty swordfish steak? Just right.

You'll Need:

- 3 Tbsp olive oil mayonnaise
- 1 Tbsp olive oil, plus more for coating the fish
- **Zest and juice of 1 lemon**
- 2 cloves garlic, finely minced
- 1 tsp smoked paprika
- 4 swordfish steaks (about 6 oz each)
- 1 tsp fennel seeds, roughly chopped
- **Salt and black pepper to taste**

How to Make It:

- Preheat a grill or grill pan over high heat. To make the aioli, combine the mayonnaise, olive oil, lemon zest and juice, garlic, and paprika in a small mixing bowl. Stir until thoroughly blended.

- Coat the swordfish with a light film of olive oil, then season on both sides with the fennel, salt, and pepper. Grill for 4 to 5 minutes, until the first side has developed some nice grill marks and the flesh pulls away easily from the grate. Flip and continue grilling for another 4 minutes, until the fish flakes with gentle pressure from your finger and an instant-read thermometer inserted into the thickest part of the steaks registers 140°F. Serve each steak with a spoonful of the aioli.

Makes 4 servings

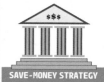

SAVE-MONEY STRATEGY

Swordfish is an excellent fish for grilling, its meatiness standing up nicely to the intense heat. But like so many great fish out there, it can be pricey, running up to $15 or more per pound. Mahi-mahi and tuna both make excellent alternatives and are usually gentler on the wallet. Even better are bluefish and mackerel, both of which are excellent for grilling and cost around $7 per pound. Plus, these two neglected fish are loaded with huge deposits of heart-healthy omega-3 fatty acids.

Per Serving:	
$4.04	280 calories 14 g fat (2.5 g saturated) 490 mg sodium

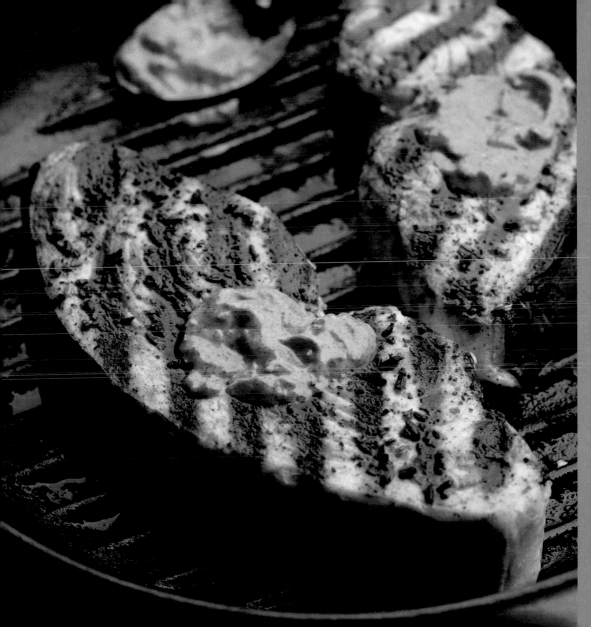

CHAPTER **8**

APPETIZERS, SNACKS & SMALL BITES

Artichoke-Lemon Crostini

Crostini means "toast" in Italian, but let's be clear now that there is a gaping chasm between toast and flame-grilled bread. The former is merely crunchy, while the latter soaks up the smoke and the char of the open flame, making it the perfect vessel for a variety of toppings—meat, vegetables, cheeses, anything really. Below and the recipes that follow are our favorite crostini, but by all means, grill the bread and top however you see fit.

You'll Need:

- 1 jar (5 oz) marinated artichoke hearts
- ¼ cup grated Parmesan
- Juice of 1 lemon
- 1 Tbsp olive oil, plus more for brushing on the bread
- 2 cloves garlic, minced
- Salt and black pepper to taste
- 4 (½"-thick) slices ciabatta or country bread

How to Make It:

- Preheat a grill or grill pan over high heat. While the grill is heating up, combine the artichoke hearts, Parmesan, lemon juice, olive oil, garlic, and a good pinch of salt and pepper in a food processor. Pulse until pureed but still slightly chunky.

- Lightly brush the bread on both sides with olive oil and grill over high heat for about 2 minutes per side, until lightly charred on the outside but still a bit soft in the center. Slather the toasts with the artichoke puree and serve.

Makes 4 servings

MEAL MULTIPLIER

When it comes to crostini, you are only limited by your imagination. Consider these just a few among the hundreds of possibilities for amazing crostini toppings.

- Grilled rounds of eggplant tossed with vinegar, red pepper flakes, and mint
- Chopped tomatoes, garlic, basil, and olive oil
- Canned white beans pureed with olive oil, garlic, and rosemary
- Fresh ricotta and grilled bell peppers

Per Serving:
$1.19

130 calories
8 g fat (1.5 g saturated)
290 mg sodium

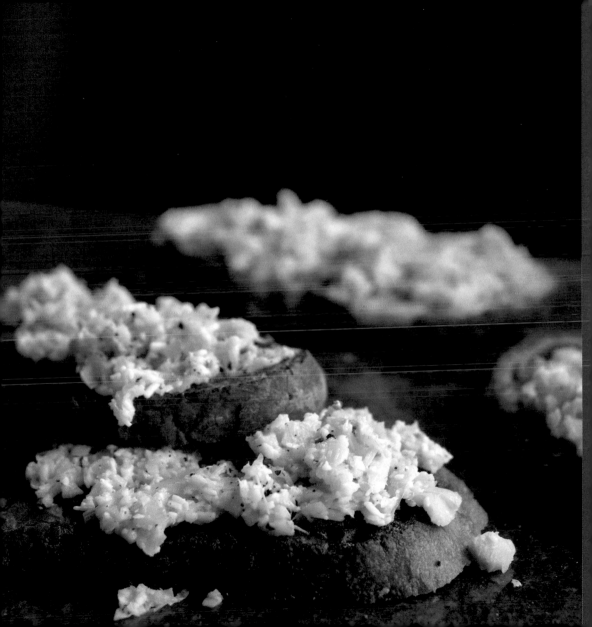

Fig & Prosciutto Crostini

We're helpless junkies for the combination of pork and fruit, and this crostini takes that enduring combination to its most delicious extreme. Strips of salty, porky, glorious prosciutto are offset by the full-throttle sweetness of ripe, juicy figs. The surrounding cast—peppery arugula, goat cheese, honey—are only there to further strengthen this sacred union.

You'll Need:

- ½ cup fresh goat cheese
- 8 fresh figs, quartered
- 2 cups arugula
- 4 slices prosciutto, cut into strips
- 1 Tbsp balsamic vinegar
- 1 Tbsp olive oil, plus more for brushing on the bread
- Salt and black pepper to taste
- 4 (½"-thick) slices ciabatta or country bread
- 1 Tbsp honey

How to Make It:

- Preheat a grill or grill pan over high heat. While the grill is heating up, combine the goat cheese, figs, arugula, prosciutto, balsamic, and olive oil. Mix until the ingredients are evenly coated and season with salt and pepper.

- Lightly brush the bread on both sides with olive oil and grill over high heat for about 2 minutes per side, until lightly charred on the outside, but still somewhat soft in the center. Divide the fig mixture among the toasts and drizzle each with a bit of honey before serving.

Makes 4 servings

Per Serving:
$2.56

260 calories
11 g fat (4 g saturated)
450 mg sodium

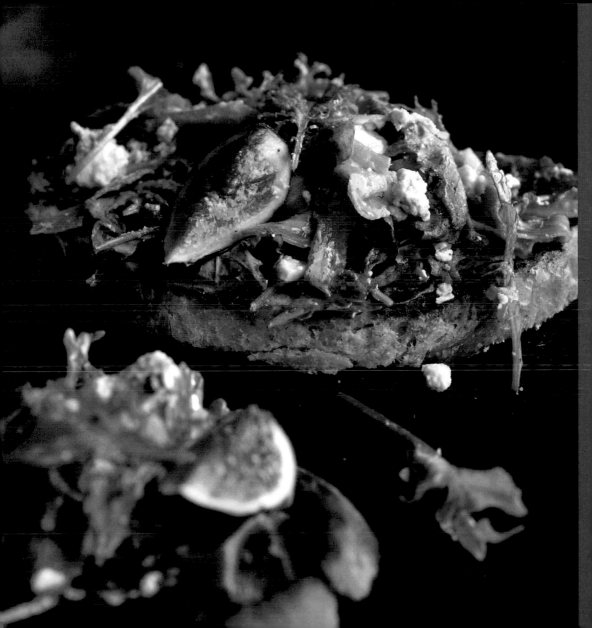

Chickpea Crostini

Every meal at Babbo, Mario Batali's flagship restaurant in New York, begins with a simple chickpea crostini that hits all the right notes to rouse the appetite—sweet, sour, salty, hot. It takes divine intervention to score a reservation at Babbo, but thankfully, one of the best parts of the meal is easy enough to re-create at home. This is our take on the first bite.

You'll Need:

- 1 **can (14 oz) garbanzo beans (aka chickpeas), drained and rinsed**
- 2 **Tbsp olive oil, plus more for brushing on the bread**
- 2 **Tbsp tapenade**
- 1 **Tbsp balsamic vinegar**
- ¼ **tsp fresh rosemary**
- 1 **pinch red pepper flakes**

Salt and black pepper to taste

- 4 **(½"-thick) slices ciabatta or country bread**

How to Make It:

- Preheat a grill or grill pan over high heat. While the grill is heating up, combine the chickpeas, olive oil, tapenade, balsamic, rosemary, and pepper flakes. Mix until the chickpeas are evenly coated. Season with salt and pepper.

- Lightly brush the bread on both sides with olive oil and grill over high heat for about 2 minutes per side, until lightly charred on the outside but still a bit soft in the center. Top each piece of bread with enough chickpea mixture to cover. You'll likely have leftover chickpeas, which can be served as a side dish or with more toasted bread. Covered, they keep in the refrigerator for up to 1 week.

Makes 4 servings

These garbanzos are amazing on their own or served alongside grilled chicken, steak, or lamb.

Per Serving:
$0.88

200 calories
8 g fat (1 g saturated)
340 mg sodium

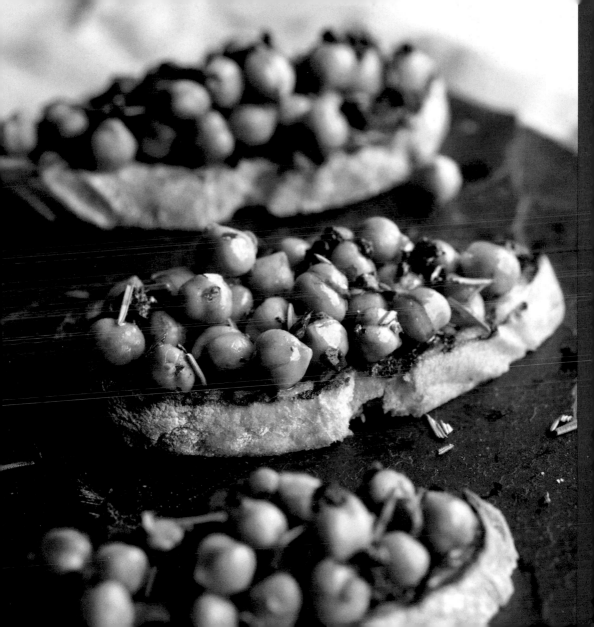

Chipotle Honey Wings

The deep fryer has one prevailing virtue: It makes food crisp. But in exchange for the crunch, you get saddled with hundreds of worthless calories every time you tussle with fried food. We think you can do better—and here's a perfect example how. Wings are never better than when they're hot off the grill, skin beautifully browned and meat suffused with smoke, which is why it's so surprising to see the same boring oil-soaked wings on every restaurant menu in America. We hope these will be all the proof you need to make the switch from the fryer to the grill.

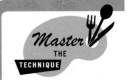

You'll Need:

- 1–2 chipotle peppers in adobo
- 2 Tbsp honey
- 2 cloves garlic, chopped
- Juice of 1 lime
- 2 lb chicken wings
- Salt to taste
- Chopped cilantro

These wings will be pretty fiery with two full chipotles. If you want to tone down the heat, stick to a single pepper.

How to Make It:

- In a blender or food processor, puree the chipotle peppers, honey, garlic, and lime juice. Reserve.

- Preheat a grill over medium-low heat. Season the wings all over with salt. Grill the wings for 5 to 7 minutes per side, until the skin is nicely browned and crispy and the meat is cooked through. Combine the wings and the sauce in a large mixing bowl and toss until the wings are thoroughly coated. Top with the cilantro.

Makes 6 servings

Per Serving:
$1.62

360 calories
24 g fat (7 g saturated)
390 mg sodium

Master THE TECHNIQUE

Crispy low-cal wings

Want the crisp without the calories? Try this simple trick: Toss the whole batch of wings in ½ tablespoon each baking powder and salt, then lay them out on a baking rack set on a sheet pan and place in the fridge overnight, being careful the wings don't come into contact with other foods. The air will help remove moisture from the skin while baking powder helps weaken protein strands. Both are key to producing crispier wings.

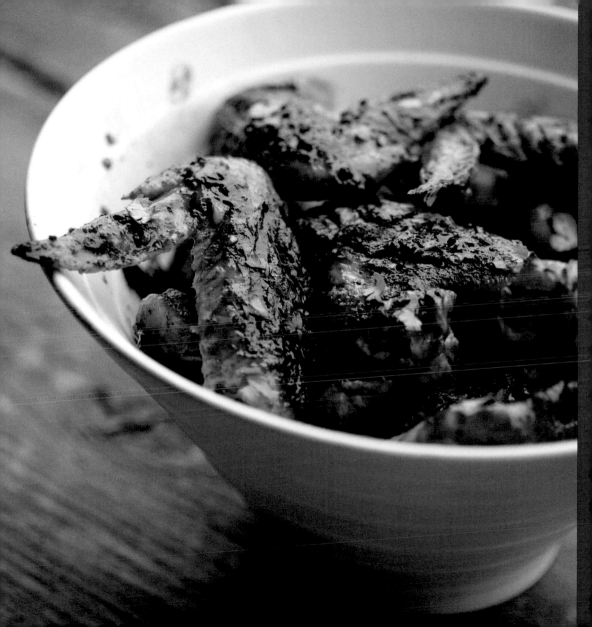

Tuna Satay Skewers

Appetizer sections are home to the densest caloric concentrations on America's menus. It's hard to find anything in the starters section that hasn't touched the deep fryer or isn't built entirely out of refined carbs and cheap fat. What you really want to start your meal with is a big dose of protein: Not only does it get your metabolism firing, protein also keeps your belly full, which helps ward off overeating later in the meal. Luckily, these grilled tuna skewers are nearly pure protein.

You'll Need:

- 1 lb ahi tuna, cut into 8 long pieces
- 8 metal skewers, or wooden skewers soaked in water 30 minutes before cooking

Salt and black pepper to taste

Peanut Sauce (page 48)

How to Make It:

- Heat a grill or stovetop grill pan until hot. Thread the tuna onto the skewers, season all over with salt and black pepper, and paint with the peanut sauce. Cook for 2 minutes per side, until charred on the outside but still pink in the center. Serve the skewers with the remaining sauce.

Makes 4 servings

LEFTOVER LOVE

Find yourself with more peanut sauce than you need for the tuna? Perfect. It will keep in the fridge for up to 3 days and is perfect for quick stir-fries on busy weeknights. Heat a wok or sauté pan over high heat; sauté chicken, beef, or pork with broccoli, asparagus, bell peppers, and onions. When the produce and protein are almost fully cooked, dump in the peanut sauce, along with a splash of water or chicken broth to thin it out. Cook for 2 to 3 minutes more. Serve sprinkled with crushed peanuts and accompanied by lime wedges.

Per Serving:
$3.32

300 calories
8 g fat (2 g saturated)
270 mg sodium

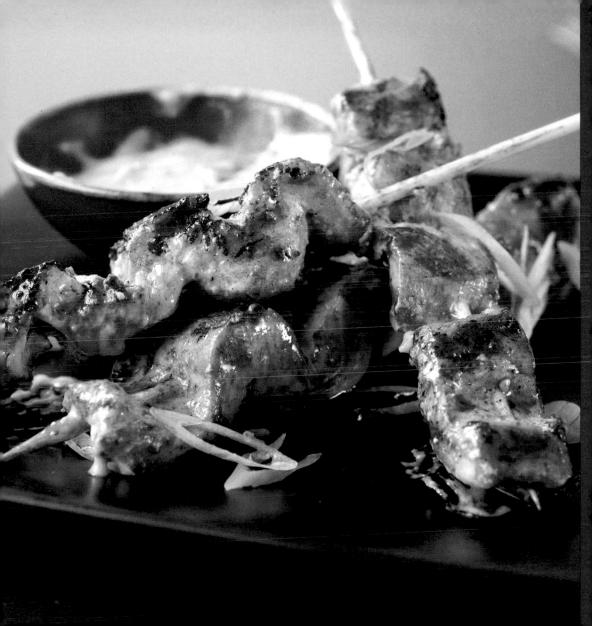

Grilled Baba Ghanoush

Think of baba ghanoush as hummus, but with eggplant standing in for chickpeas. Most recipes for this Middle Eastern specialty call for the eggplant to be baked in the oven, which misses the point entirely: This dip is all about the sweet-smoky combination that comes from grilled eggplant. This is the perfect appetizer to put out to tame raging appetites while you move on to the meatier matters of grilling.

You'll Need:

1 large eggplant

Olive oil for rubbing on the eggplant

2 Tbsp tahini

Juice of 1 lemon

2 cloves garlic, chopped

¼ tsp cumin

Salt and black pepper

Chopped fresh parsley (optional)

4 whole-wheat pitas

Tahini is a paste made from ground sesame seeds. Can't find it? Peanut butter will work in a pinch.

How to Make It:

- Preheat a grill over medium heat. Prick the eggplant all over with a fork and rub with a thin coating of olive oil. Grill, turning occasionally, for about 15 minutes, until the skin is charred and the inside is very soft. Allow the eggplant to cool for at least 5 minutes before handling. (This step can be done up to a day ahead.)

- Peel back the charred skin and scoop out the soft innards of the eggplant, using a spoon to scrape off every last bit of flesh from the skin (it's quite alright if a bit of charred skin makes it into the mix). Pulse the eggplant in a food processor with the tahini, lemon juice, garlic, and cumin until smooth. Season with salt and pepper. Transfer to a serving bowl and top with chopped parsley, if you like.

- Heat the pitas on the grill, in a toaster, or in the oven until very warm and soft. Cut into wedges and serve with the baba ghanoush.

Makes 4 servings

Per Serving:
$0.93

200 calories
5 g fat (1 g saturated)
250 mg sodium

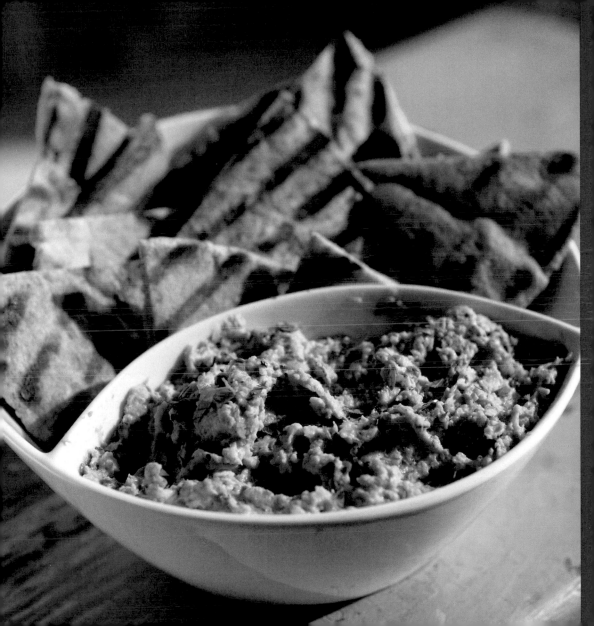

Grilled Meatballs
with Smoky Tomato Sauce

We wanted to keep the essential awesomeness of meatballs and red sauce intact but ditch about 80 percent of the calories, so we nixed the mountain of spaghetti and turned to our friend Old Smoky for the solution.

You'll Need:

MEATBALLS

½ lb ground sirloin

½ lb ground pork

¼ cup bread crumbs

¼ onion, minced

¼ cup grated Parmesan

1 egg, beaten

1 clove garlic, minced

½ tsp fennel seeds

½ tsp salt

SMOKY TOMATO SAUCE

1 lb Roma tomatoes, tops removed, halved

1 small onion, sliced

Olive oil

1 clove garlic, minced (or 2 cloves Grilled Garlic, page 50)

Salt and black pepper to taste

How to Make It:

● Preheat a grill over medium heat. While the grill heats up, make the meatballs: Combine the sirloin, pork, bread crumbs, onion, Parmesan, egg, garlic, fennel seeds, and salt in a large mixing bowl. Gently roll the mixture into golf ball–sized orbs, being careful not to overwork the meat (which will give you tough, chewy meatballs).

● To make the tomato sauce, drizzle the tomatoes and onion with enough olive oil to lightly coat. Place on one side of the grill and cook for about 10 minutes, until the onions are very soft and the tomato skins begin to blister. Peel off the tomato skins and puree the rest in a blender with the onion, garlic, 1 tablespoon olive oil, and salt and pepper.

● While the tomatoes and onions are grilling, place the meatballs on the other side of the grill and cook on all sides for 8 to 10 minutes, until they are charred and firm to the touch.

● Serve the meatballs with the tomato sauce and slices of grilled bread, if you like.

Makes 4 servings

Per Serving:
$2.04

350 calories
21 g fat (7 g saturated)
540 mg sodium

MEAL MULTIPLIER

Pork and beef are traditional meatball fodder for a reason, but limit yourself to them and you're missing out on a world of exciting possibilities. Combine any of the following with bread crumbs and eggs for a tasty departure from the standard meatball:

● Finely minced tuna with toasted pine nuts and raisins

● Ground chicken with minced ginger and scallion, served with Mango Chutney (page 200)

● Ground lamb with garlic, red pepper flakes, and chopped fresh mint, served with the same tomato sauce used on this page

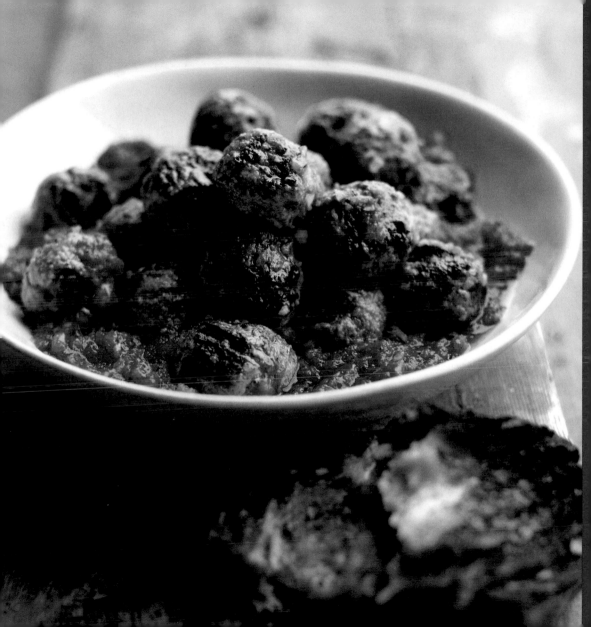

Ham & Pineapple Quesadillas

Most quesadillas in America are made either in a skillet or, worse, the micro-wave, while the best cooking implement goes entirely overlooked. The grill not only adds a smoky char and a lasting crisp to a quesadilla, it also allows you to cook two or three at a time, making this one of the quickest, easiest recipes in the entire book. The inspiration here comes from that uniquely American take on pizza, the Hawaiian pie. Try dipping wedges into warm marinara to complete the effect.

You'll Need:

4 (8" diameter) tortillas

1 cup shredded Jack cheese

1 cup shredded Swiss cheese

4 slices deli ham, cut into thin strips

1 cup chopped pineapple

Pickled jalapeño peppers (optional)

Canola oil for brushing

Pico de Gallo (page 46), Smoky Tomato Sauce (page 258), or your favorite store-bought salsa for serving

How to Make It:

● Preheat a grill or grill pan over medium heat. Place two tortillas on a large cutting board or clean kitchen surface. Evenly divide the cheeses, ham, pineapple, and jalapeños (if using) between them. Top each with another tortilla.

● Brush the top tortillas lightly with oil, then place directly on the grill, oiled side down. (If you're using a grill pan, you'll need to cook one quesadilla at a time.) Lightly brush the tortillas now facing up with oil. Grill, turning 45 degrees midway through, for 4 to 5 minutes. Flip the quesadillas and grill on the other side, turning 45 degrees midway through, for another 4 to 5 minutes, until the tortillas are lightly toasted and the cheese is fully melted. (The cheese will melt better if you close the lid while cooking.) Cut into wedges and serve with pico de gallo or salsa.

Makes 4 servings

Per Serving: **$1.77**

370 calories
18 g fat (10 g saturated)
620 mg sodium

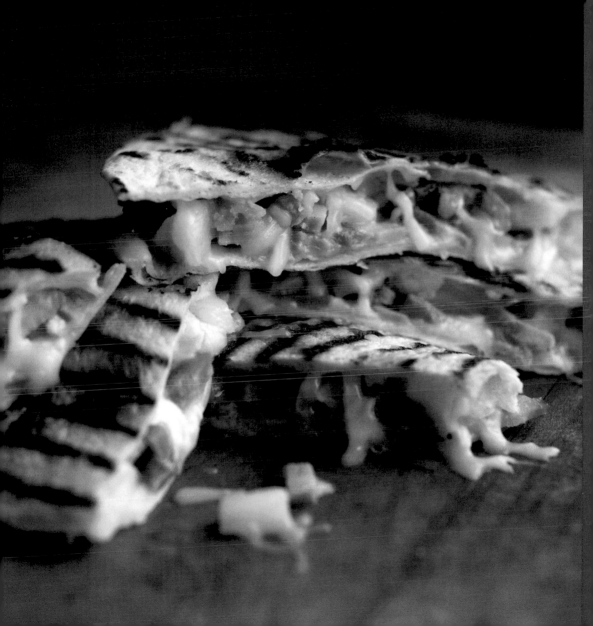

Tomato Bread (2 Ways)

It seems so basic, but when the tomatoes are ripe and the bread is good, few combinations are as satisfying. In Spain, they smash ripe tomatoes directly on the bread to create one of the country's iconic dishes. The other take is a nod to the South, where thick-cut tomatoes team up with mayo for a summer treat.

Spanish Style

You'll Need:

- 2 **very ripe large tomatoes, halved**
- 2 **Tbsp olive oil, plus more for brushing on the bread**

Coarse sea salt to taste

- 4 **(½"-thick) slices ciabatta or country bread**
- 1 **clove garlic, peeled and halved**

It's helpful to have two types of olive oil on hand: one normal bottle for cooking, one nice bottle for drizzling on raw or cooked foods. Both of these recipes are best with high-quality oil.

How to Make It:

- Using a large box grater, grate the flesh side of the tomatoes through the largest holes until everything but the skin has passed through. Stir the olive oil into the tomato pulp and season with salt.

- Preheat a grill or grill pan over high heat. Brush the bread on both sides with olive oil and grill over high heat for about 2 minutes per side, until lightly charred on the outside, but still a bit soft in the center. While the bread is still hot, rub one side with a cut garlic clove. Spoon the tomatoes over the toasts and top with a few flakes of coarse salt.

Makes 4 servings

American Style

You'll Need:

- 4 **(½"-thick) slices ciabatta or country bread**
- 2 **Tbsp olive oil, plus more for brushing**
- 1 **clove garlic, peeled and halved**
- 3 **very ripe medium heirloom tomatoes (preferably different colors), sliced**
- 2 **Tbsp chopped fresh chives**

Coarse sea salt and black pepper to taste

How to Make It:

- Preheat a grill or grill pan over high heat. Lightly brush the bread on both sides with olive oil and grill over high heat for about 2 minutes per side, until lightly charred on the outside, but still a bit soft in the center. While the bread is still hot, rub one side with a cut garlic clove.

- Layer the tomatoes across the bread, varying colors if you're lucky enough to find a variety of heirlooms. Top with the chives and 2 tablespoons olive oil and season with salt and pepper.

Makes 4 servings

Per Serving: **$1.56**
130 calories
8 g fat (1 g saturated)
120 mg sodium

Per Serving: **$1.82**
130 calories
8 g fat (1 g saturated)
120 mg sodium

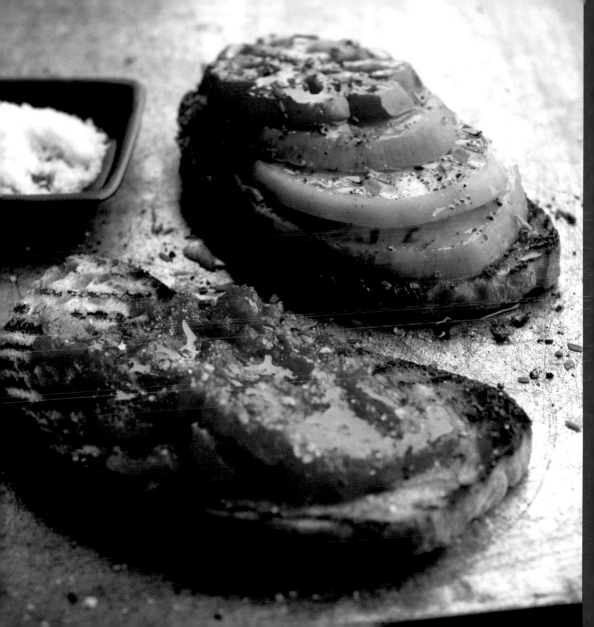

Oysters
with Garlic Butter and Tabasco

If there is one unconventional grilled food that everybody should try once, it's the grilled oyster. As the shell heats up from the bottom, the oyster begins to cook gently in the bath of garlic, butter, and brine. It ends up somewhere between the soft, slippery texture of a raw oyster and the creamy, slightly chewy effect of a cooked one. A bit of bubbling garlic butter and a shake of Tabasco take the experience over the top. Be sure to have a cold beer, or a glass of sparkling wine, close at hand.

You'll Need:

12 oysters, shucked

2 Tbsp salted butter, cut into small pieces

2 cloves garlic, very finely minced

Tabasco to taste

Lemon wedges

How to Make It:

- Preheat a grill or grill pan over medium heat. Divide the butter and garlic among the oysters. When the grill is hot, place the oysters directly on the grate, shell side down. Grill for about 5 minutes, until the butter has fully melted and the oysters have begun to firm up. Serve with hot sauce and lemon wedges.

Makes 4 servings

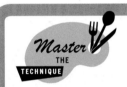

Master THE **TECHNIQUE**

Shucking oysters

Place the oysters in the freezer for 15 minutes; the cold helps to loosen the muscle that holds the shell closed. Using a towel to hold the oyster, insert an oyster knife (or any thin blade—like a paring knife) in the oyster's back hinge. Rotate the knife 90 degrees, rocking it back and forth to pop the top open. Slide the knife across the oyster to sever the connective tissue, being careful not to lose the precious oyster liquor in the shell.

Per Serving:
$3.12

80 calories
7 g fat (3 g saturated)
130 mg sodium

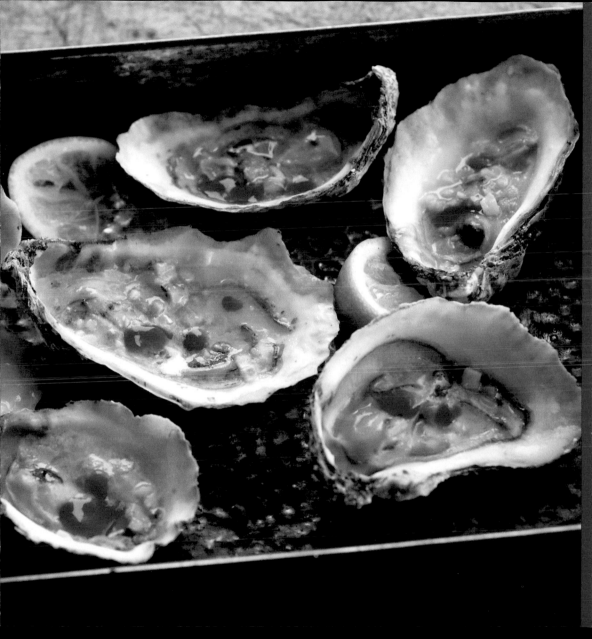

Grilled-Corn Guacamole

Normally our guacamole ethos boils down to this: Less is more. It's tough to watch people pollute the enduring union of avocado, salt, and citrus with high-calorie intruders like mayonnaise and sour cream. But this recipe, like so many great ones out there, was born out of serendipity, the result of having some leftover grilled corn and a handful of cherry tomatoes. It's not better than classic guac, it's just different—in the best possible way. Serve with tortillas warmed on the grill, tucked into tacos, or spooned over the top of grilled chicken or fish. Or with tortilla chips, of course.

You'll Need:

- 1 ear corn
- 2 medium Hass avocados, pitted and peeled
- 1 clove garlic, minced

Salt to taste

- 1 cup cherry tomatoes, halved
- 1 handful cilantro, chopped

Juice of 1 lime

How to Make It:

- Preheat a grill over medium heat. Peel the corn husk back, being careful so it remains attached to the base of the cob, and remove the silk inside. Re-cover the ear with the husk and soak in cold water for 5 minutes.

- Grill the corn for 10 minutes, turning a quarter-turn every few minutes. Peel back the husk and place the corn back on the grill. Grill, turning occasionally, for 5 minutes more, until the kernels are nicely browned. When the corn is cool enough to handle, use a knife to cut the kernels from the cob.

- Combine the avocado, garlic, and a few good pinches of salt in a mixing bowl. Use a fork to mash the avocado until you have a consistency somewhere between smooth and chunky. Fold in the corn kernels, tomatoes, cilantro, and lime juice.

Makes 4 servings

Per Serving:
$1.69

200 calories
15 g fat (2.5 g saturated)
325 mg sodium

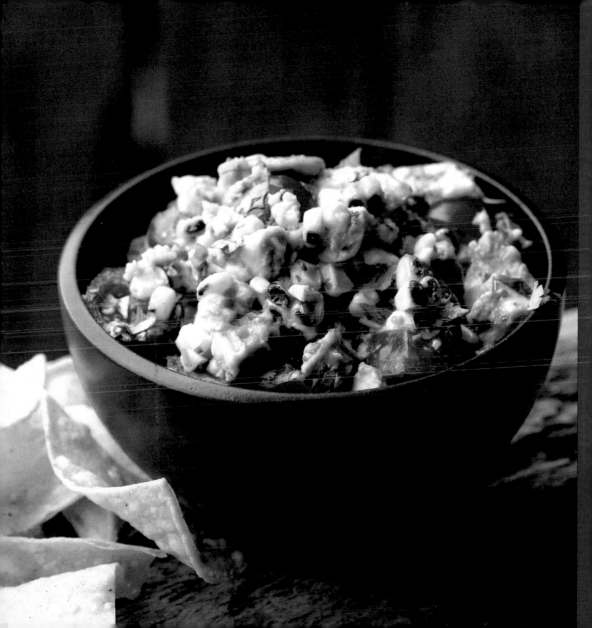

Grilled Raisin-Walnut Bread
with Ricotta and Grapes

By themselves, grilled grapes are the world's healthiest dessert. Paired with ricotta, fresh rosemary, and cracked black pepper, they create something that straddles the sweet-savory world in a deeply delicious way. It's the kind of dish that people will question at first, but as they bite down, their eyes will open wide and eventually sink into the backs of their heads—a powerful reminder that experimentation in the kitchen is always a good thing.

You'll Need:

1 **medium bunch (about ½ lb) red grapes**

4 **(½"-thick) slices raisin-walnut bread**

1 **cup part-skim ricotta**

1 **tsp chopped fresh rosemary**

Black pepper to taste

Want to turn this into dessert? Omit the black pepper and drizzle on a light stream of honey instead.

How to Make It:

● Preheat a grill over high heat. Place the grapes directly on the grate and grill for about 10 minutes, until the skins are blistered and the insides are hot and juicy. While the grapes grill, grill the bread, turning, until lightly browned and crisp.

● Spread the ricotta in a thick layer on the slices of bread. Remove the grapes from the stems and arrange on top of the ricotta, along with the rosemary and a generous amount of freshly cracked black pepper.

Makes 4 servings

A more traditional bread like ciabatta will work fine. So will cinnamon-swirl bread sold by makers like Sun-Maid.

Per Serving:
$1.71

200 calories
6 g fat (3.5 g saturated)
180 mg sodium

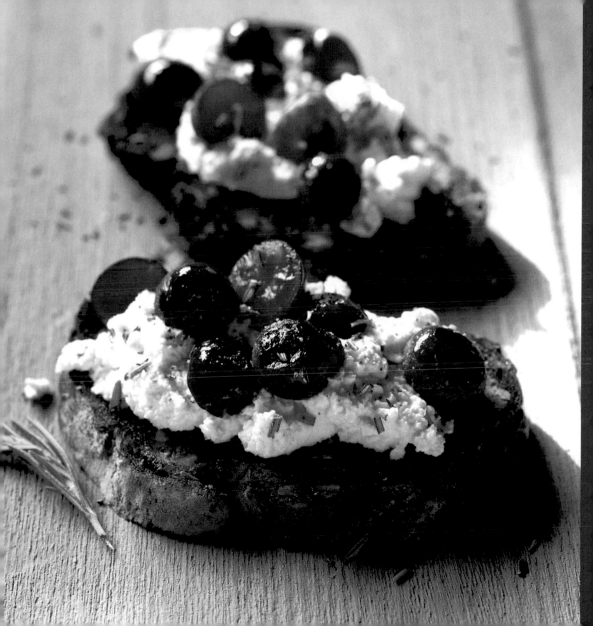

Chorizo Tostadas

Buy a box of tostada shells in the supermarket and you'll get a few flat, dry pieces of additive-addled corn that look more like flying saucers than dinner. But put a fresh corn tortilla on the grill until it perfectly straddles the tender-crispy spectrum and you have the base for something spectacular. You can vary this recipe dozens of different ways, but the mix of spicy chorizo, fresh avocado, and crumbled cheese is as good a place to start as any.

You'll Need:

- 6 oz fresh Mexican-style chorizo
- 1 avocado, peeled and pitted
- 1 cup Tomatilla Salsa (page 204 or store-bought)
- 4 corn tortillas
- ½ Tbsp canola oil for brushing
- ½ cup Cotija cheese

Cotija is a dry, crumbly Mexican cheese available in Latin markets. If you can't find it, feta or even fresh goat cheese works nearly as well.

This recipe makes more salsa than you'll need. Use the leftovers to slather on sandwiches or for topping fried eggs in the morning.

How to Make It:

- Remove the chorizo from its casing and cook in a medium-sized sauté pan set over medium heat for 7 to 8 minutes, until just cooked through. Remove to a plate lined with paper towels to absorb the excess fat.

- Place the avocado in a mixing bowl and mash with a fork until smooth. Stir in the tomatillo salsa.

- Preheat a grill over low heat. Brush the tortillas on both sides with oil and grill for 3 to 4 minutes, until the bottoms are crispy and browned. Flip, top with the chorizo, and continue grilling for another 3 to 4 minutes, until the bottoms begin to crisp. Top the tostadas with the avocado salsa and the crumbled cheese.

Makes 4 servings

MEAL MULTIPLIER

Crunchy grilled tostadas are the perfect vehicles for dozens of Latin-inspired toppings. Here are three other combinations worth trying:

- Refried beans, pepper Jack cheese, and grilled chicken
- Grilled strips of zucchini, mushrooms, and jalapeños, topped wtih Tomatillo Salsa
- Mashed avocado, finely chopped raw ahi tuna, lime juice, and arugula
- Grilled Scallop Ceviche (page 276)

Per Serving:
$1.87

310 calories
18 g fat (8 g saturated)
740 mg sodium

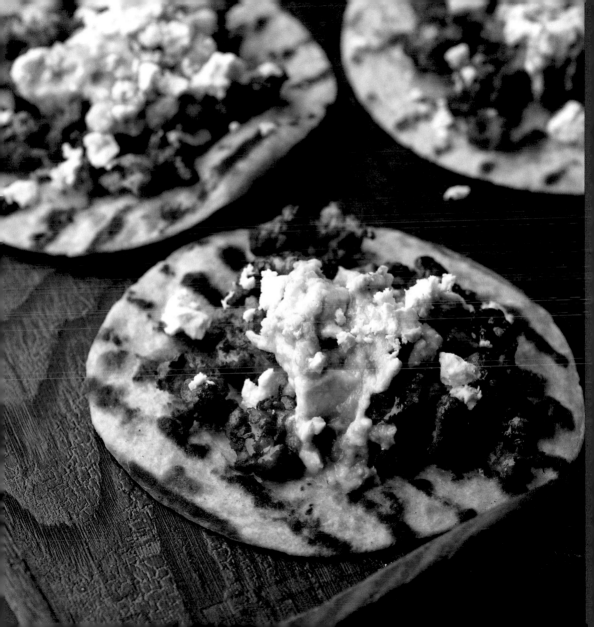

Sweet & Spicy Ahi

Ahi tuna is one of the greatest grill ingredients of all—lean, meaty, and incredibly simple to cook. The key to great ahi is a screaming hot flame, which allows you to sear the outside while leaving the center raw—a nod to its role as a star of the sushi bar. As such, it takes well to Asian flavors like ginger, soy, and rice wine vinegar. Serve this as is for an impressive appetizer, or with a bit of steamed brown rice for an ultra-lean dinner.

You'll Need:

- ¼ cup rice wine vinegar
- ¼ cup soy sauce
- 1 Tbsp honey
- 1 Tbsp minced ginger
- 1 jalapeño pepper, minced
- ¼ cup chopped cilantro
- ¼ cup peanut oil
- 1 English cucumber, sliced into thin rounds
- 1 lb ahi tuna (2–3 fillets)

Salt and black pepper to taste

How to Make It:

- Combine the rice wine vinegar, soy sauce, honey, ginger, jalapeño, and cilantro in a medium mixing bowl. Slowly drizzle in the oil, whisking to fully incorporate. Add the cucumber and let soak at least 10 minutes before you cook the tuna.

- Preheat a grill or grill pan over high heat. Season the tuna all over with salt and pepper. Place on the hottest part of the grill and grill for 2 minutes per side, until grill marks have developed but the center is still raw. (If you like your tuna cooked through, cook for 4 minutes per side.)

- Slice the tuna into thin pieces and divide among four plates. With a slotted spoon, place a pile of cucumbers on each plate. Drizzle the remaining sauce over the tuna.

Makes 4 servings

Per Serving:
$3.83

280 calories
15 g fat (2 g saturated)
820 mg sodium

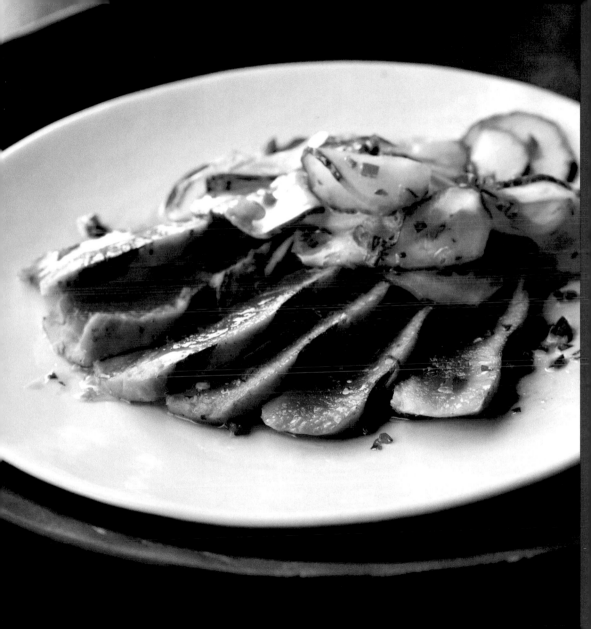

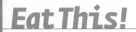

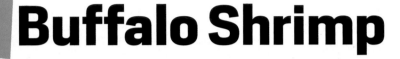

Buffalo Shrimp

Deep-fried chicken wings coated in butter and dipped in blue cheese can be a bit of a one-note affair: fat on fat on fat. By trading lean shrimp for the wings, using a yogurt-based blue cheese sauce in lieu of the blue cheese, and, most importantly, turning to the grill instead of a vat of bubbling oil, we've trimmed 75 percent of the calories from the classic bar food while adding new dimensions to its enduring appeal. We think you'll approve.

You'll Need:

- ¼ cup plain Greek yogurt
- ¼ cup olive oil mayonnaise
- 2 Tbsp crumbled blue cheese
- Juice of ½ lemon
- 1 lb medium shrimp, peeled and deveined
- Salt and black pepper to taste
- Metal skewers, or wooden skewers soaked in water for 30 minutes
- 2 Tbsp butter
- 1 Tbsp hot sauce (we like Frank's RedHot)

How to Make It:

- Combine the yogurt, mayonnaise, blue cheese, and half the lemon juice in a small bowl. Reserve.

- Preheat a grill or grill pan over high heat. Season the shrimp with salt and pepper and thread on the skewers. Grill the shrimp for 1 to 2 minutes per side, until pink and just firm.

- Melt the butter in a large sauté pan. Stir in the hot sauce and remaining lemon juice and remove from the heat. Strip the shrimp from the skewers and add to the pan, tossing until evenly coated with the sauce. Serve with the blue cheese sauce for dipping.

Makes 4 servings

Per Serving:
$2.42

230 calories
12 g fat (5 g saturated)
230 mg sodium

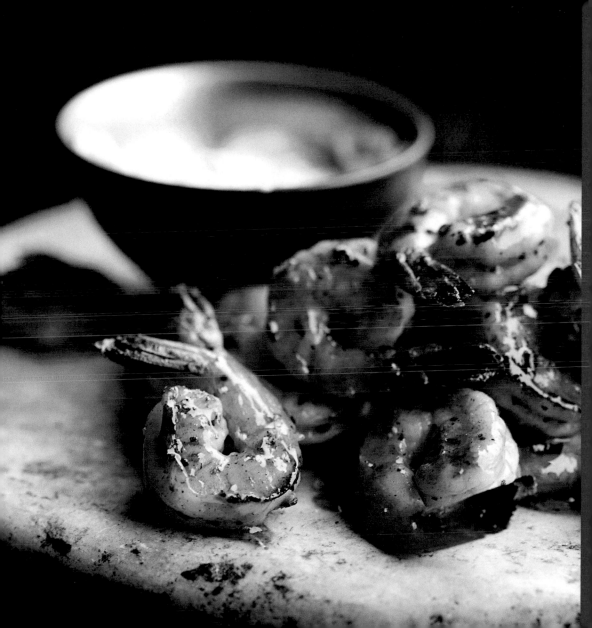

Grilled Scallop Ceviche

All signs point to Peruvian food being one of the next big international cuisines to make an impression on North American eating. At the heart of the Peruvian kitchen is ceviche, a simple dish of raw seafood marinated in lime juice and onion until the citric acid effectively "cooks" the fish. This isn't a traditional ceviche since the scallops are cooked first, but the grilling adds a new dimension to the original formula, while the lime juice, onions, and cilantro help retain the classic ceviche flavors. If there is a healthier dish anywhere in the world, we haven't found it.

You'll Need:

1 lb medium sea scallops

Salt and black pepper to taste

2 medium oranges (preferably blood oranges), peeled and segmented

½ English cucumber, thinly sliced

1 small avocado, peeled, pitted, and cubed

1 small red onion, thinly sliced

½ jalapeño pepper, minced

2 Tbsp olive oil, plus more for coating the scallops

Juice of 2 limes

½ cup chopped cilantro

Grilled bread or grilled corn tortillas

If you can't get your hands on scallops, shrimp make for a fine substitute.

How to Make It:

• Preheat a grill or grill pan over high heat. Drizzle the scallops with just enough olive oil to coat, then season on both sides with salt and pepper. When the grill is very hot, add the scallops and grill for about 2 minutes, until nice grill marks have developed and the flesh easily pulls away from the grill. Flip and cook for another 2 minutes, until the scallops are firm but gently yielding to the touch.

• Slice the scallops in half horizontally, then combine with the oranges, cucumber, avocado, onion, and jalapeño. Drizzle in the 2 tablespoons olive oil, the lime juice, and cilantro, and season with salt and pepper. Serve with grilled bread or corn tortillas.

Makes 4 servings

Per Serving:
$3.93

340 calories
16 g fat (2 g saturated)
390 mg sodium

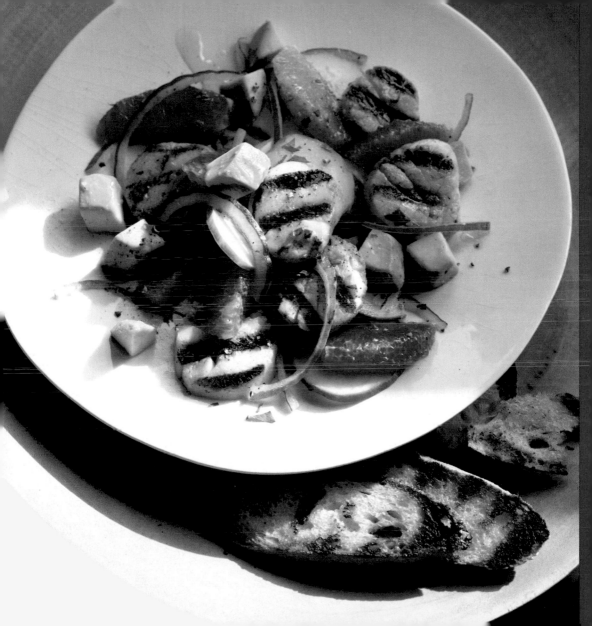

Vietnamese-Style Chicken Wings

Down a small side street in downtown Ho Chi Minh City, an open-air restaurant called Ban Xeo 46A houses hungry revelers who line up until the early hours of the morning to eat crispy crepes, spring rolls, and what may be the greatest chicken wings on the planet. No, they're not doused in Texas Pete and drowned in blue cheese dressing, but rather gently coated with a perfectly balanced sweet-salty mix of sugar and fish sauce. This recipe is, we hope, a faithful interpretation of the original, but with the smoke of the grill standing in for the oil of the fryer.

You'll Need:

2 lb chicken wings

½ cup fish sauce

¼ cup sugar

2 cloves garlic, minced

Black pepper to taste

½ cup chopped fresh cilantro or mint

How to Make It:

- Combine the wings, fish sauce, sugar, garlic, and black pepper in a sealable plastic bag. Seal and refrigerate to marinate for at least 2 hours (or up to 8 hours).

- Preheat a grill over medium heat. Remove the wings from the bag, reserving the marinade. Grill the wings for about 5 minutes per side, until the skin is nicely browned and crispy and the meat pulls easily away from the bone.

- While the wings cook, place the marinade in a saucepan over medium heat and bring to a simmer. Cook for about 10 minutes, until reduced by half. When the wings are done, toss with the sauce and garnish with the fresh herbs.

Makes 6 servings

Per Serving: **$1.80**	340 calories 24 g fat (7 g saturated) 670 mg sodium

SECRET WEAPON

Fish Sauce

Made from fermented oily fish, fish sauce tends to pack a stiff aroma. But this funky condiment forms the backbone of much of Southeast Asian cuisine and, despite it's strong nose, adds a pleasantly salty, sweet punch of flavor to a variety of dishes and sauces. Try marinating steak or vegetables in a 50-50 mix of fish sauce and olive oil and you'll be won over instantly. Find a bottle in large grocery stores or Asian markets.

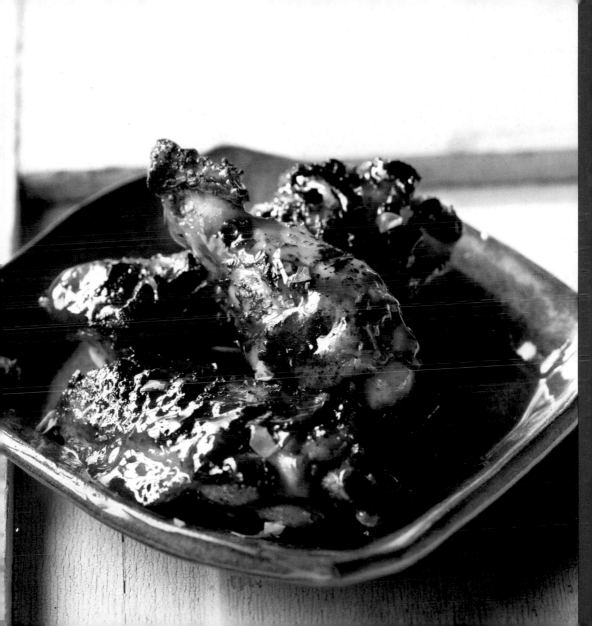

Smoking Gazpacho

It's tough to improve on a dish that's been around for hundreds of years. Gazpacho was invented by Spaniards as a way to cool off and nourish during the oppressive heat of the Andalusian summer. But the heat of the grill brings out the best in the vegetables that compose this cold soup, making for a more intensely flavorful gazpacho than those made with raw vegetables alone. Like most soups, this one is best made at least a few hours ahead, giving the flavors time to make friends while they chill out in the refrigerator.

You'll Need:

3 **large tomatoes (about 1½ pounds)**

1 **medium onion, halved**

1 **green bell pepper, stemmed, seeded, and quartered**

1 **small hothouse cucumber, roughly chopped**

1½ **cups low-sodium tomato juice**

¼ **cup olive oil, plus more for drizzling**

2 **Tbsp sherry vinegar**

2 **cloves garlic, peeled**

A few shakes **Tabasco sauce**

Salt to taste

Garlic Croutons

How to Make It:

● Preheat a grill over high heat. When hot, grill the tomatoes, onion, and bell pepper, turning, for about 12 minutes, until their skins are lightly blistered and their flesh very soft.

● Combine the grilled vegetables with the cucumber, tomato juice, olive oil, vinegar, garlic, Tabasco, and salt in a blender and puree until mostly smooth (a few light chunks in gazpacho is a good thing). Place the gazpacho in the refrigerator to chill for at least 1 hour before serving.

● Serve each bowl of gazpacho with a crouton and an extra drizzle of olive oil.

Makes 4 servings

Per Serving:
$1.46

200 calories
14 g fat (2 g saturated)
560 mg sodium

Garlic Croutons

You'll Need:

1 **baguette**

Olive oil for drizzling

2 **cloves garlic, halved**

How to Make It:

● Preheat a grill over medium heat. Use a bread knife to slice the baguette on the diagonal into ¼"-thick slices. Drizzle the bread with olive oil and place on the grill. Cook for about 3 minutes per side, until brown and crunchy. Rub one side of each slice with a piece of garlic and serve. Keeps for up to 1 week, covered, in the pantry.

Makes about 20 croutons

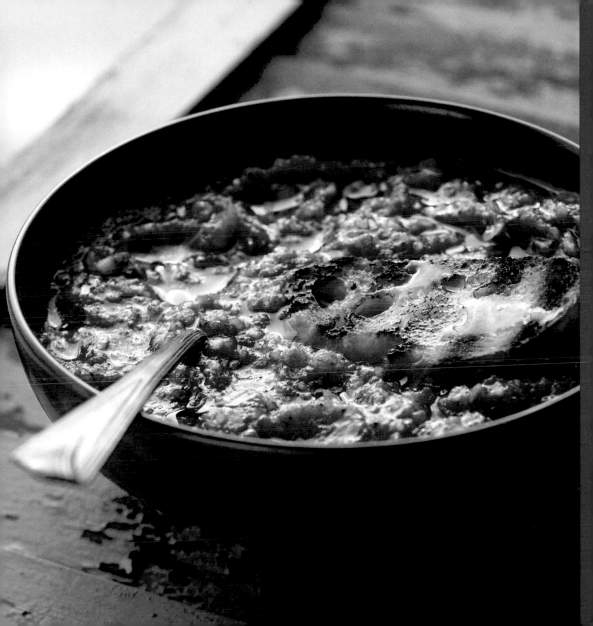

SALADS

CHAPTER **9**

You Can Grill

THAT?

Grills were made for more than steaks and burgers. These unusual ingredients also benefit from the smoke-and-fire treatment.

Spinach

Both full-grown spinach and arugula can be cooked directly on the grill grate. Thoroughly clean the leaves and leave the stems intact (it will make them easier to handle on the grill). Place over a medium fire and grill for 3 to 5 minutes, until the leaves begin to wilt and crisp around the edges. Dress the greens with a drizzle of olive oil, the juice of a lemon, some shaved Parmesan cheese.

Lettuce

Firm heads of lettuce like iceberg, cabbage, or—our favorite—radicchio, take well to the transformative powers of the grill. Halve or quarter the heads and drizzle with olive oil. Grill over high heat until the outer leaves are blackened and wilted and the center is softened. Serve radicchio drizzled with balsamic, dress cabbage with Honey-Dijon Vinaigrette (page 49), and anoint iceberg wedges with crumbled bacon, fresh tomatoes, and blue cheese dressing.

Edamame

Most people only know edamame as those green little pods they pick at before their sushi arrives, but tossed onto the grill and cooked until nicely charred, they become a whole different animal. Grill them over medium heat directly on the grate or in a grill basket for about 10 minutes, until the pods begin to blacken. Toss with coarse sea salt, sesame seeds, chili powder, or any other spice that gets you going.

Avocado

Grilled guacamole? Absolutely. Halve the avocado lengthwise and remove the pit. Place directly on the grate of a hot grill, cut side down, and grill for about 5 minutes, until nice grill marks have developed. From here, you can cube the avocado for salad, mash it for a smoky guacamole, or fill each half with tuna or chicken salad for an incredible twist on the classic.

Watermelon

Nothing wrong with a hunk of juicy watermelon as is, but like with all fruit, the grill helps to concentrate its sweetness and intensity. Cut thick watermelon steaks, drizzle with a bit of olive oil, and grill over high heat, turning once. Your mission is to sear the outside while keeping the center close to raw, creating a lovely hot-cold contrast. This should take about 8 minutes. Grilled watermelon can be eaten as is right off the grill (sprinkled with a bit of coarse sea salt), or put to use in a salad of arugula, goat cheese or feta, and toasted almonds.

Cake

Angel food cake, biscuits, and banana bread all benefit from a turn on the grill, not just because they come off hot, but also because the grill crisps the surface while keeping the interior warm and moist. Grill slices of banana bread over medium-high heat, turning, for 8 minutes, until crisp. While the bread grills, make a sauce by simmering ½ cup butter with ½ cup brown sugar. When sticky and dark, stir in ½ cup coffee. Top the banana bread with a scoop of cool Greek yogurt and a few spoons of the coffee caramel.

Cheese

Halloumi is a Middle Eastern cheese famous for its ability to stand up to high heat, but plenty of other cheeses can also take the heat. Provolone, mozzarella, and even a wheel of brie can be grilled until hot and gloriously gooey. Keep the cheese cold until the grill is ready to go, then place it on the grate and grill for 6 to 8 minutes, turning, just until the surface of the cheese browns and begins to melt. You can use grilled cheese to top a sandwich or anchor a salad, but the best move is to serve it as is, with slices of grilled bread rubbed with garlic for scooping.

Bacon

Yes, grilled bacon. It's best to use thick-cut bacon, as it stands up better to the heat than the scrawny stuff produced by most national brands. Grill over a low flame, turning, for about 12 minutes, until the fat renders and the meat crisps up. Use grilled bacon in a BLT or as a burger topping, or turn it into pig candy: Rub the bacon with brown sugar and a bit of cayenne before going on the grill; during the final 5 minutes of cooking, brush on thin coats of maple syrup. Mmmm, candied bacon.

Sizzling Caesar Salad

This is no gimmick: Grilled Caesar salad is a revelation. Standard Caesar qualifies as one of those faux-healthy foods we implore people to avoid ordering in restaurants, but when grilled at home, it's a whole different story.

You'll Need:

DRESSING

Juice of 1 lemon

2 Tbsp red wine vinegar

1 Tbsp olive oil mayonnaise

1 clove garlic, minced

2 anchovies (soak in milk for 10 minutes if you want to mellow the flavor)

1 tsp Worcestershire sauce

6–8 turns of a black-pepper mill

½ cup olive oil

2 heads romaine lettuce •

Olive oil for coating the lettuce

¼ cup finely grated Parmesan

Garlic Croutons (page 280)

How to Make It:

- To make the dressing, combine the lemon juice, vinegar, mayonnaise, garlic, anchovies, Worcestershire, and pepper in a food processor or blender. With the motor running, slowly drizzle in the olive oil until a thick, creamy dressing is formed.

- Preheat a grill over high heat. Peel off the dark outer leaves of the romaine (if using hearts of romaine, no peeling necessary). Halve each head vertically, leaving the stems intact to hold the lettuce together. Drizzle with just enough olive oil to coat the cut sides. Place the lettuce, cut side down, on the hottest part of grill and cook for 3 to 5 minutes, until the leaves have begun to wilt and char.

- Divide the lettuce among 4 plates, drizzle with enough dressing to lightly coat, and top with the Parmesan and a few croutons.

Makes 4 servings

Most grocery stores now sell bags of romaine hearts, which are ideal for this recipe.

Per Serving:
$1.66

310 calories
26 g fat (4 g saturated)
460 mg sodium

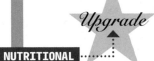

Upgrade

NUTRITIONAL

The main nutritional knock against Caesar salad is that, beyond the lettuce itself, there's nothing particularly healthy about it. In the worst hands, that's true, but there are many ways to bolster a Caesar, making it both more substantial and more nutritious. Here are three tasty additions that will boost the basic grilled Caesar recipe:

ı Grilled or shredded rotisserie chicken and sundried tomatoes

ı Chopped olives, marinated artichoke hearts, and roasted red peppers

ı Grilled shrimp, grilled corn kernels, and grilled strips of poblano peppers

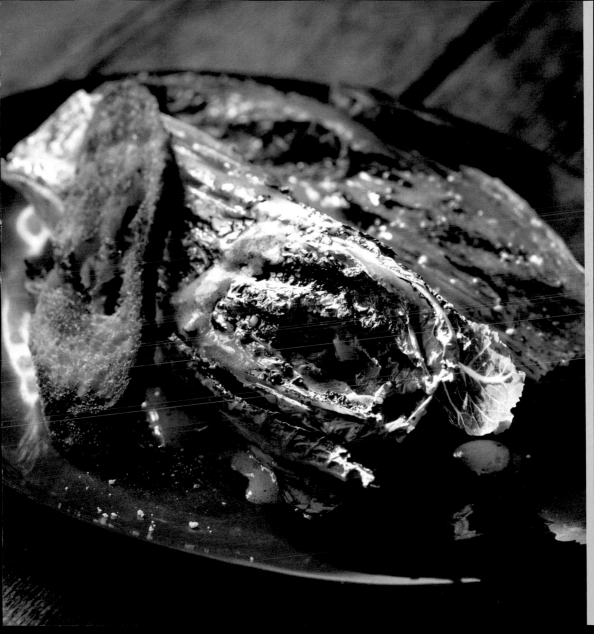

Grilled Peach Salad

No fruit can take the heat quite like a peach can. The sear of the flame does something magical to stone fruit, concentrating its sweetness and acidity, transforming its flesh into something creamy and luxurious. A perfect summer peach hot off the grill is a special enough on its own, but when paired with crunchy almonds, salty prosciutto, and tangy crumbles of goat cheese, it makes for one of the greatest salads you can eat.

You'll Need:

1 shallot, minced

2 Tbsp balsamic vinegar

½ Tbsp chopped fresh rosemary leaves (optional)

½ Tbsp honey

3 Tbsp olive oil

Salt and black pepper to taste

2 peaches, halved and pitted

16 cups mixed baby greens

4 slices prosciutto, torn into strips

½ cup fresh goat cheese

¼ cup chopped almonds

How to Make It:

● Preheat a grill or grill pan over medium heat.

● In a mixing bowl, combine the shallot, balsamic, rosemary (if using), and honey. Let the shallot soften in the vinegar for at least 5 minutes. Slowly drizzle in the olive oil, whisking to incorporate. Season with salt and pepper and reserve.

● When the grill is hot, place the peaches directly on the grate, cut side down. Grill, rotating the fruit 45 degrees midway through, for 4 to 5 minutes, until the flesh is nicely caramelized. Flip the peaches and grill on the rounded sides for a few minutes, just until the bottoms begin to soften.

● Slice the peaches into ¼" pieces. Combine with the greens, prosciutto, goat cheese, and almonds in a large mixing bowl. Whisk the vinaigrette one last time, then add a few tablespoons at a time to the salad, tossing, until the ingredients are lightly coated.

Makes 4 servings

Per Serving:
$2.37

310 calories
21 g fat (6 g saturated)
530 mg sodium

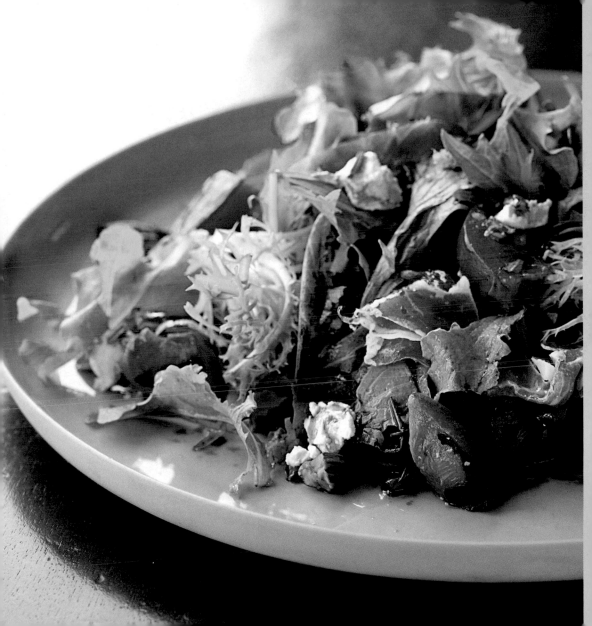

Grilled Salmon Salad

For most people, the idea of a salad starts and stops with lettuce. But why confine yourself to leaves? Salads can be made from any combination of meat, fish, and vegetables bound together with dressing. This muscular salad brings together a full dinner's worth of protein and vegetables, playing tastes and textures off each other for the greater good of your taste buds.

You'll Need:

- 1 shallot, thinly sliced
- 2 Tbsp red wine vinegar
- 1 lb salmon fillet (preferably in a single piece)
- ½ lb green beans, tips removed
- ¼ cup olive oil, plus more for coating the fish and beans
- Salt and black pepper to taste
- ½ Tbsp Dijon mustard
- 20 cherry tomatoes, halved
- 2 Tbsp capers, rinsed

How to Make It:

- Preheat a grill over medium heat. Combine the shallot and red wine vinegar in a bowl and set aside.

- Coat the salmon and the green beans with olive oil and season with salt and pepper. Place the salmon on the grill, skin side down. Grill for 5 to 6 minutes, until the skin firms up and pulls away from the grill. Flip and continue grilling for 2 to 3 minutes longer, until the thickest part of the fish flakes with gentle pressure from your finger. While the salmon grills, cook the green beans in a grill basket or directly on the grill grate, turning, for 7 to 8 minutes, until soft.

- Stir the mustard into the reserved vinegar mixture. Slowly whisk in the ¼ cup olive oil. Break the salmon into large flakes. In a bowl, combine the salmon with the green beans, tomatoes, and capers. Pour the vinaigrette over the top, season with salt and pepper, and toss to thoroughly combine.

Makes 4 servings

Per Serving:
$3.53

310 calories
21 g fat (3 g saturated)
400 mg sodium

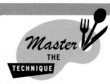

Master THE
TECHNIQUE

Protein-based salads

This style of salad works especially well with left-over meat or fish, such as an extra rotisserie chicken from the market, leftover Thanksgiving turkey, or a neglected tuna steak from last night's dinner.

ı Shredded chicken or turkey, mandarin slices, almonds, and broccoli florets

ı Sliced pork tenderloin, peaches, green beans, pecans, and crumbled blue cheese

ı Grilled tuna, roasted red peppers, olives, sundried tomatoes, and pine nuts

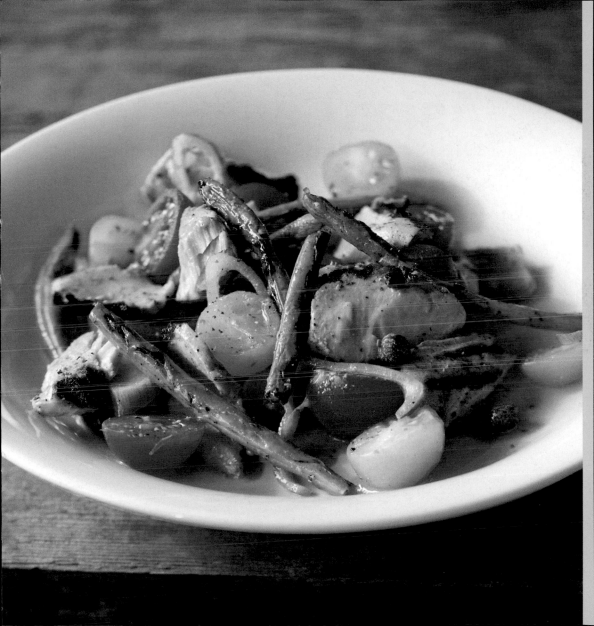

Asian Beef Salad
with Sriracha-Honey Dressing

Restaurant salads suffer from a double dose of shamefulness: They are not only boring and sloppily executed, they also come with more calories and fat than your average bacon cheeseburger. A frightening example: You'd be better off eating three full orders of Applebee's Asiago Peppercorn Steak than tussling with the tame-sounding Oriental Grilled Chicken Salad. Disgraceful. Here, we harbor the big flavors of the East—sweet, spicy, tart, cool—but leave all the excessive calories out of the equation. A generous portion of lean flank steak and creamy cubes of avocado make sure this salad truly satisfies.

You'll Need:

1 lb flank steak

Salt and ground black pepper to taste

1 tsp sriracha or other hot sauce

2 tsp honey

½ Tbsp low-sodium soy sauce

Juice of 1 lime

¼ cup canola oil

1 bag watercress (if your market doesn't stock watercress, a head of Bibb lettuce will work fine)

1 pint cherry tomatoes, sliced in half

1 small red onion, thinly sliced

½ English cucumber, thinly sliced

1 avocado, peeled, pitted, and chopped

Handful of fresh cilantro leaves

How to Make It:

- Preheat a grill or grill pan over medium-high heat. Season the flank steak all over with salt and pepper and cook until medium rare, about 3 to 4 minutes per side. Allow the steak to rest for at least 5 minutes before slicing thinly across the natural grain of the meat.

- While the meat rests, combine the sriracha, honey, soy sauce, and lime juice with a pinch of pepper in a mixing bowl. Slowly drizzle in the oil, whisking to combine.

- In a large salad bowl, combine the watercress, tomatoes, onion, cucumber, avocado, cilantro, and sliced steak and slowly drizzle in the dressing, tossing the ingredients gently with each addition, until everything is lightly coated.

Makes 4 servings

Per Serving:
$4.39

430 calories
31 g fat (6 g saturated)
475 mg sodium

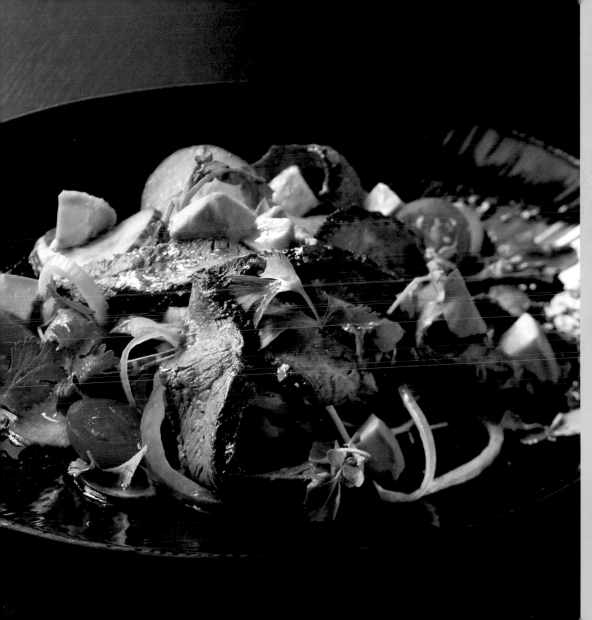

Eat This!

Panzanella

This salad, a staple throughout Tuscany, is a powerful example of the importance of eating foods in their proper season. Make this bread-and-tomato salad in the winter and it might fail to win you over. But try it in August, when tomatoes are juicy and peppers and cucumbers crisp and sweet, and it's a revelation. Serve it next to a hunk of juicy grilled chicken and it will become one of your backyard standbys.

You'll Need:

- 1 loaf ciabatta or country bread, sliced into ½"-thick pieces
- 2 cloves garlic, halved
- 2 large tomatoes (preferably heirloom), chopped
- 1 medium cucumber, seeded and sliced
- 1 large red or yellow bell pepper, stemmed, seeded, and chopped
- ½ medium red onion, thinly sliced
- 15–20 fresh basil leaves, roughly chopped
- 3 Tbsp olive oil, plus more for drizzling
- 2 Tbsp red wine vinegar

Salt and black pepper to taste

How to Make It:

- Preheat a grill or grill pan over high heat. Lightly drizzle the bread with olive oil and grill for about 3 minutes per side, until nicely browned and crisp. Rub both sides of the bread lightly with a garlic clove half, then cut the bread into cubes.

- Toss the toasted bread with the tomatoes, cucumbers, bell peppers, onion, and basil in a large bowl. Drizzle in the olive oil and vinegar. Season with salt and pepper.

Makes 4 servings

MEAL MULTIPLIER

Panzanella may traditionally be a summertime salad, but the idea of tossing grilled bread with vegetables can be carried through all four seasons. Simply replace the tomato, cucumber, and peppers with any of the following combinations and proceed with the recipe.

ı Fall: Brussels sprouts and butternut squash
ı Winter: Carrots and cauliflower
ı Spring: Asparagus, radish, and cubes of avocado

Per Serving:
$2.86

260 calories
11 g fat (2 g saturated)
500 mg sodium

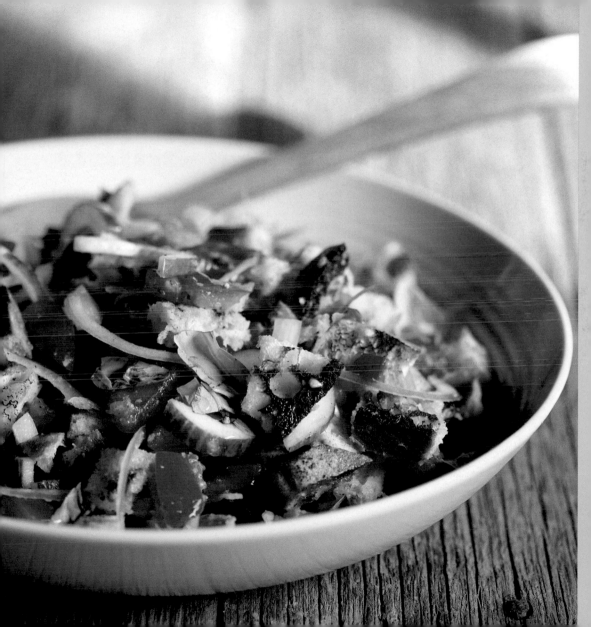

Grilled Halloumi & Strawberry Salad

Halloumi, a firm sheep and goat's milk cheese with a lightly salty bite, is popular in the kitchens of the Middle East. More than anything, halloumi is known for its ability to stand up to high heat without melting, making it a killer weapon in the grill master's arsenal. It works best when paired with something sweet, like these strawberries, which helps cut through the richness of the cheese.

You'll Need:

- 2 cups sliced strawberries
- 3 Tbsp balsamic vinegar
- 1 medium shallot, thinly sliced

Freshly cracked black pepper

- ½ lb halloumi, cut into 4 rectangles
- 3 Tbsp olive oil, plus more for coating the cheese
- 16 cups baby spinach, arugula, or mixed baby greens
- ¼ cup smoked almonds

How to Make It:

- Preheat a grill or grill pan over medium-high heat. Combine the strawberries, vinegar, shallot, and pepper in a large mixing bowl. Let the shallots and strawberries macerate in the vinegar for at least 10 minutes.

- Coat the cheese with a light film of olive oil. Grill for 2 minutes, until grill marks have developed, then rotate 45 degrees and grill for another 2 minutes. Flip the cheese and repeat the process until the cheese is lightly charred and warm throughout.

- Drizzle the 3 tablespoons of olive oil into the bowl with the strawberries. Add the spinach and almonds and toss. Divide the salad among 4 plates and top each with a piece of grilled cheese.

Makes 4 servings

Per Serving:
$2.94

420 calories
28 g fat (9 g saturated)
970 mg sodium

SECRET WEAPON

Halloumi

For those looking to cut carbohydrates from their diet, halloumi serves as a protein-packed replacement for quick-burning starches. Try it in place of grilled bread for any of the crostini recipes in Chapter 8, as a stand-in for croutons in salads, or even as a pancake surrogate in the morning: Sauté in a pan until crispy, then top with fresh fruit and a light drizzle of maple syrup. Find halloumi at Middle Eastern grocers, Whole Foods Markets, or online at Igourmet.com.

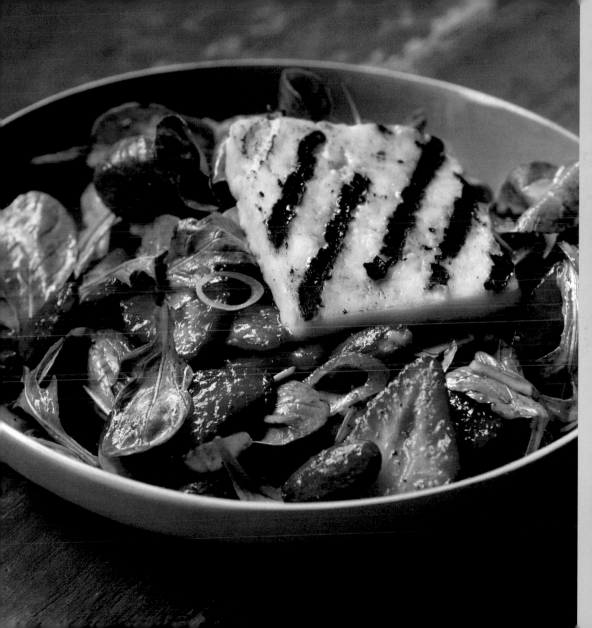

Blackened Chicken & Mango Salad

Calorie for calorie, there is not a more nutrient-dense recipe in this book. This salad has it all: fiber, healthy fat, lean protein. Oh, and it's delicious!

You'll Need:

- 1 lb boneless, skinless chicken breasts
- 1 Tbsp chili powder
- Salt and black pepper to taste
- 1 ear corn, shucked and blanched in boiling water for 5 minutes
- 1 Tbsp honey
- ½ Tbsp chipotle pepper puree
- Juice of 1 lime
- 1 clove garlic, minced
- 3 Tbsp canola oil, plus more for coating the chicken
- 1 head Bibb lettuce
- 1 mango, peeled, pitted, and chopped
- 1 avocado, peeled, pitted, and chopped
- 1 cup black beans
- 1 small red onion, thinly sliced

How to Make It:

- Preheat a grill or grill pan over high heat. Coat the chicken breasts with canola oil then season with the chili powder and salt and pepper.

- Grill the chicken for about 5 minutes per side, until nicely charred, firm to the touch, and cooked through. At the same time, grill the ear of corn, turning, for 8 to 10 minutes, until the kernels are nicely browned. Let the chicken rest for 5 minutes before slicing into thin strips. Use a knife to separate the toasted corn kernels from the cob.

- Combine the honey, chipotle, lime juice, and garlic in a bowl. Slowly add the oil, whisking constantly to incorporate. Season with a few pinches of salt and pepper.

- In a large mixing bowl, combine the chicken, corn, lettuce, mango, avocado, black beans, and onion. Slowly add the dressing a tablespoon at a time, tossing, until it lightly coats all ingredients.

Makes 4 servings

Per Serving:	440 calories
$3.69	22 g fat (2.5 g saturated)
	490 mg sodium

SAVE-MONEY STRATEGY

Chicken breasts are excellent sources of lean protein and take well to the grill, but they typically cost up to twice as much as less-popular chicken thighs. Considering that a 4-ounce serving of thigh has just 6 calories more than the breast and is usually a good deal juicier, it's a perfect substitute for those looking to save a few dollars on dinner.

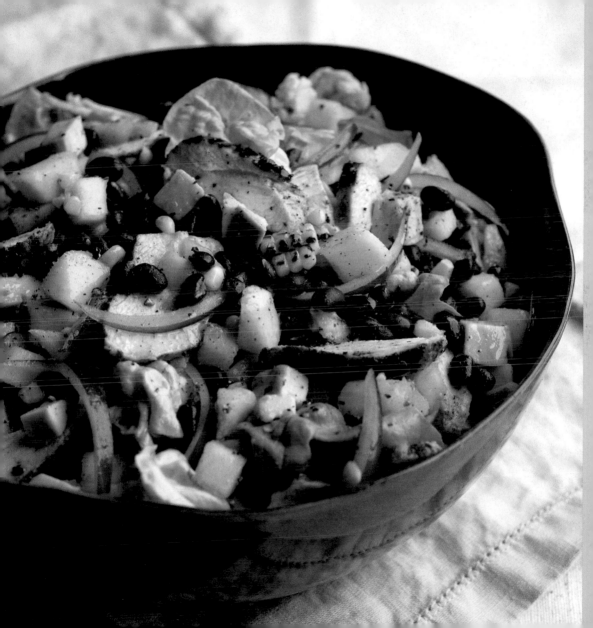

Grilled Calamari Salad

Squid is one of the most abundant forms of seafood in the global market, yet few Americans have ever enjoyed it in any other way than deep-fried. This recipe is proof positive that the grill produces better calamari than the fryer.

You'll Need:

- 1 lb squid, cleaned, tentacles reserved for another use
- ½ Tbsp peanut or canola oil

Salt and black pepper to taste

Juice of 1 lime

- 1 Tbsp fish sauce
- 1 Tbsp sugar
- ½ Tbsp chili garlic sauce (preferably sambal oelek)
- 4 cups watercress

Watercress isn't always easy to find. Baby arugula, or even a few big handfuls of fresh basil leaves, can easily take its place here.

- 1 small cucumber, peeled, seeded, and cut into matchsticks
- 1 medium tomato, chopped
- ½ red onion, very thinly sliced
- ¼ cup roasted peanuts

How to Make It:

- Preheat a grill over high heat. Toss the squid bodies with the oil and generously season with salt and lots of black pepper. When the grill is very hot, add the squid and grill for about 5 minutes, until lightly charred all over.

- Combine the lime juice, fish sauce, sugar, and chili sauce in a mixing bowl and whisk to blend. Slice the grilled squid into ½" rings. In a salad bowl, toss the squid, watercress, cucumber, tomato, onion, and peanuts with the dressing. Divide the salad among 4 plates.

Makes 4 servings

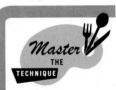

Master **THE** `TECHNIQUE`

Cooking calamari

Grilling squid ranks right up there next to tying your shoes and making your bed in the difficulty category, yet most people are terrified of the prospect. Purchase whole squid bodies (available fully cleaned, fresh or frozen, at any decent fish market or quality grocery store) and either grill them whole over high heat for no more than 5 minutes, or cut them into rings and sauté in olive oil for the same amount of time. When the calamari turns taught and firm, it's done.

Per Serving: **$3.04**

220 calories
8 g fat (1.5 g saturated)
590 mg sodium

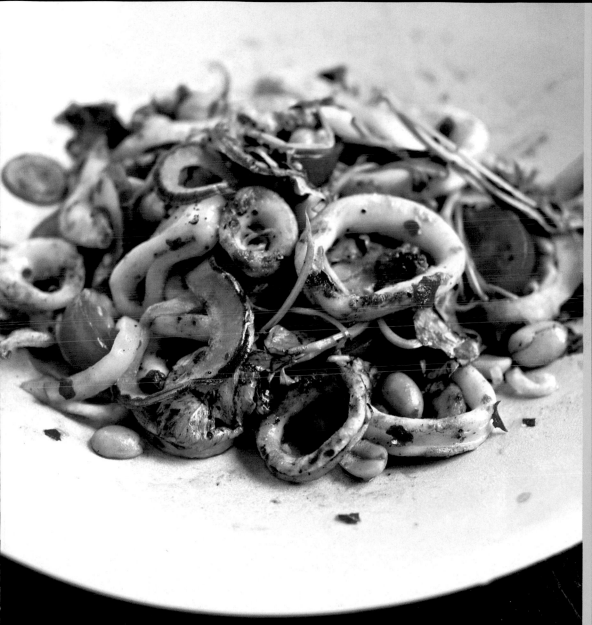

Tuna Niçoise

Tuna salad is a food industry euphemism for fish awash in a sea of mayo. But this French-inspired tuna salad is the real deal. Tucked within the leaves are vitamin-dense green beans, lycopene-loaded cherry tomatoes, and omega-3-packed tuna, providing a perfect balance of protein, fiber, and healthy fat.

You'll Need:

4 eggs

Salt and black pepper to taste

1 lb red potatoes, quartered into ½" chunks

½ lb green beans, ends removed

2 tuna steaks (6 oz each)

16 cups baby mixed greens (8-oz bag)

¼ cup Honey-Dijon Vinaigrette (page 49)

1 pint cherry tomatoes, sliced in half

¼ cup chopped black or green olives (kalamata and Niçoise are best)

How to Make It:

● Bring a large pot of water to a gentle simmer. Carefully lower in the eggs. Cook for 8 minutes (this should yield creamy, not chalky, yolks) and remove with a slotted spoon. Transfer to a bowl of cold water.

● Salt the same pot of water and add the potatoes. Cook for 15 to 20 minutes, until tender but not mushy. Right before the potatoes are done, toss in the green beans and cook for 3 to 5 minutes, until crisp-tender. (You can cook the green beans in their own pot, but why waste the water and the energy?)Drain both vegetables together.

● Heat a grill or grill pan over high heat. Season the tuna with salt and pepper. When the grill is very hot, cook the tuna for 2 minutes per side, until browned on the outside but still pink in the middle. Remove, rest for a few minutes, then slice into thin strips.

● Peel the eggs and slice in half. Toss the greens with enough vinaigrette to just lightly cover. Divide among 4 chilled plates or bowls. In individual piles around the lettuce, arrange the potatoes, tomatoes, olives, green beans, and eggs. Top with slices of tuna and drizzle with extra vinaigrette, if you like.

Makes 4 servings

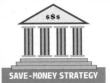

SAVE-MONEY STRATEGY

Fresh tuna is an amazing product that takes well to quick pan-searing and high-heat grilling. Trouble is, it can set you back up to $20 a pound. If you're looking to cut the cost of this dinner by about 60 percent (and speed things up a bit), ditch the fresh fish and reach for a high-quality can of tuna instead (our favorite brand is Ortiz from Spain). If you'd like to cut costs but still want to fire up the grill, use chicken breasts, thighs, or pork tenderloin in place of the tuna.

Per Serving:	350 calories
$5.17	11 g fat (3 g saturated)
	370 mg sodium

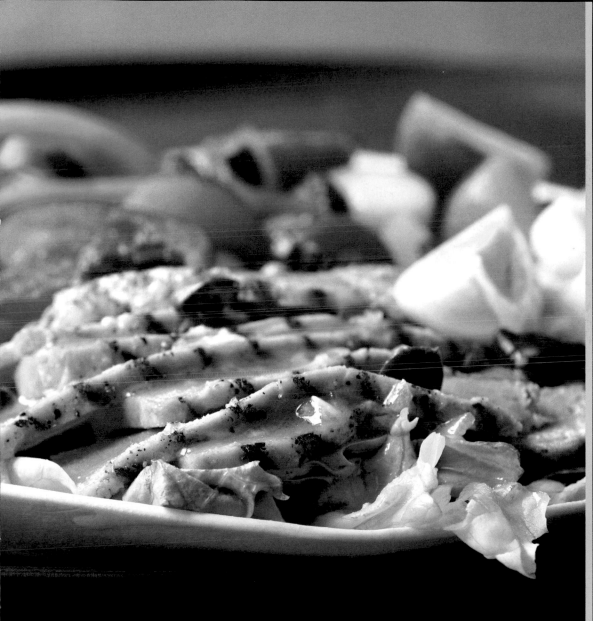

Watermelon-Tomato Salad

Nothing to grill here at all. In fact, this recipe is only marginally more challenging than pouring yourself a bowl of cereal. But the results speak for themselves: sweet, refreshing watermelon made all the better when paired with the acidity of tomato, the saltiness of feta, and the bite of basil. A lovely summer salad meant to go with anything you pull off the grill.

You'll Need:

8 cups cubed watermelon

2 lbs tomatoes, chopped into ½" chunks

½ cup feta cheese

1 cup chopped fresh basil

3 Tbsp olive oil

2 Tbsp balsamic vinegar

Salt and black pepper to taste

How to Make It:

- In a large mixing bowl, combine the watermelon, tomatoes, feta, and basil. Drizzle in just enough olive oil and balsamic to lightly coat the ingredients and season with salt and pepper.

Makes 6 servings

This salad tastes—and looks—best with a mixture of heirloom tomatoes: red, yellow, green.

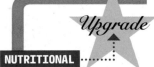

Upgrade

NUTRITIONAL

Watermelon might taste like dessert, but it's no nutritional slouch. Beyond containing a healthy dose of vitamins A and C, watermelon is also one of the produce world's greatest sources of lycopene. This potent antioxidant, found commonly in red foods like tomatoes and strawberries, has been found to provide a strong defense against a variety of cancers, including breast, prostate, lung, and others.

Per Serving:
$2.60

180 calories
10 g fat (3 g saturated)
375 mg sodium

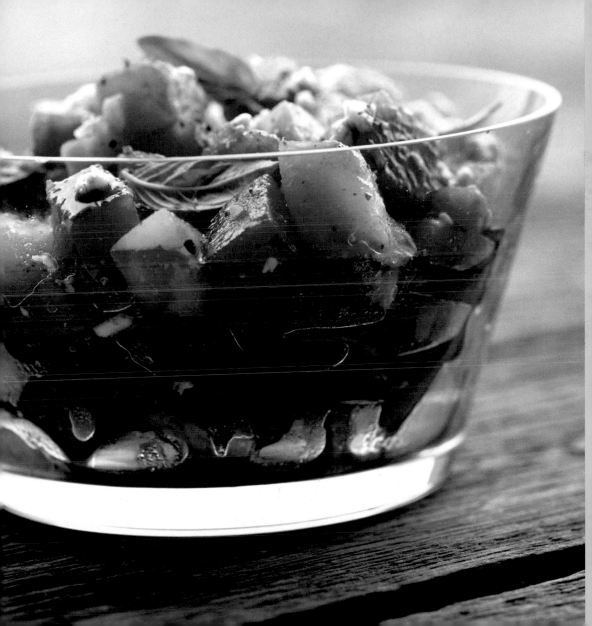

VEGETABLES

How to GRILL any Vegetable

To maximize flavor and texture, every vegetable demands its own specific treatment. Here's your grilling game plan for getting the most out of everything veggie, from asparagus to zucchini.

Asparagus

HEAT: High
TIME: 10 minutes

Trim the bottom inch off the spears and toss in a good amount of olive oil, salt, and black pepper. To prevent asparagus from rolling and slipping through the cracks, line up groups of 6 to 8 spears and run skewers through the top and bottom ends. Grill over high heat, turning once, for 3 to 4 minutes per side, until lightly browned and just tender all the way through. Asparagus turns from tender to mushy very quickly, so watch them carefully.

Broccoli/ Cauliflower

HEAT: Low
TIME: 10 to 15 minutes

If you like your broccoli or cauliflower al dente, then simply break the heads into smaller florets, rub them with oil, skewer them, and grill over low heat for 15 minutes. But if you want the florets tender from head to stem, you'll need to blanch them first. Bring a pot of water to a boil, drop in large pieces of either (or both), and boil for 3 minutes. Drain and

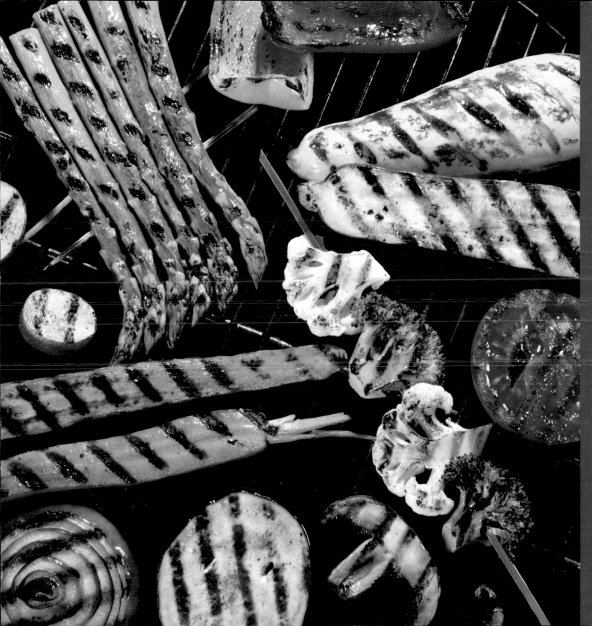

rinse with cold water for 30 seconds. Grill over low heat on skewers, in a grilling basket, or directly on the grate until lightly charred and tender, about 10 minutes. Cauliflower is incredible rubbed in curry powder, while broccoli just needs olive oil before, grated Parmesan and lemon juice after.

Carrots

HEAT: Low
TIME: 20 minutes
Wash and peel the carrots; if the carrots are thick, halve them lengthwise. Toss with olive oil, salt, and pepper (cumin and coriander are also excellent carrot spices). Place directly on the grate and grill over low heat for about 20 minutes. Grilled carrots take well to sauces: Try Barbecued Carrots (page 334), or brush on bottled teriyaki or hoisin at the end of grilling. Save brushing with sauce for the last 10 minutes of cooking,

otherwise a sugary sauce will burn before the carrots are tender.

Eggplant

HEAT: High
TIME: 8 to 10 minutes for slices, 15 minutes for whole eggplant
Whether using smaller Japanese eggplant or darker, larger Italian eggplant, slice the vegetable into ½"-thick rounds, coat with a light film of oil, and season with salt and pepper. Grill over high heat for 4 to 5 minutes per side, until lightly charred and softened. For dips and purees, grill eggplant whole for about 15 minutes, until the skin is charred and the flesh is very soft.

Mushrooms

HEAT: Medium-high
TIME: 8 to 12 minutes
While mushrooms have a high water content, they can dry out if grilled too long, so it's best to grill

them over a medium-high flame until lightly charred and just cooked through, about 8 minutes for shiitake caps, 12 minutes for whole portobellos. If you want to grill smaller button or cremini mushrooms, run a skewer lengthwise through the caps. Or make individual mushroom packets by seasoning ½" chunks of mushrooms with olive oil, chopped garlic, salt, and pepper and enclosing in foil packets, then grilling for 10 minutes.

Onions

HEAT: Medium
TIME: 6 to 10 minutes
Onion rings can go directly on the grill, but you're bound to lose at least a quarter of your product to the fire. Instead, peel the onions and slice into ¼"-thick pieces. Skewer with toothpicks to secure the slices and grill over medium heat for 3 to

4 minutes per side, until soft and browned. If you want a deeply caramelized onion, turn the heat down and grill the onions for up to 10 minutes per side.

Peppers

HEAT: Medium
TIME: 10 minutes for quarters, 25 minutes for whole peppers
If you plan on peeling the peppers, it's best to place whole peppers on the grill and close the lid. If you want chunks of grilled peppers for sandwiches or fajitas, cut whole peppers into quarters, removing the stem, seeds, and white, flavorless ribs inside. Grill whole peppers in a covered grill over medium heat, turning once or twice, for about 25 minutes, until the skin is black and blistered (peel off the skin before eating). Grill pepper quarters or pieces, turning, for about 5 minutes per side.

Potatoes

HEAT: Medium
TIME: 15 minutes for wedges or slices, 30 to 40 minutes for whole potatoes
Grilled potatoes are best when parboiled, then finished on the grate. Cook them in a large pot of boiling water until just tender, about 10 minutes, then drain. Cut into slices or wedges and rub with oil, salt, and pepper. Grill over medium heat, turning, for about 15 minutes, until brown and crispy all over. For an incredible "baked" grilled potato, prick whole russet potatoes with a fork, wrap in foil, and place directly in the hot embers of a charcoal fire (or on the grate of a gas grill). Grill, rotating them 45 degrees every 10 minutes or so, for 40 minutes, until very tender.

Tomatoes

HEAT: High
TIME: 5 to 10 minutes
The sweet and smoky intensity of a grilled tomato plays great as a side dish to meat, just as it forms a powerful base for sauces, soups, and salsas. Halve the tomatoes, rub with oil, and place cut side down on the grate. Grill over high heat for 5 minutes, until caramelized. Serve as is, or, if building a sauce or salsa, flip the tomatoes and continue grilling for another 5 minutes, until the skins blister. Peel off the skins and pulverize.

Zucchini

HEAT: High
TIME: 6 to 8 minutes
You'll lose tiny rounds through the grates, so it's best to slice zucchini lengthwise into ¼" thick planks. Lay them at a 45-degree angle across the grate to maximize caramelization. Grill over high heat, turning, for 6 to 8 minutes. The same rules apply for summer squash.

Spicy Steak Fries

The number one most consumed vegetable in America is the french fry, a woeful reality for a populace already starved for something green in its diet. But the potatoes themselves (a vegetable rife with powerful antioxidants) aren't to blame; it's the cauldron of bubbling fat. We should call this recipe Freedom Fries, since these spicy, crispy grilled potatoes liberate you from the nutritional tyranny of the oil-soaked spud. Serve these next to a juicy steak and a glass of red wine for an all-world dinner.

You'll Need:

2 large russet potatoes, thoroughly washed

Salt to taste

1 Tbsp canola oil

1 tsp smoked paprika

1 tsp chili powder

½ tsp garlic powder

⅛ tsp cayenne pepper

¾ tsp salt

½ tsp black pepper

How to Make It:

- Place the potatoes in a pot, cover with water, and season with salt. Cook over high heat for 12 to 15 minutes, until tender but still firm. Drain.

- Preheat a grill over medium heat. When the potatoes are cool enough to handle, cut each lengthwise into 8 wedges. Toss with the oil and all the spices. Place the potato wedges on the grill and cook, turning once, for about 12 minutes, until brown and crispy.

SAUCE selector

What's a fry without something to dunk it in? Here are five quick DIY sauces you can serve alongside these grilled spuds:

- Ketchup spiked with curry powder, smoked paprika, or chipotle peppers
- Olive oil mayonnaise cut with lemon, minced garlic, and chopped fresh parsley
- Greek yogurt mixed with sriracha hot sauce, garlic, and lime juice
- Peanut Sauce (page 48)
- Chimichurri (page 47)

Per Serving:
$0.53

180 calories
4 g fat (0.5 g saturated)
450 mg sodium

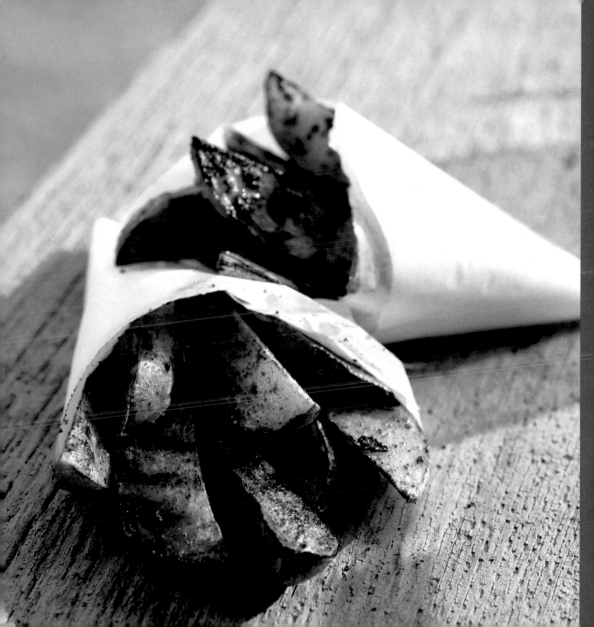

Grilled Corn
with Miso Butter

One of the great pleasures of summer is eating candy-sweet fresh corn any way you can get it. That pleasure is intensified threefold by the transformative powers of the grill, which teases out every last milligram of natural sugars locked inside those kernels. Remember: Just like meat or fish, corn can be overcooked, turning from sweet and juicy to dry and chewy in a flash. Allowing the corn to steam inside the husks first helps cut the risk substantially.

You'll Need:

- 4 ears corn
- ¼ cup (½ stick) butter, softened at room temperature
- ¼ cup white (shiro) miso

How to Make It:

- Peel the corn husks back, being careful so they remain attached to the base of the cobs, and remove the silk inside. Re-cover the ears with the husks and soak in cold water for 5 minutes.

- Mix together the butter and miso until they form a uniform spread. Set aside.

- Preheat a grill or grill pan over medium heat. Grill the corn for 10 minutes, turning a quarter-turn every few minutes. Peel back the husks and place the corn back on the grill. Cook, turning occasionally, for about 5 minutes, until the kernels are nicely browned. Slather each cob with the miso butter.

Makes 4 servings

$$(\Psi + \mathsf{I})^2$$

MEAL MULTIPLIER

Other delicious ways to anoint a cob of grilled corn:

- Drizzle with Chimichurri (page 47).
- Brush with mayonnaise thinned with lime juice, then top with chili powder and grated Parmesan.
- Brush with softened butter mixed with chopped cilantro, garlic, and minced jalapeño.

Per Serving:
$0.78

190 calories
11 g fat (5 g saturated)
340 mg sodium

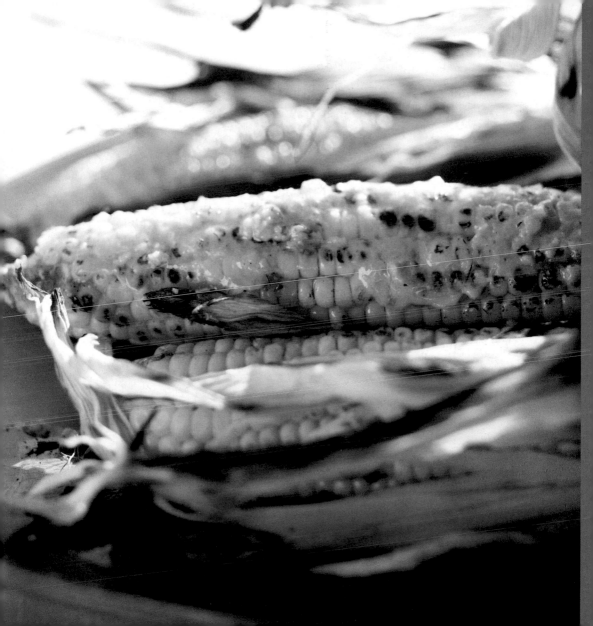

Grilled Asparagus
with Romesco

Grilled asparagus with a drizzle of olive oil, a shake of salt, and a squeeze of lemon represents one of the simplest and most delicious expressions of a vegetable's potential, especially when done in the early months of spring when asparagus is sweet and tender. But we thought we'd take it one small step further, adding to the mix the Spanish sauce called romesco. Made from roasted peppers and toasted almonds, it brings a sweet and smoky dimension to asparagus—and, for that matter, anything savory you pull from the grill. One dip and you'll be slayed.

You'll Need:

1 **bunch asparagus,** woody ends removed

2 **Tbsp olive oil**

Salt and black pepper to taste

Romesco (page 50)

How to Make It:

● Preheat a grill or grill pan over medium heat. Toss the asparagus with the olive oil and salt and pepper. Grill, turning once midway through, for about 8 minutes, until lightly charred and just tender (but not mushy!). If you're serving this as an appetizer, place the asparagus on a large platter with the romesco in the center for dipping. If intended as a side with dinner, divide the asparagus among 4 plates and pass the romesco at the table.

Makes 4 servings

Per Serving:
$1.49

180 calories
11 g fat (1.5 g saturated)
380 mg sodium

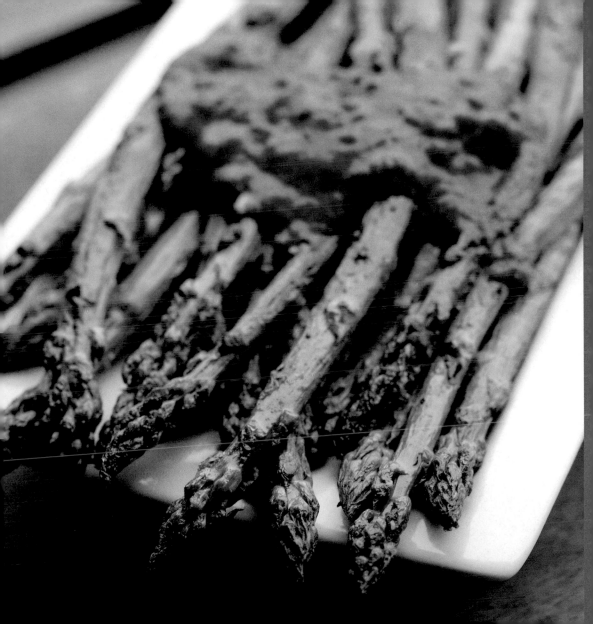

Blackened Cauliflower Steaks
with Worcestershire Aioli

We're unabashed fanatics of blackened food, since the quick and easy blackening technique brings huge flavors to meat and fish without tacking on calories (in fact, if anything, the antioxidant-rich spices boost the overall nutritional value of blackened food). But why limit the fun to fish and fowl? Hearty vegetables like portobello caps, zucchini planks, and, above all, cauliflower, are perfect for the blackening treatment.

You'll Need:

2 Tbsp olive oil mayonnaise

Juice of ½ lemon

2 tsp Worcestershire sauce

1 clove garlic, minced

1 head cauliflower

½ Tbsp canola oil

1 Tbsp Magic Blackening Rub (page 51, or store-bought blackening seasoning)

How to Make It:

- Preheat a grill or grill pan over medium heat. For the aioli, combine the mayonnaise, lemon juice, Worcestershire, and garlic and reserve.

- Cut away the green branches from the cauliflower, but leave the stem fully intact (it will help hold the steaks together). Remove the last inch from each side of the cauliflower head so that you're working with only the most substantial part (save those florets for another use). Cut the cauliflower into four ½"-thick steaks. Drizzle the steaks lightly with the oil, and cover both sides of each with the blackening seasoning.

- Grill the steaks for 4 to 5 minutes per side, until the spices blacken and the cauliflower is tender all the way through. Serve with the aioli drizzled on top.

Makes 4 servings

Per Serving:
$0.56

100 calories
5 g fat (0.5 g saturated)
290 mg sodium

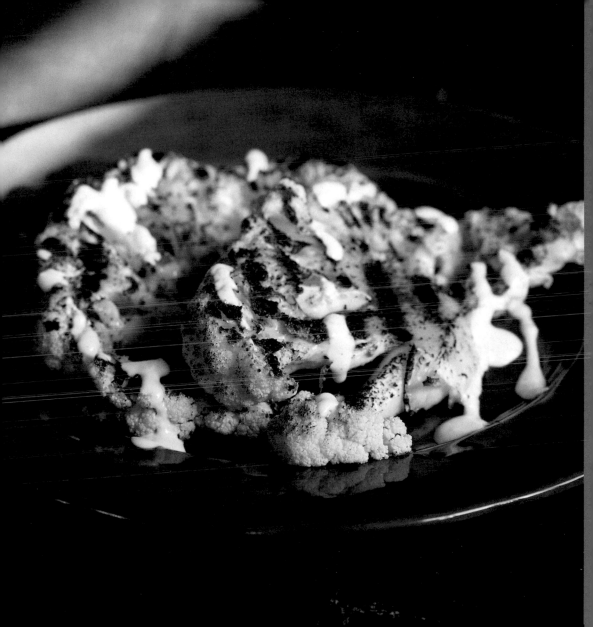

Brussels & Bacon

Brussels sprouts used to be the vegetable that nobody wanted to eat, the one kids and adults alike pushed around on their plates until fate or a hungry animal under the table intervened. But recent years have seen brussels become one of the best-selling vegetables in the restaurant world, an easy way for chefs at trendy restaurants to stretch profit margins. Why the big change? Smart cooks stopped boiling and steaming brussels and started using high-heat cooking techniques to bring out the best in the vegetable. They also discovered pork fat does a lot to make a sprout more sexy. This recipe honors both advancements.

You'll Need:

- 1 lb brussels sprouts, bottoms removed

Olive oil for coating

Salt and black pepper to taste

- 4 strips thick-cut bacon, cut into ¾" pieces
- 4 metal skewers, or wooden skewers soaked in water for 30 minutes
- 1 Tbsp maple syrup

How to Make It:

- Bring a pot of water to a boil. Add the brussels sprouts and cook for about 7 minutes, until barely tender. Drain. Toss with enough olive oil to lightly coat and season with salt and pepper.

- Preheat a grill or grill pan over medium heat. Thread the brussels and bacon onto the skewers, alternating between the two. Grill, turning once, for about 5 minutes per side, until the sprouts have browned and the bacon is cooked through and crispy. Use a spoon to drizzle a very light stream of maple syrup over each skewer before serving.

Makes 4 servings

Per Serving:
$1.18

260 calories
21 g fat (6 g saturated)
340 mg sodium

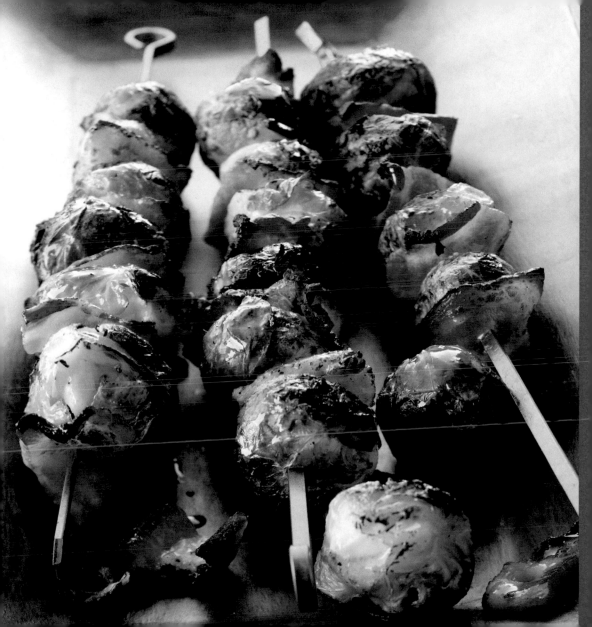

Miso Tofu Bowls

Sometimes the best way to approach cooking tofu and vegetables is to think, "What would a carnivore do?" That's why we cut tofu into thick steaks and marinate it in a powerful miso sauce that doubles as a dressing for the finished product. This is tofu for vegetarians and meateaters alike.

You'll Need:

- ¼ cup white miso
- ¼ cup sugar
- 2 Tbsp soy sauce
- 2 Tbsp rice wine vinegar
- ¼ cup water
- 2 cloves garlic, minced
- 2 Tbsp minced ginger
- 1 block firm tofu (12 oz), sliced into ¼"-thick steaks
- 1 head broccoli, florets broken into 1" pieces
- Oil for coating
- Salt and black pepper to taste
- Metal skewers, or wooden skewers soaked in water for 30 minutes
- 4 cups cooked brown rice
- Toasted sesame seeds for garnish

How to Make It:

- Combine the miso, sugar, soy sauce, vinegar, water, garlic, and ginger in a mixing bowl and whisk until smooth. Place the tofu steaks in a sealable plastic bag and pour the miso marinade over the top. Seal the bag and marinate in the refrigerator for at least 1 hour (or up to 1 day).

- Preheat a grill or grill pan over medium heat. Toss the broccoli with the oil and season with salt and pepper. Thread the broccoli onto the skewers, running the sharp point through each stalk to hold it in place.

- Remove the tofu from the bag, reserving the marinade. Grill the tofu, turning once, for about 10 minutes, until caramelized and lightly crisp on the outside. Cook the broccoli, turning, for about 12 minutes, until the florets are browned and the stalks have softened.

- Divide the rice among 4 bowls. Top with the tofu and broccoli, then drizzle some of the leftover marinade over the top. Garnish with sesame seeds.

Makes 4 servings

Per Serving:	
$1.74	390 calories 7 g fat (1 g saturated) 820 mg sodium

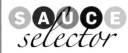

SAUCE selector

Tackling tofu

Grilled tofu, when done properly, can satisfy even the most relentless carnivore. That means cooking it over a medium flame until the outside is crispy and the center warm and creamy. It also means starting with a powerful marinade, which can be brushed on during or after cooking as well. Try one of these other options as an alternative to the miso:

- Equal parts Asian-style chili sauce such as sriracha, lime juice, and honey
- Horseradish Steak Sauce (page 198)
- Rub with Blackening Rub (page 51) and top with Smoky Aioli (page 242)

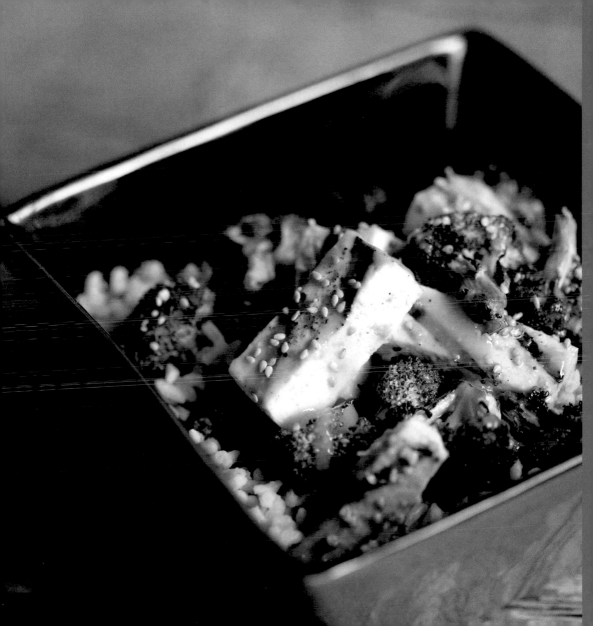

Grilled Portobellos
with Tomato and Mozzarella

Ah, the portobello mushroom, the one vegetable nearly every backyard chef has turned to at least once in his career. It can be a satisfying alternative to a steak, but it nearly always emerges from the grill as an overcooked afterthought, a half-hearted attempt to appease the meatless crowd. With a bit of finesse, though, the portobello's potential is limitless, especially when that finesse involves filling its generous cap with one of the culinary world's greatest triumvirates: tomatoes, basil, and mozzarella.

You'll Need:

- 4 **portobello mushrooms, cleaned, stems removed**
- 1 Tbsp olive oil
- 2 Tbsp balsamic vinegar
- Salt and black pepper to taste
- 2 **medium tomatoes, chopped**
- ¾ cup chopped fresh mozzarella
- 2 Tbsp prepared pesto

How to Make It:

- Preheat a grill over medium-low heat. Use a spoon to lightly scrape away some of the gills on the underside of the mushroom caps (this will create extra space for the filling). Place the mushrooms in a shallow baking dish, drizzle with the olive oil and balsamic vinegar, and season with salt and pepper. Combine the tomatoes, mozzarella, and pesto in a mixing bowl.

- Grill the portobellos, gill side down, for 2 minutes, then flip and fill each cap with the tomato mixture. Close the grill and grill for another 8 to 10 minutes, until the mushrooms are soft and lightly charred and the mozzarella has melted.

Makes 4 servings

$$(\math{Y}+\math{I})^2$$

MEAL MULTIPLIER

Three more fillings to reinvent the stuffed mushroom:

- Toasted fresh bread crumbs mixed with fresh rosemary, garlic, and crumbled goat cheese
- Fresh chicken or turkey sausage sautéed with onions, minced garlic, and a ladle of your favorite bottled tomato sauce
- Grilled shrimp or chicken tossed with olives, capers, roasted red peppers, and feta cheese

Per Serving:	
$1.92	270 calories 17 g fat (7 g saturated) 345 mg sodium

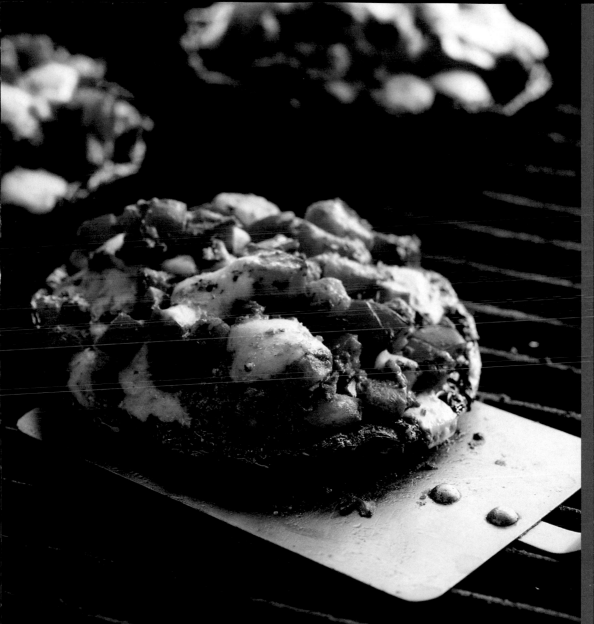

Stuffed Peppers

Oven-baked stuffed peppers have long been a simple, healthy solution to the dinner dilemma. But why use an oven when you can get better results with a grill? With the top closed, the peppers soften and caramelize and absorb those toasty notes of a real fire. No empty carb fillers here, just the pure flavors of sautéed spinach, sundried tomatoes, and chicken sausage.

You'll Need:

- 1 Tbsp olive oil
- ½ medium onion, minced
- 2 cloves garlic, minced
- 2 links uncooked chicken sausage, casings removed
- 1 bag (10 oz) frozen spinach, thawed
- 2 Tbsp chopped oil-packed sundried tomatoes
- ½ cup crumbled feta cheese
- Salt and black pepper to taste
- 4 large red, yellow, or green bell peppers

Dry sundried tomatoes are considerably cheaper, but they need to be reconstituted in warm water for 15 minutes before chopping.

How to Make It:

- Heat the olive oil in a large skillet or sauté pan over medium heat. Add the onion and garlic and cook until soft, about 3 minutes. Add the sausage and continue cooking for about 5 minutes, until the fat has rendered out and the meat is cooked through. Drain any excess fat. Stir in the spinach and sundried tomatoes and cook for another 3 minutes, until the tomatoes are softened and the spinach is wilted. Remove from heat, stir in the feta, and season with salt and pepper.

- Preheat a grill over medium-low heat. Carefully remove the tops of the peppers so the stems are still intact. Remove the seeds from inside. Distribute the stuffing among the peppers, packing them tight so that the stuffing doesn't fall out during cooking. Place the tops of the peppers back on, securing them with toothpicks.

- Place the peppers on the grill, cut side up. Close the grill and cook for about 10 minutes, until the bottoms are lightly charred and softened. Carefully place the peppers on their sides and cook, turning occasionally, for another 10 minutes, until the flesh is tender but the peppers still hold their shape.

Makes 4 servings

Per Serving:
$3.38

240 calories
11 g fat (4.5 g saturated)
620 mg sodium

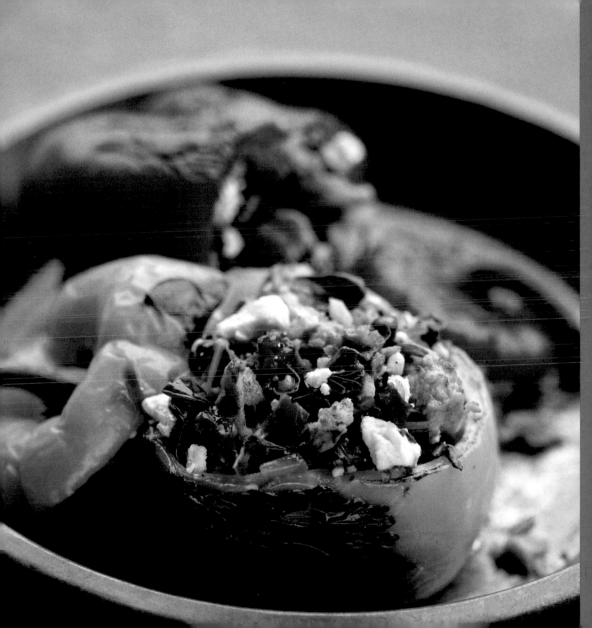

Onion-Stuffed Onions

No vegetable is more vital to everyday cooking than the onion, the base of countless sauces, stocks, roasts, and stir-fries. For all the work the onion puts in as a selfless supporting actor, it rarely takes on a leading role. This recipe is all about the onion, a tribute to its versatility and overall deliciousness. Slow-cooked onions are combined with mushrooms, stock, and cheese, then stuffed into an onion and grilled. It's like eating French onion soup infused with the smoke of the grill and served inside a caramelized-onion bowl.

You'll Need:

- 6 medium red onions
- 1 Tbsp butter
- Salt and black pepper to taste
- ¼ lb button mushrooms, chopped
- ¾ cup red wine
- ¾ cup chicken stock
- 1 cup shredded reduced-fat Swiss cheese
- 1 tsp chopped fresh rosemary
- 4 Tbsp dried bread crumbs

How to Make It:

- Use a paring knife and a spoon to scoop out the centers of 4 of the 6 onions, leaving the base and a few outer layers of onion intact. Dice the scooped-out onions and the remaining 2 onions.

- Heat the butter in a saucepan over medium heat. Add the diced onions and a pinch of salt and cook, stirring occasionally, for 5 minutes, until softened and translucent. Add the mushrooms and continue cooking for another 5 minutes. Stir in the wine and stock and simmer for about 15 minutes, until the liquid has thickened around the onions. Remove the pan from the heat and stir in the cheese, rosemary, and a generous amount of pepper.

- Preheat a grill over medium-low heat. Fill the 4 onion shells with the onion mixture and top with the bread crumbs. Place on the grill, close the lid, and grill for about 20 minutes, until the onion shells are very soft but still hold their shape.

Makes 4 servings

Per Serving:
$1.66

270 calories
11 g fat (7 g saturated)
350 mg sodium

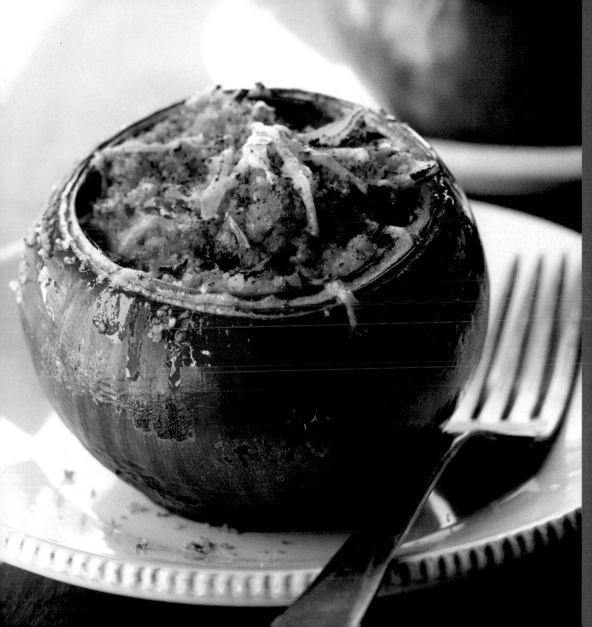

Baby Artichokes
with Mint Vinaigrette

Regular artichokes require more prep work than some cooks at home are willing to do. Baby artichokes, on the other hand, are tender enough that they can basically be cooked as is, with minimal peeling and trimming. That makes them perfect candidates for the grill, where a steady medium flame turns the artichoke hearts soft and sweet and the outer petals beautifully crisp. The dressing here works like a marinade in reverse, suffusing the artichokes with friendly flavors *after* the cooking process.

You'll Need:

- 12 baby artichokes
- 3 Tbsp olive oil, plus more for coating the artichokes
- Salt and black pepper to taste
- Juice of 1 lemon
- ¼ cup chopped fresh mint
- 2 cloves garlic, finely minced
- ¼ tsp red pepper flakes

How to Make It:

- Preheat a grill over medium heat. Split the artichokes in half and peel off the first layer of tough outer layers of leaves. Drizzle with enough olive oil to coat, then season with salt and black pepper. Grill the artichokes, cut side down, for about 10 minutes, until lightly charred and soft. Flip and grill for another 8 to 10 minutes, until tender all the way through.

- Peel off any burnt dark outer leaves. Combine the artichokes with the 3 tablespoons olive oil, lemon juice, mint, garlic, and red pepper in a large mixing bowl. Serve immediately, or allow to sit and marinate for an hour or two before serving.

Makes 4 servings

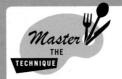

Master
THE
TECHNIQUE

Prepping artichokes

Can't find baby artichokes in your local market? You can follow the recipe with normal artichokes, only you'll need to prep them more carefully. This means trimming the spiky half-inch top of the vegetable, removing a few outside layers of leaves, then splitting them in half and scooping out the purple choke with a spoon. Grill them for 25 to 30 minutes, using low heat to ensure they'll cook all the way through before burning.

Per Serving:
$1.56

170 calories
10 g fat (1.5 g saturated)
320 mg sodium

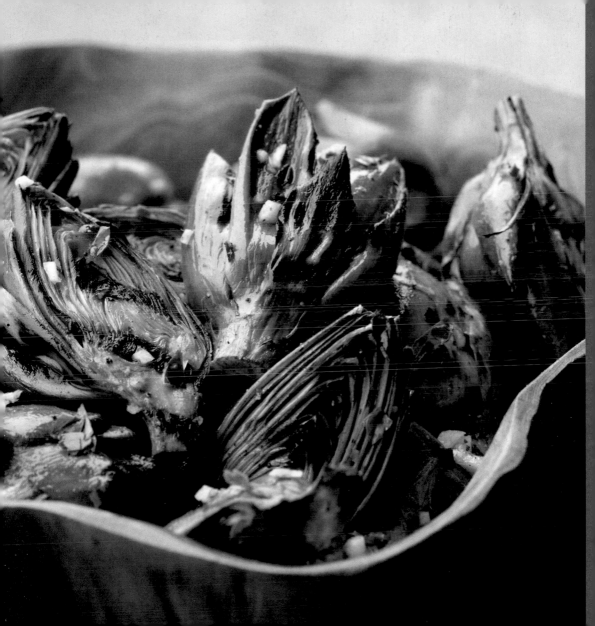

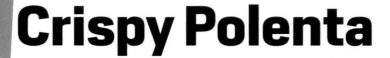

Crispy Polenta

Unless you use a stick of butter to fatten it up, boiled cornmeal can make for a drab side dish. But polenta has a second life as a firm, grilled triangle that can be flavored or topped however you like. Pour soft, cooked polenta into a shallow dish, allow it to firm up, then cut it into triangles. Cooked on the grill until hot and crisp, polenta makes a great side to Grilled Whole Fish (page 220) and Chicken Under a Brick (page 158), but it also works beautifully as a substitute for bread in crostini and bruschetta recipes.

You'll Need:

- 1 cup dried polenta
- 2 Tbsp butter
- ¼ cup grated Parmesan
- 2 tsp chopped fresh rosemary
- Salt and black pepper to taste

How to Make It:

- Prepare the polenta according to package instructions, stirring in the butter, Parmesan, and rosemary at the last moment. Season with salt and pepper.

- Pour the polenta into a shallow 8" x 8" square or 11" x 7" rectangular dish, using a spatula to spread it out evenly, as if making a cake. The polenta should come about ½" up the sides of the dish. Leave on the countertop or in the refrigerator until it cools and hardens, at least 30 minutes. (This step can be done a day or two ahead of time.)

- Preheat a grill or grill pan over medium heat. Remove the polenta from the dish in one piece. Cut into triangles, squares, or whatever shape you prefer. Grill the polenta pieces, turning, for about 5 minutes per side, until crisp and grill marks have developed on both sides.

Makes 6 servings

MEAL MULTIPLIER

Use one of these toppings to punch up the potential of grilled polenta.

- Chopped tomatoes, garlic, basil, and olive oil
- Grilled Japanese eggplant tossed with mint, red pepper flakes, olive oil, and vinegar
- Ricotta cheese and roasted red peppers
- Any of the crostini recipes in Chapter 8

Per Serving: **$0.37** | 150 calories
6 g fat (3 g saturated)
380 mg sodium

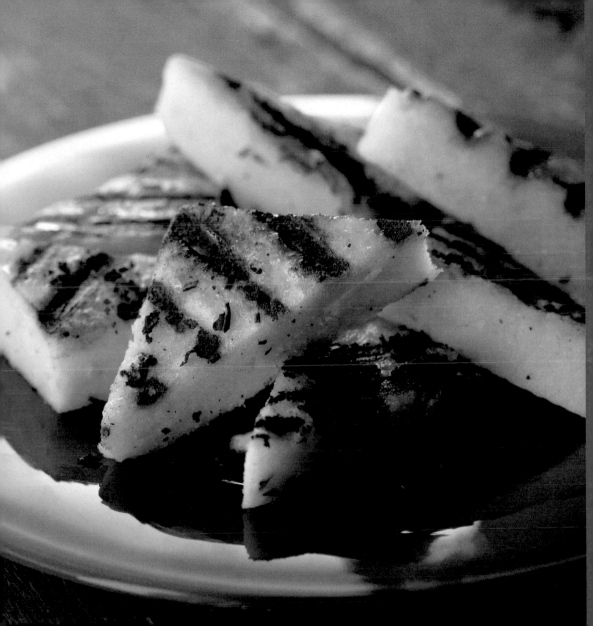

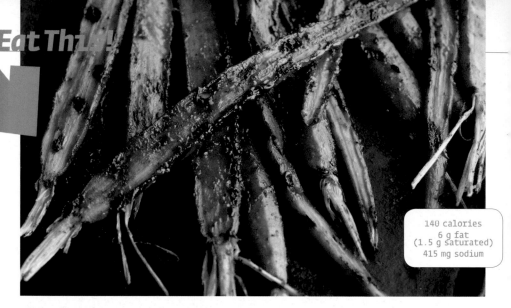

140 calories
6 g fat
(1.5 g saturated)
415 mg sodium

Barbecued Carrots

Sometimes it's best to pretend your vegetables are meat. This recipe treats the orange root vegetable just like a pork shoulder or a chicken drumstick: First, you coat the carrots in a spice rub, then you glaze them with a sweet-spicy barbecue sauce until the centers are soft and the edges crisp and caramelized. Beats boiling, steaming, or sautéing any day. Test out the same treatment on any firm root vegetables: turnips, parsnips, sweet potatoes.

You'll Need:

8   **medium carrots, peeled and cut in half lengthwise**

1   **Tbsp olive oil**

½   **Tbsp All-Purpose Barbecue Rub (page 50)**

½   **cup Classic Barbecue Sauce (page 45)**

How to Make It:

- Preheat a grill over medium heat. Toss the carrots with the olive oil and the rub. When the grill is hot, add the carrots and grill, turning occasionally, for 10 to 15 minutes (depending on the size of your carrots), until the outsides are deeply browned and the flesh is tender throughout. In the final 5 minutes of cooking, use a brush to continuously glaze the carrots with the sauce.

Makes 4 servings

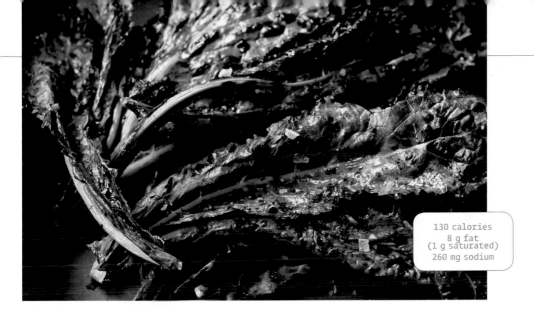

Crack Kale

If you're wondering why it's called Crack Kale, you won't be by the time you finish making this recipe. Cooked slow over a low flame, the water inside the kale evaporates as the stems and leaves turn crispy like potato chips.

You'll Need:

- 1 **bunch kale, bottom 2" of stems removed**
- 2 **Tbsp olive oil**

Coarse sea salt and black pepper to taste

How to Make It:

- Preheat a grill over low heat. Toss the kale with the olive oil, salt, and pepper. Spread out over the grill grate, being sure that the kale doesn't overlap. Cook, turning once midway through, until the kale darkens and turns very crispy, about 15 minutes total. Sprinkle with more sea salt.

Makes 4 servings

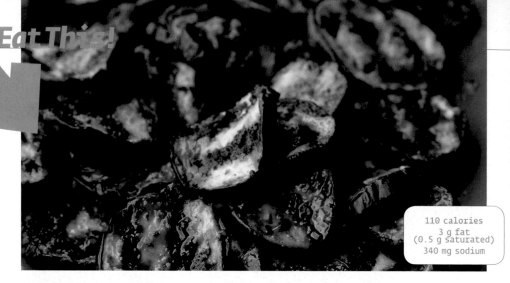

110 calories
3 g fat
(0.5 g saturated)
340 mg sodium

Miso-Glazed Eggplant

Eggplant handled the wrong way can turn into a sponge for salt and oil, but when cooked over high heat on a roaring grill, the flesh turns sweet and smoky without absorbing excess fat or salt. Slender, light purple Japanese eggplant (smaller and less bitter than the dark Italian orbs more commonly available in American supermarkets) can be found in markets like Whole Foods or Asian markets (though regular eggplant will work in a pinch). The sweet-salty miso paste, a traditional sauce used in Japanese kitchens, caramelizes on the surface of the eggplant slices, turning them into little coins of vegetable candy.

You'll Need:

- 2 Tbsp white (shiro) miso
- 1 Tbsp honey
- 1 Tbsp peanut, vegetable, or canola oil
- ½ Tbsp rice wine vinegar
- ½ Tbsp soy sauce
- 2 medium Japanese eggplant, cut into ⅓"-thick slices

How to Make It:

- Preheat a grill or grill pan over medium heat.

- Combine the miso, honey, oil, vinegar, and soy sauce in a small bowl. Lay the eggplant slices on a baking sheet and brush the tops with the miso mixture. Place on the grill, miso side down, and grill for 3 to 4 minutes, until nicely caramelized. Brush the tops with the miso mixture, flip, and cook for another 3 to 4 minutes, until the miso has formed a deep brown crust on the eggplant. Brush one last time with the mixture before serving.

Makes 4 servings

Cole Slaw

130 calories
8 g fat
(1 g saturated)
200 mg sodium

Crunchy, cool, and suffused with vinegar tang, this slaw has nothing to do with those soupy, mayo-drenched, oversweetened versions you find in most supermarket deli cases. Great as a side, but also perfect for topping sandwiches.

You'll Need:

- 2 Tbsp Dijon mustard
- 2 Tbsp mayonnaise
- 2 Tbsp vinegar (red wine, white wine, or cider)
- 2 Tbsp canola oil
- Salt and black pepper to taste
- ½ head green cabbage, very thinly sliced
- ½ head red cabbage, very thinly sliced
- 3 carrots, cut into thin strips
- 1 tsp fennel seeds
- Pickled Jalapeños

How to Make It:

- Mix the mustard, mayonnaise and vinegar in a bowl. Slowly whisk in the oil. Season with salt and pepper.
- Combine the cabbages, carrots, fennel seeds, jalapeños (if using), and dressing in a large bowl. Toss so that everything is evenly coated and season with more salt and pepper.

Makes 6 servings

Grilled Potato Salad

250 calories
12 g fat
(2.5 g saturated)
460 mg sodium

There will always be a time for a mayo-heavy potato salad, calories be damned, but we're firm believers that the standard formula could use some readjustment. As rich as it sounds, the use of an olive oil dressing makes this salad a good deal healthier than the standard.

You'll Need:

- 2 lb medium Yukon gold potatoes
- 2 medium yellow onions, sliced into ¼"-thick rings and skewered with toothpicks
- ¼ cup white or red wine vinegar
- 1 Tbsp Dijon mustard
- ½ Tbsp sugar
- ¼ cup olive oil, plus more for coating the potatoes and onions
- Salt and black pepper to taste
- 4 strips bacon, cooked and crumbled
- ½ cup crumbled blue cheese
- ½ cup chopped fresh parsley

Cut 75 calories per serving by eliminating the bacon and blue cheese. Even without these two, it's still a superlative potato salad.

How to Make It:

- Place the potatoes in a large saucepan of water and season with a few pinches of salt. Bring to a boil over high heat and cook for about 15 minutes, until the potatoes are just tender. Drain and slice into ¼"-thick disks.
- Preheat a grill over medium-high heat. Drizzle the potatoes and the onion slices with enough olive oil to coat. Grill the potatoes for about 5 minutes per side, until the surface is browned and crisp. At the same time, grill the onions for about 4 minutes per side, until lightly caramelized and soft.
- Combine the vinegar, mustard, and sugar. Whisk in the ¼ cup olive oil. Season with salt and pepper. Combine the potatoes, onions, bacon, blue cheese, and parsley in a large mixing bowl. Toss with the dressing.

Makes 6 servings

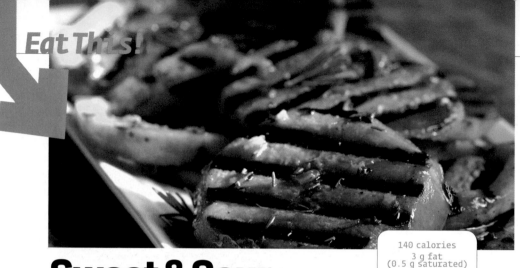

140 calories
3 g fat
(0.5 g saturated)
210 mg sodium

Sweet & Sour Butternut Squash

"Sweet and sour" conjures images of mediocre Chinese takeout, but most food cultures across the world play with the combination in some way or another. This particular version comes from the Italian love of agrodolce: the sweetness from honey, the sour from red wine vinegar, plus a bit of garlic, rosemary, and red pepper to liven it all up. Tossed with hot, caramelized pieces of butternut squash, it creates an incredible side dish.

You'll Need:

¼ cup red wine vinegar

2 Tbsp honey

2 cloves garlic, minced

1 tsp chopped fresh rosemary

Pinch red pepper flakes

1 medium butternut squash, peeled and cut into ⅓"-thick slices

Olive oil for coating the squash

Salt and black pepper to taste

How to Make It:

● Preheat a grill or grill pan over medium heat. Bring the vinegar, honey, garlic, rosemary, and red pepper flakes to a simmer in a small saucepan. Simmer for 5 minutes, until the mixture is thick and syrupy.

● Toss the squash with enough olive oil to coat and season with salt and black pepper. Grill the squash, turning, for 12 to 15 minutes, until lightly browned on both sides and soft and tender throughout. Toss with the vinegar-honey syrup.

Makes 4 to 6 servings

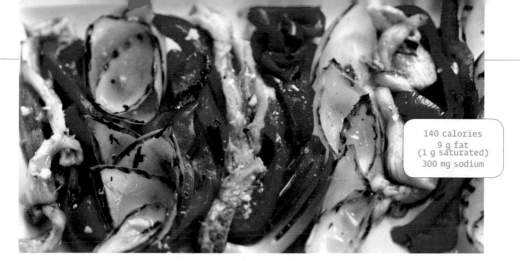

Grilled Vegetable Salad

This amazingly simple, satisfying grilled salad (called escalivada) hails from Catalonia, where eggplant, onion, and red pepper are the most common faces in vegetable stands and supermarkets. But the idea can work with any combination of vegetables: zucchini, asparagus, fennel, carrots, squash, and more. It's about the interplay of smoke and the different types of natural sweetness found in slow-cooked vegetables. Cook them until soft, dress with a bit of vinegar, good olive oil, and coarse salt, and eat with gusto.

You'll Need:

- 1 **medium eggplant**
- 2 **medium yellow onions, halved**
- 2 **red bell peppers**
- 2 **Tbsp olive oil, plus more for coating the vegetables**
- 1 **Tbsp sherry vinegar or red wine vinegar**
- 2 **cloves garlic, minced**

Coarse sea salt

How to Make It:

- Preheat a grill over medium heat. Drizzle the eggplant, onions, and bell peppers with enough olive oil to lightly coat. Grill, turning the vegetables occasionally, for about 20 minutes, until the outsides of the vegetables pick up a deep char and the insides are completely soft.

- Place the eggplant and peppers in a large bowl and cover with plastic wrap. Let steam for 5 minutes, which will help when stripping off the charred skin. Remove any of the heavily charred exterior pieces of the onions. Peel the eggplant and bell peppers. Cut the vegetables into thin strips (for the onions, separating the individual petals should suffice). On a large serving plate, organize each vegetable into individual piles so that they look like the stripes on a flag. Sprinkle with the 2 tablespoons olive oil, the vinegar, garlic, and salt.

Makes 4 servings

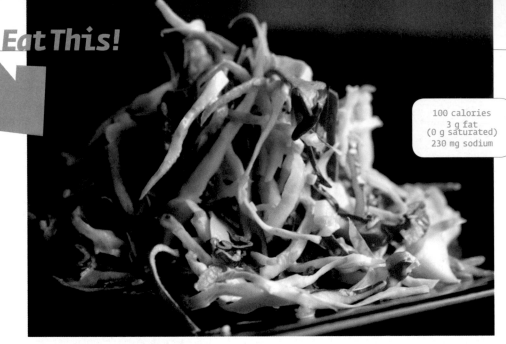

100 calories
3 g fat
(0 g saturated)
230 mg sodium

Asian Slaw

Most coleslaws turn out to be a bowl of mayonnaise dressed with a bit of cabbage, a formula for a nutrition disaster—not to mention a tide of drab, palate-numbing fat. Our Eastern-inspired take on the Western classic uses the big flavors of lime, sesame, and chili sauce to phase out the reliance on mayo, making for both a lighter and more flavorful slaw that goes as well on sandwiches as it does by itself.

You'll Need:

Juice of 1 lime

1 Tbsp olive oil mayonnaise

1 Tbsp sugar

1 tsp Asian-style chili sauce like sriracha

1 tsp sesame oil

8 cups shredded cabbage (preferably a mix of purple and napa cabbage)

1 large carrot, peeled and grated

1 Tbsp sesame seeds

How to Make It:

● In a large salad bowl, mix together the lime juice, mayonnaise, sugar, chili sauce, and sesame oil. Add the cabbage, carrots, and sesame seeds and toss to combine. Season with salt and pepper.

Makes 4 to 6 servings

Cowboy Beans

Baked beans, both the type that come in cans and those that come from the kitchens of barbecue shacks, are usually one step away from candy, bombed as they are with brown sugar, molasses, and honey. Too bad, since beans really are A-list eats. To preserve their health status and maximize deliciousness, we mitigate the sugar surge and build flavor instead with a few of our all-time favorite foods: cayenne, beer, and bacon.

You'll Need:

4 strips bacon, chopped into small pieces

1 medium onion, minced

2 cloves garlic, minced

1 cup dark beer

2 cans (16 oz each) pinto beans, rinsed and drained

¼ cup ketchup

1 Tbsp chili powder

1 Tbsp brown sugar

Pinch of cayenne pepper

How to Make It:

● Heat a large pot or saucepan over medium heat. Add the bacon and cook until it's just turning crispy, 3 to 5 minutes. Add the onion and garlic and sauté until translucent, another 3 minutes. Stir in the beer, beans, ketchup, chili powder, brown sugar, and cayenne. Simmer until the sauce thickens and clings to the beans, about 15 minutes.

Makes 6 servings

Grilled Cauliflower with Fish Sauce Vinaigrette

In most American households, cauliflower is eaten in one of two ways: steamed or boiled. Too bad, since besides being boring ways to eat most vegetables, both methods actually concentrate cauliflower's sulfurous undertones. Grilling mellows the gases and teases out cauliflower's natural sugars, creating something infinitely more enjoyable than the soggy florets most people are accustomed to. Tack on a punchy dressing and suddenly the prospect of eating your veggies is looking a whole lot more enjoyable.

You'll Need:

¼ cup warm water

1 Tbsp sugar

¼ cup fish sauce

Juice of 1 lime

12–15 fresh mint leaves, chopped

1 small red chile pepper, minced

1 head cauliflower, cut into large pieces

1 Tbsp canola, vegetable, or peanut oil

Salt and black pepper to taste

How to Make It:

● Combine the water and sugar in a small mixing bowl and stir to dissolve the sugar. Add the fish sauce, lime juice, mint, and minced chile. Reserve.

● Preheat a grill or grill pan over medium heat. Toss the cauliflower with the oil and season with salt and pepper.

Place the florets in a vegetable grill basket (or directly on the grate) and grill, turning occasionally, for 12 to 15 minutes, until the cauliflower is browned on the outside and just tender all the way through. Toss in a large mixing bowl with the vinaigrette.

Makes 4 servings

DESSERTS

GRILL
THIS
NOT
THAT!

Sundae Matrix

The grill does magical things to fruit, softening its flesh, concentrating its natural sweetness, and transforming it into something that feels like dessert on its own. Trick it out with ice cream and a few toppings and you have a world-class sundae on your hands. As decadent as it may seem, a scoop of ice cream combined with fresh fruit and a few toppings comes in under 300 calories—pretty impressive considering how indulgent these sundaes taste.

Four Quick Recipes

Mix and match fruit, ice cream, and add-ons however you like; there are literally hundreds of different paths to deliciousness. These four here just happen to be among our favorites.

CHOOSE A FRUIT

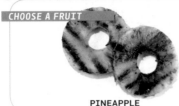

Other stone fruits like apricots and plums work just as well on the grill.

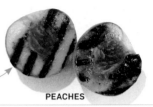

PINEAPPLE

PEACHES

CHOOSE AN ICE CREAM

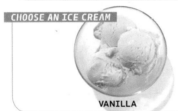

As always, our ice cream brand of choice is Breyers, which makes low-calorie products with a minimum number of ingredients. Using Breyers instead of a "premium" brand like Häagen-Dazs or Ben & Jerry's will save you nearly 150 calories per scoop.

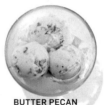

VANILLA

BUTTER PECAN

CHOOSE A TOPPING

A hot shot of concentrated espresso is best, but even a pour of good strong coffee can be an excellent—and unexpected—addition to a sundae. Both provide a huge rush of virtually calorie-free antioxidants.

HERSHEY'S SYRUP GENUINE

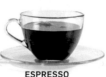

CHOCOLATE SYRUP

ESPRESSO

ADD SOME CRUNCH

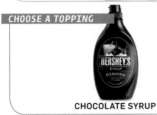

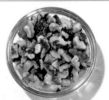

CHOPPED ROASTED PEANUTS

CRUSHED WALNUTS

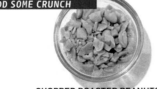

AFFOGATO
Grilled figs + vanilla ice cream + espresso + chocolate-covered espresso beans

PEACHES AND CREAM
Grilled peaches + butter pecan ice cream + Sauternes + granola

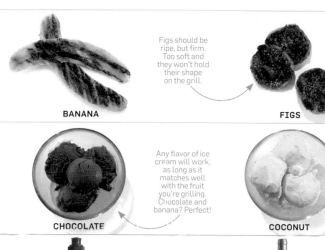

BANANA

Figs should be ripe, but firm. Too soft and they won't hold their shape on the grill.

FIGS

Any flavor of ice cream will work, as long as it matches well with the fruit you're grilling. Chocolate and banana? Perfect!

CHOCOLATE

COCONUT

A splash of Vin Santo, port, or Sauternes adds a sophisticated touch to a sundae.

DULCE DE LECHE

SWEET WINE

CHOCOLATE-COVERED ESPRESSO BEANS

GRANOLA

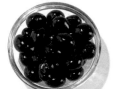

PIÑA COLADA
Pineapple + coconut ice cream + dulce de leche + coconut flakes

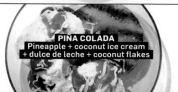

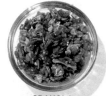

THE ELVIS
Grilled banana + peanut butter ice cream + chocolate sauce + crushed peanuts

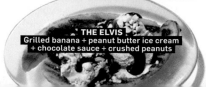

Sundae Basics

Rule 1
Grill fruit with the same attentiveness with which you grill steak. You don't want to blast the fruit so the heat melts it into mush. You want fruit that is caramelized and soft on the outside, but with a bit of bite in the center. For most fruit, that means 10 minutes tops on the grill.

Rule 2
The interplay of hot and cold is what makes this dessert so special. Have the ice cream at the table, slightly softened, ready to be scooped shortly after the fruit comes off the grill.

Rule 3
Use salty (roasted peanuts, granola) and bitter (espresso, a drizzle of olive oil) ingredients to cut through the sugar of the fruit and ice cream; it makes for a more interesting dessert.

Rule 4
Use small bowls and spoons. A study from Cornell University found that people who used both ate 30 percent less ice cream than people who used big bowls and spoons.

Grilled Banana Splits

This isn't just some gimmicky way to cram a popular dessert into a book about grilling: There truly is something transformative about the way the banana emerges from the grill grate. The warm caramelized fruit adds a layer of sexiness to the classic split, especially in the way the heat of the banana plays off the chill of the ice cream. Salted peanuts add crunch and contrast while chocolate doubles down on the decadence. And yet all of this can be yours for the low, low price of just 320 calories!

You'll Need:

- 2 **bananas, unpeeled**
- 2 **Tbsp light brown sugar**
- 4 **scoops vanilla ice cream**
- 4 **Tbsp chocolate sauce, heated**
- 4 **Tbsp roasted and salted peanuts, roughly chopped**

For the best possible splits, the bananas should be ripe, but not soft.

How to Make It:

- Preheat a grill or grill pan over medium-high heat. Cut the bananas in half horizontally, being sure to leave each half in the peel. Coat the cut sides of the bananas with the brown sugar, using your fingers to press the sugar into the flesh of the fruit. Place the bananas on the grill, cut side down, and grill for about 3 minutes, until the sugar caramelizes and forms a deep-brown. Flip and grill for another 2 to 3 minutes, until the bananas are warmed all the way through but not mushy.

- Remove the peels from the bananas and place each half in the bottom of a bowl. Top with a scoop of ice cream, a good drizzle of hot chocolate sauce, and a handful of crushed peanuts.

Makes 4 servings

Per Serving:
$0.96

320 calories
12 g fat (5 g saturated)
38 g sugars

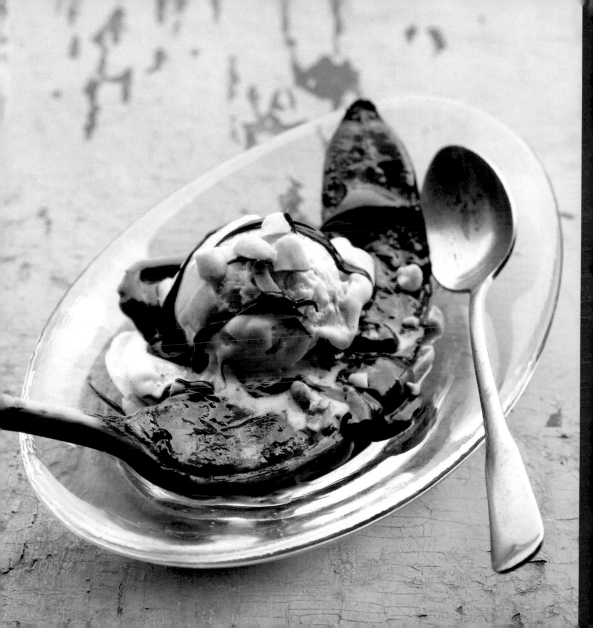

Stone Fruit Pizzas

After graduating from college, one of us (we won't say who) decided to go into the grilled pizza business. The plan was to set up shop in the farmers' markets of Southern California. At a final tasting to decide which vendors won a slot and which were sent packing, this dessert pizza won over the panel of judges and caused a small riot among passing pedestrians.

You'll Need:

½ **cup balsamic vinegar**

1 **Tbsp honey**

Pizza Dough (page 110)

2 **lbs mixed stone fruits (peaches, plums, apricots), halved and pitted**

Olive oil, for brushing

1 **cup low-fat ricotta or mascarpone cheese**

Mascarpone, a creamy, spreadable Italian cheese, makes for a great dessert pizza. It's more caloric than ricotta, so be mindful of the portion size if using.

If making the dough expressly for these pizzas, cut the salt by half and triple the amount of sugar.

How to Make It:

● Preheat a grill using a two-zone fire (see "Go High and Low," page 40), one zone high and the other low. Close the lid so that the heat can effectively build up. While the grill heats up, simmer the balsamic and honey in a small saucepan set over medium-low heat for about 10 minutes, until the liquid has reduced by about three-fourths.

● Cook the fruit on the hottest part of the grill, flesh sides down, for about 5 minutes, until caramelized and soft. Flip and grill for another 2 to 3 minutes, until the bottoms are soft. Remove and slice into ¼" pieces.

● Divide the dough into two equal balls. On a well-floured surface, use a rolling pin to stretch each ball into 12" circles.

● Place one of the dough circles on a lightly floured pizza peel. Brush the top with oil and slide it directly onto the hot part of the grill. Cook for about 30 seconds, until the dough begins to brown, then use a pair of tongs to rotate it 45 degrees. Grill for another 30 seconds, creating diamond-shaped grill marks on the crust. Flip the dough and place, raw side down, on the cooler side of the grill. Working quickly, spread half of the cheese on the pizza, then top with half of the grilled fruit slices. Close the grill top and let the pizza grill for 2 to 3 minutes. Use your tongs to rotate the pizza 45 degrees and continue grilling for another minute or two, until the crust is crisp beneath. Repeat with the other pizza. Drizzle the balsamic over the tops of the pizzas.

Makes 6 servings

Per Serving:
$1.81

350 calories
4.5 g fat (2 g saturated)
16 g sugars

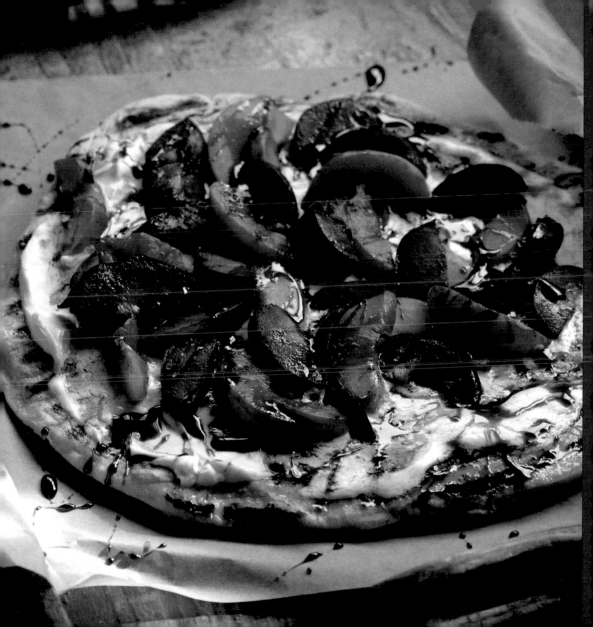

Banana-Nutella Panini

Sandwiches have always been defined as savory affairs, but there's no reason you can't bookend your dessert with two slices of bread the same way you would your lunch. Toast those pieces of bread until the sandwich is crispy on the outside and hot on the inside, and the appeal of a handheld dessert is all the more obvious. There are few better partnerships on the planet than banana and chocolate—so, really, there's no way this recipe could go wrong.

You'll Need:

- **4 Tbsp chocolate-hazelnut spread**
- **8 slices whole-wheat bread**
- **2 very ripe bananas, sliced**
- **2 Tbsp butter, melted**

The most widely available version is Nutella, but we prefer Nocciolata, which has a much more respectable ingredient list.

How to Make It:

- Preheat a grill or grill pan over medium heat. Divide the chocolate spread among 4 slices of the bread, pave completely with the banana slices, and top with the remaining pieces of bread. Brush both sides of each sandwich with a light coating of melted butter (which will help the sandwiches brown and crisp easily).

- Place the sandwiches on the grill and top with a light object—a clean pot or pan works great—that applies just enough pressure to weigh down the sandwiches and help them crisp. Grill for 3 to 4 minutes, until the bottoms are nicely toasted; flip and repeat. Cut the sandwiches in half on the diagonal and serve.

Makes 4 servings

MEAL MULTIPLIER

More additions to your dessert-sandwich repertoire:

- Peanut butter, banana, and honey
- Mascarpone or ricotta cheese and strawberries
- Marshmallow spread and dark chocolate chips (think s'mores)

Per Serving:
$1.12

340 calories
13 g fat (5 g saturated)
20 g sugars

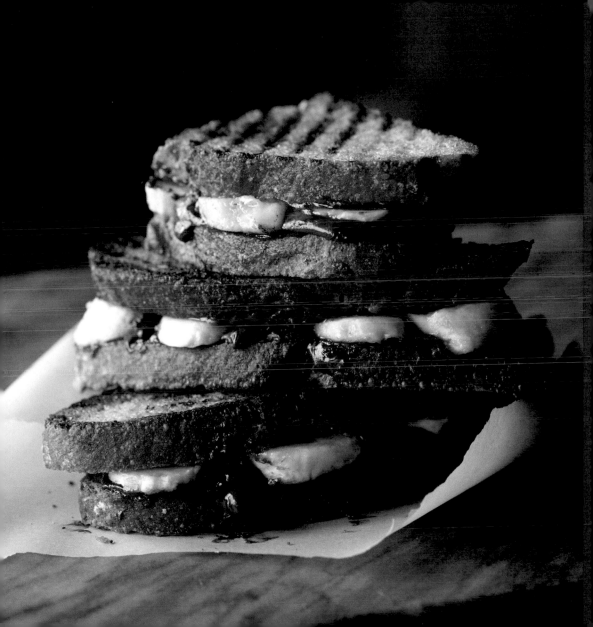

Grilled Apples à la Mode

When it comes to grilling fruit, peaches and pineapples tend to get most of the love. But if pie-eating has taught us anything, it's that apples become exponentially more delicious when cooked. We like to skip the fussy, calorie-dense crust in favor of a crunchy, sweet stuffing baked directly inside the apple. The heat of the grill softens and sweetens the fruit from the outside while it melts the butter and toasts the pecans within. Hot off the grill, with a scoop of vanilla ice cream melting over the top, this apple rivals a slice of warm homemade apple pie à la mode any day.

You'll Need:

- 4 medium baking apples (Golden Delicious, Roma, etc.)
- ¼ cup brown sugar
- 2 Tbsp cold butter, chopped into small pieces
- ¼ cup chopped pecans or walnuts
- ¼ cup raisins
- ¼ tsp cinnamon
- 4 scoops vanilla ice cream

How to Make It:

- Preheat a grill over medium-low heat. Using a paring knife and spoon, and working from the top of the apple, scoop out the core and center part of the fruit, leaving a firm base and a ½" shell of apple around the middle section.

- Combine the brown sugar, butter, pecans, raisins, and cinnamon in a mixing bowl. Pack each apple full with the mixture. Place the apples directly on the grill grate and close the lid. Grill for about 25 minutes, until the fruit is soft all the way through. Serve each apple with a scoop of ice cream over the top.

Makes 4 servings

Per Serving:
$1.70

390 calories
17 g fat (8 g saturated)
51 g sugars

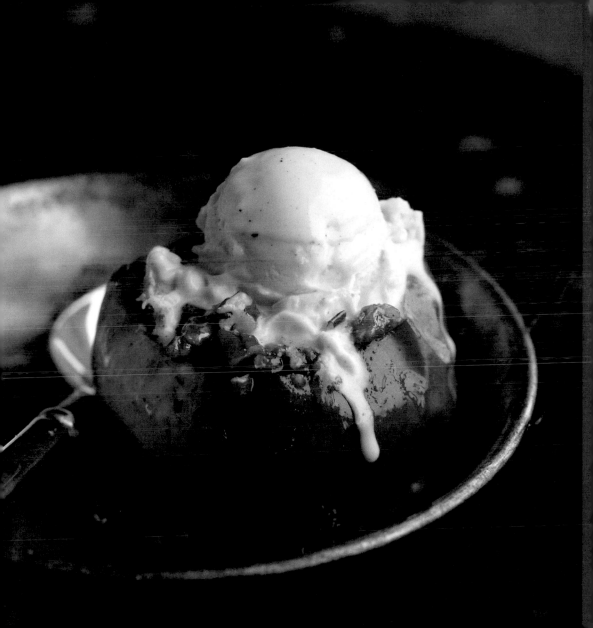

Strawberry Shortcake

Why take a classic—one as basic and beloved as strawberry shortcake—and mess with it on the grill? The short answer: Why not? The long answer: The grill helps caramelize sugars, amplify texture, and gives the dish a hot-cold component that makes it more compelling—and delicious—than the original. This version is special for other reasons, as well. Strawberries come alive in a marinade of balsamic and cracked pepper (a classic Italian pairing that is hard not to love once you try it), and the fresh whipped cream is laced with a shot of balsamic, giving it an addictive tang that brings the whole dessert together.

You'll Need:

- 1 cup whipping cream
- 4 Tbsp balsamic vinegar
- 1 small carton strawberries, stemmed and sliced
- A few pinches of black pepper
- 4 (1½"-thick) slices angel food cake

How to Make It:

- Preheat a grill or grill pan over medium heat. Use an electric beater to beat the cream until it forms soft peaks (it should cling to the beaters, but not get stuck inside them). Add 2 tablespoons of the balsamic and continue beating until the whipped cream has a uniform color. (Alternatively, this can be done by hand with a whisk and a cold metal bowl. Makes for a good workout.)

- Combine the remaining 2 tablespoons balsamic with the strawberries and pepper in a bowl. Allow them to marinate while you grill the angel food cake.

- Grill the cake slices for 3 to 4 minutes per side, until well browned and crispy on the outside. Divide among 4 plates or bowls, top with the strawberries and spoon the whipped cream over the top.

Makes 4 servings

Per Serving:
$2.16

220 calories
12 g fat (7 g saturated)
6 g sugars

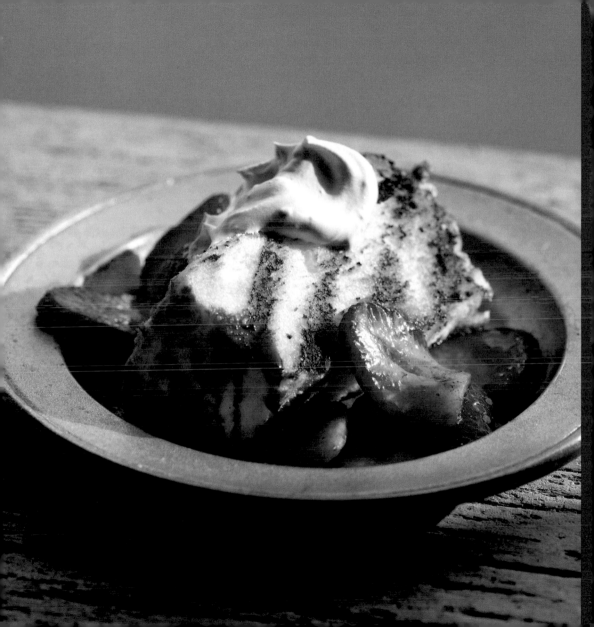

S'mores
Chocolate–Peanut Butter & Chocolate-Caramel

In the 80-odd years since the first known recipe for s'mores surfaced in an obscure Girl Scout publication, very little has changed with the campfire classic; it had the same three ingredients back then as it does now: graham crackers, chocolate, marshmallow. Admittedly, it's tough to improve upon the time-tested formula, but with the original as our inspiration and the grill as our muse, we think these two new iterations would do the Girl Scouts proud.

You'll Need:

- 8 large marshmallows
- 8 metal skewers, or wooden skewers soaked in water for 30 minutes
- 2 Tbsp dulce de leche
- 16 chocolate wafer cookies (like Nabisco Famous Chocolate Wafers)
- 2 Tbsp smooth peanut butter

Dulce de leche is a special type of caramel popular in Latin America. It's now widely available in the states, but if you can't find it, standard caramel sauce will do.

How to Make It:

- Preheat a grill over medium heat. Place a marshmallow at the end of each skewer. (If everyone wants to toast their own marshmallows, pass them around to guests.) Grill the marshmallows, turning, for about 3 minutes, until lightly brown and toasted all over. If using a charcoal grill, remove the grate and roast the marshmallows close to the coals; if using a gas grill, you can place directly on the hot grate.

- Spread ½ tablespoon of dulce de leche on each of 4 cookies and spread ½ tablespoon of peanut butter on each of another 4 cookies. Top each with a toasted marshmallow and another cookie. If you like, place the s'mores directly on the grill just long enough to warm, 1 to 2 minutes.

Makes 4 servings

Per Serving:
$1.02

330 calories
13 g fat (3 g saturated)
29 g sugars

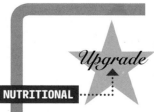

Upgrade

NUTRITIONAL

While swapping in peanut butter for chocolate in this recipe constitutes a step up in the nutrition status of the s'more, there are even greater strides that can be made while not sacrificing the overall feeling of decadence. Try pairing slices of banana with the peanut butter, slices of apple or pear with dulce de leche, or, in a riff on the classic s'mores construction, thick slices of strawberry with antioxidant-rich dark chocolate.

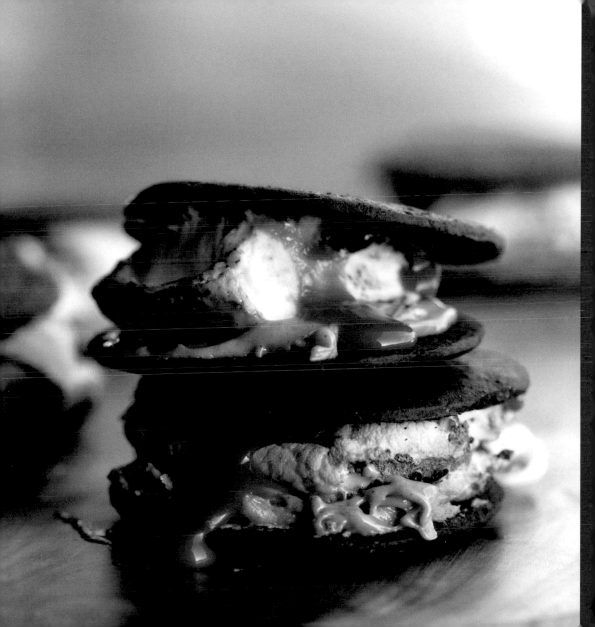

Index

Outwitting
Squirrels

Outwitting Squirrels

101 *Cunning Stratagems to Reduce Dramatically the Egregious Misappropriation of Seed from Your Birdfeeder by Squirrels*

Second Edition
Revised & Even Craftier

BILL ADLER, JR.

CHICAGO
REVIEW
PRESS

Library of Congress Cataloging-in-Publication Data

Adler, Bill.
  Outwitting squirrels.

    1. Bird feeders.   2. Squirrels—Control.
3. Squirrels—Humor.   4. Mammals—Control.
5. Mammals—Humor.   I. Title.
QL676.5.A34   1988   639.9'78   88-20283
ISBN 1-55652-302-5

10   9

To my parents,
whom I constantly tried to outwit as a child,
and who, sometimes,
lovingly let me get away with it.

Contents

Acknowledgments

The perennial fear among writers with acknowledgments is that you're going to leave someone out. With a book like *Outwitting Squirrels: 101 Cunning Stratagems to Reduce Dramatically the Egregious Misappropriation of Seed from Your Birdfeeder by Squirrels*, however, the danger is just the opposite: I might mention somebody who's too embarrassed to be associated with this book.

Still, I couldn't have done it alone. My thanks go first to squirrels who volunteered to let me test the squirrelproofness of various feeders on them. Second, I want to thank the hundreds of birds who patiently waited out these squirrels while the squirrels prevented them from getting to the seed.

A number of humans also gave invaluable assistance. I want to thank Peggy Robin, who let me use her backyard as a proving ground for feeders. Peggy's criticisms and suggestions when *Outwitting Squirrels* was still tucked inside my word processor helped make this a better book.

George Petrides, proprietor of The Wild Bird Center, was a fountain of information about birds, squirrels, and people who feed both. As I was interviewing people for this book, nearly everyone said I have to talk to Professor Vagn Flyger, one of the country's foremost squirrel experts. I did, and I appreciate his lending me his knowledge for *Outwitting Squirrels*. Heidi Hughes, who owns The Wild Bird Company, had many valuable things to say about feeding birds, especially about keeping birds safe from human-inspired hazards. Liz Cummings at the U.S. Fish and Wildlife Service offered numerous perspectives into the personalities of particular species.

Richard Mallory, publisher and editor of the *Dick E. Bird News*, graciously allowed me to reprint articles and illustrations from his wonderful newspaper. His insight into squirrels and birds was a valuable resource.

A number of wild bird product companies and distributors graciously offered me their years of experience in dealing with squirrels. I want to thank Marlene Couter of Duncraft, Olin Looker of Looker Products, Dr. Stephen Clarke of Clarke Products, Thomas Post of The Audubon Workshop, Richard Clarke of The Bird House, and Marie Gellerstedt of Nixalite of America.

My thanks also go to Richard Swain for letting me republish his essay, "The Squirrel and the Fruitcake," here.

My friend and neighbor Stephanie Faul originally got me interested in feeding birds several years ago. She had no idea it would lead to this.

It's hard to write a book as fun and informative as *Outwitting Squirrels* without wanting to read sections to people as you go along. Several friends graciously listened to paragraph after paragraph—not all polished at the time—as I progressed. These friends include Marta Vogel, Mitch Schultz, and Carol Dana.

Thanks also to: Janet Levy, Joseph Argentieri, Nancy A. Keep, Pam Price, Dan Clemmensen, John Robertson, E. George Strasser, Lanny Chambers, John Duke, Caroline Lloyd, Michael Timko, Dorothy B. Sindel, Kris Campbell, Kristen J. Ingram, Colby F. Jordan, A. Dale Rhoads, Gregg Bassett, Jerry Blinn, and Iris Rothman.

And of course, this book never would have been published if it weren't for Linda Matthews of Chicago Review Press, who was willing to risk having an entire species vow never to use Chicago Review Press as their publisher. This book benefited greatly from Linda's suggestions and experience.

Introduction

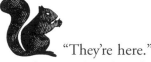 "They're here."

That may be a line from the movie *Poltergeist*, but it's also the horror cry of tens of millions of Americans who feed birds as they prepare to defend their feeders from hordes of squirrels. Each day, tons of birdseed is poured into birdfeeders to attract and benefit beautiful winged creatures—cardinals, doves, chickadees, goldfinches—and each day, tons of birdseed is pilfered by marauding squirrels. If there's one thing that birders have in common it is their enemy: the squirrel.

Mention squirrels to any bird feeder and you will inspire a half-hour monologue about how these cunning little mammals managed to overcome the most inventive, dangerous-looking, and expensive antisquirrel systems. Sometimes you have to believe that if the creativity and energy that bird feeders put into thwarting squirrels were directed toward world peace or eliminating traffic jams, we'd have no more earthly problems.

People who feed birds have tried every possible antisquirrel concoction their imaginations can conjure. Every situation seems to demand its own solution. Defensive options range from water cannons to giving squirrels feeders of their own. From barbed wire and electrified feeders to coating birdfeeders with Ben Gay and Teflon, to baffling the top and bottom side of feeders so that birds can barely get in—nothing seems to work.

Until now. Until *Outwitting Squirrels: 101 Cunning Stratagems to Reduce Dramatically the Egregious Misappropriation of Seed From Your Birdfeeder by Squirrels.* For the first time, the sum of humankind's knowledge about squirrels and how to defeat them is available in one place.

Writing *Outwitting Squirrels* was one of the most pleasurable experiences I've had as an author. There are few topics that lend themselves to both a serious examination and playfulness. While researching *Outwitting Squirrels* I talked with dozens of people in the bird business and with ordinary birders who have extraordinary squirrel problems. I was impressed by the inventiveness and persistence of the bird feeders who tried to keep squirrels at bay—and impressed by the squirrels. I was entertained by people's stories about squirrels. I believe that reading *Outwitting Squirrels* will be as much fun for you as writing it was for me.

Who are we, the people who feed wild birds and scream and flail our arms at squirrels? Where do we fit in the range of what "normal" Americans do? You'll be pleased to know that birdfeeding and squirrel yelling are common practices. We bird feeders participate in the most popular hobby in America after gardening. There are eighty million Americans who dish out meals to birds. We spend over $500 million a year on birdseed, $54 million on birdfeeders, $25 million on bird-baths, and $17 million a year on bird books. There's a tremendous amount of interest and money involved with feeding birds. And wherever there are birdfeeders, there are squirrels.

As annoying and frustrating as squirrels are, they are humorous as well. After all, squirrels think that the birdseed is for them and there's no power on earth that will convince them otherwise.

So while *Outwitting Squirrels* gives concrete, useful information that birders can use to stop squirrels from poaching, it's also a funny and philosophical book. Funny, because every time a human constructs another barrier, squirrels break through. Funny, also, because bird feeders spend hundreds of hours and dollars trying to keep these small animals away—and the squirrels have nothing better to do all day long than break into feeders. Philosophical because there must be some overall significance to this human-bird-squirrel triangle. Right?

Maybe there's a meaning to these antisquirrel antics, and maybe not. But there is one essential fact to keep in mind when it comes to squirrels: we are smarter and stronger than squirrels. We can win against squirrels. We will win against squirrels. And along the way, we're going to have plenty of fun.

Author's Notes on the Second Edition

I caught myself feeding a squirrel the other day.

Indeed a lot has changed since 1987, when I first wrote *Outwitting Squirrels*.

I have not become soft on squirrels. There is nothing in the behavior of squirrels that has changed my opinion that squirrels are just common thieves shrouded in fur, with cute, fluffy tails. If you feed birds—beautiful, majestic, creatures of the wind—then you must also curse squirrels. And work to outwit them.

But first, let me explain what appears to be a transgression on my part. I can understand that my offering peanuts to squirrels (actually a single squirrel, but I'll get to that in moment) looks as if I have joined Evil itself. In fact, it does send shivers down my spine to see anyone offering a nut to one of these creatures.

But since 1987 a lot has happened to me. Namely, I have children.

Certainly I agree that small children and squirrels don't mix (squirrels bite, they carry fleas, and they teach bad manners), but it's hard to resist your five-year-old daughter when she looks out the kitchen window and pleads, "Daddy, it's Bushy's cousin. Can we give him a peanut?" Karen's a redhead and that makes it even harder to say no to her. (Karen's preschool has a feeding station set up for its resident squirrel, Bushy, so this one, to Karen, had to be Bushy's cousin. I intend to talk with the school's head soon about teaching their pupils squirrelfeeding.)

So I gave Bushy's cousin a peanut. Karen and her little sister Claire squealed with delight. They jumped up and down and insisted that I lift them on top of the counter so that they could get a better look at Bushy's cousin. Then Karen said, "Could he have another peanut? He looks so hungry." And Claire, her two-and-a-half-year-old sister said, "Cn he 'nother pinut? He hukgry." I complied. One nut led to another and soon I was shuffling in and out in my slippers all winter, giving this squirrel unearned peanuts. Karen and Claire loved it. They stuck their noses right against the window and watched the squirrel pick the nut up in his little handlike claws and nibble it to nothingness. At first Bushy's cousin was apprehensive (he must have heard about Karen and Claire's reputation for chasing their grandmother's cat around her house), but after a short time, Bushy's cousin realized that the glass between him and them was impenetrable—he was safe.

Eventually we ran out of peanuts, though my kids had a great time. And I have to admit, it was a little more enjoyable than sitting with them and watching Barney videos. Still, the nuts cost about three dollars, which could have gone a long way toward feeding the blue jays who also were in need of food. When we ran out of peanuts, Karen suggested peanut butter. (I guarantee she didn't learn that from me!) So for the next few days, Bushy's cousin dined on Carr's crackers with peanut butter. As you can imagine, once children like something, they never want it to end, or so it seems to us adults. But eventually, Karen and Claire lost interest in Bushy's cousin, and we went back to Barney, who, despite all his flaws, doesn't raid birdfeeders.

In the spirit of things, I guess it's important to come completely clean about my squirrel affairs. There was one other time, I forget exactly when, but I think it was in 1990, that I was caught in the act of feeding a squirrel. Squirrels, plural, actually—and I was caught on film. It happened like this: Our local CBS affiliate was doing a program on rogue squirrels, and they asked if I would like to be interviewed. Naturally, the program wouldn't be any good without squirrels, so I had to conjure up a few, which is in itself no problem, because all one has to do is toss out a few peanuts and squirrels will come running. That's what I did: tossed out a few nuts and a horde of squirrels came running. All of a sudden every squirrel for miles was in my yard. There was a feeding frenzy. If I had been swimming off the coast of Australia and had done a similar thing with sharks around, I wouldn't be here today—or at the very least, I'd be typing with my elbows. That's how ferocious these squirrels were. Just the faintest whiff of peanut aroma and they become aggressive, maniacal varmints. The filming went well, though some of the squirrels seemed to consider the possibility that I was keeping a stash of peanuts in my pant legs. The show filmed me on the deck in my backyard, and to facilitate getting more nuts we kept the kitchen door open. You probably know where this is heading. The next thing I knew I was chasing a squirrel around my kitchen using a roll of paper towels to urge him to seek safety outside. And the camera man was hot on my heels.

How humiliating. But perhaps more than anything this incident has increased my resolve to perpetuate the good research around the world that has gone into outwitting squirrels. Since the Internet was developed in 1987 it, more than any single other instrument, has improved our capability to thwart squirrels by facilitating the rapid exchange of information about squirrels. Information can be transmitted through the Net faster than squirrels can run. Although there have been reports of squirrels chewing through phone lines to sabotage our lines of communications, I don't think that squirrels have yet learned how valuable the Internet has become. (One Netzian disagreed. To one of my queries he wrote, "Go ahead. Put all your best tricks on the Internet where the International Squirrels Who Raid Birdfeeders Association can download them for research in ways to overcome them!")

I've learned a lot about squirrels over the past years. For example, did you know that squirrels in some areas of the country are smarter than others? One person who read the original *Outwitting Squirrels* wrote that her metal feeder with a spring-loaded door works "brilliantly for Tennessee squirrels, but there are a few high-IQ Washington, D.C. ones that have figured out a way to suspend themselves spread-eagle across the top of the feeder with one paw free to reach down, exert pressure, and help themselves to the seed." Makes sense to me that squirrels would be better at being squirrelly when in close proximity to so many politicians.

I have long felt that this is more than a matter of squirrels versus birds. Ultimately, both squirrels and birds will thrive, and neither really needs humans. (Though who would squirrels harass if we weren't here—cats?) But I believe that our battle against squirrels must endure, because if we can't figure out a way to outwit squirrels, how can we ever expect to get a man or woman to Mars?

Misadventures With Squirrels

I'm getting low on bird food and I don't know what the squirrels will do without my birdfeeder to raid.

—Sandy Rovner, the *Washington Post*

It could happen to anyone. Of that I'm now sure. And it could happen to anyone in the most innocent, innocuous way. Oh, yes, I know—because it happened to me. Once I was like most people—caring, tolerant, even curious of the natural world—but that is a distant part of my past now. I really can't remember what I used to be like—before. I can only hope that by writing this chapter I can warn others before they, too, are obsessed, are controlled by a single, overriding hatred of squirrels (at least when they come in proximity to birdfeeders).

My apartment building doesn't allow pets, except for "grandfathered" pets: those that were here before this rule was instituted. (It was my lot to live in the apartment below Dusty, a four-legged, tap-dancing dog who likes to wake his owner by practicing his Fred Astaire routine at 6 A.M.) I never actually wanted a cat or a dog, figuring that owning

1

one would be a reasonably large hassle for an apartment dweller, but as soon as I learned of this no-pets rule, I decided I needed one.

When I visited a friend's apartment and saw a birdfeeder attached to her window, surrounded by all sorts of colorful and (to my eye) exotic birds, I knew that's what I had to have. A feeder would be perfect—I would not have just one pet, but dozens. I wouldn't have to walk them, change their litter box, or vacuum my clothing every morning. Most importantly, I could have these pets and not get evicted. My friend gave me her Duncraft bird catalog, and through the miracles of modern credit, my feeder arrived in less than a week.

I opened the box quickly, followed the instructions carefully (soak the two suction cups in warm water for three minutes, then rub them with your finger to increase their sticking power), added a quart of Safeway wild bird food mix from the ten-pound supply I had already purchased in anticipation, slapped the feeder on the window, and waited. It was five in the afternoon in February. I kept waiting for my birds to arrive.

Nobody told me that birds don't come to feeders after dark.

But the next day was amazing. My feeder brought a sunset-red cardinal, two doves, a couple of finches, a chickadee, a tufted titmouse, a warbler, a junco, and a white-breasted nuthatch. (I know this because I also bought the *Audubon Society Field Guide to North American Birds*.) I'd never seen anything like this before—beautiful birds with beautiful songs coming to my window every handful of seconds. I'd just sit at my desk and look at them, or sometimes I'd walk over to the window for a closer view. A few birds like the tufted titmouse and the chickadee didn't mind my standing so close to them; others would fly back to the nearby tree and wait for my departure. It didn't bother me that some of these birds wouldn't let me come close; after all, they provided so much enjoyment and required so little in return—just sunflower seeds. On the rare occasion when a minute or two passed without a bird stopping by, I'd become terribly disappointed.

One afternoon something happened that changed my world forever. It inspired a quest that has been driving me for nearly two years; the same quest that motivates eighty million other Americans. That February afternoon, I returned from an errand, opened my door and saw *a squirrel* in my feeder. My birdfeeder! The whole squirrel—tail and everything—was inside the feeder, a rectangular lucite compartment attached to my window with suction cups.

Nothing has been the same since.

For the rest of the afternoon I stood guard over the feeder, protecting my birds from this gray rodent. Every time it approached, I flailed my arms, banged on the window—and the squirrel ran away. Unfortunately, it didn't take too many hours before the squirrel learned that the window was solid, and that despite my gestures and noise, I remained safely inside.

The squirrel, being a city creature and all, decided that it could stand the noise if it could eat. Sort of like dining at an outdoor café along a major street.

So I urgently developed a new strategy: I opened the window and yelled at the squirrel, who, recognizing the implications of an open window, bolted away. He returned; I opened the window. Now mind you, this was still winter, so I wasn't too crazy about opening my window every fifteen minutes or so to shake my fist at the squirrel, but what choice did I have? Anyway, the technique worked. This squirrel, which somehow managed to climb up two flights to my apartment, was defeated. I was victorious.

I was wrong.

The next morning it was back. Not only was it back, but the squirrel brought a friend. Still worse, my birds weren't around, apparently figuring that they ought to yield right-of-way to the gray animal with claws. But a squirrel was only a dumb animal, I thought, and it would only take a modicum of ingenuity and effort to thwart the squirrel's invasion. So I moved the feeder to a higher pane on my window, a couple of feet above the air conditioner. Sanguine over my success, I left the apartment for lunch.

When I returned, I discovered that I wasn't the only one who had been dining. Leaping a half dozen more inches from the air conditioner had posed no problem for the squirrel; in fact, he appeared to enjoy this spate of pre-lunch exercise.

All right, I thought, I'll let the squirrel get into the feeder, but for one purpose only: to watch how and from exactly what spot on the air conditioner he leaps. If I could learn the squirrel's technique, I knew that I could develop a counter to it.

This was the beginning of war.

In the meantime, I wasn't going to sit back and do nothing; my birds were counting on me. A trip to the hardware store would produce some useful ideas, I thought. I was right. At the store I found an item that I was certain would mean the squirrel's downfall, something that, despite the squirrel's long lineage extending back through generations of birdfeeder raiders, he wouldn't be able to overcome.

Before I tell you what that item was, I need to mention one other aspect of the squirrel's behavior. I noticed early on that Mr. Squirrel was adept at climbing brick walls. Very adept. In fact, it was the brick wall that the squirrel needed in order to invade my feeder. The wall was its attack route: a kind of Normandy beach of the squirrel world. Obviously, I couldn't remove the brick wall, but I could do something even better, thanks to a miracle-product of the 1980s: spray-can Teflon.

With the glee of a sixteen-year-old on prom night, I coated the walls around and below the air conditioner with a visible film of Teflon. Although I had to lean out the window precariously to reach every spot, it was worth the risk.

And I wasn't disappointed. The first squirrel that leapt onto the Teflon-coated brick was as surprised as I was overjoyed. The moment his claws caught the Teflon-coated surface he scrambled furiously to keep hold, his little legs moving rapidly in circles, as if he were being chased by a cat. It was a fun, funny, fantastic sight: here was Mr. Squirrel, so certain that he could scale any surface (except glass, but he already knew about that), especially brick, and now ordinary brick was refusing to cooperate. The squirrel's world turned topsy-turvy; the squirrel had no basis on which to compare or comprehend this new reality created by Teflon. From this moment on, there would be no rules that Mr. Squirrel could depend on.

Finally, Teflon had a valuable application.

As you can tell, that wasn't the end of the war between me and the squirrels. Teflon was great while it lasted, but unfortunately spray Teflon has one negative property: it comes off brick when it rains. Another alternative was brewing in my mind—spraying the squirrel with Teflon—but I wasn't ready for anything like that. Yet.

"Okay. I can live with a temporary setback," I said to myself. "I have more tricks up my sleeve. If only I could think of them."

Frequently, the best inventions stem not from trips to the hardware store, nor are they Rube Goldberg contraptions that are the product of weeks of imagining. Rather, they result from making use of what's around. The common, uncomplicated things. And that's precisely what I did.

Anyone who works in his apartment can tell you that there's a grave danger lurking for those who spend the day in this environment: the refrigerator. The refrigerator is the ultimate seductress for the work-at-home crowd; it is the force that moves waist size to increase faster than age. Not wanting to impersonate the individual whose girth resembles that of the golden arches at McDonald's, I opted to stock my fridge with Perrier water, a nice, non-caloric alternative to sweet drinks. But all those empty bottles! What a pain to throw away!

Yes, indeed, all those empty bottles provided the means to thwart Mr. Squirrel's birdfeeder rampages. You see, in order to jump into the feeder on the window, the squirrel had to leap from the top of my air conditioner. And he couldn't jump from just anywhere on the air conditioner: the angle had to be just right for him to get into the feeder. I'm a two-liter-a-day Perrier drinker; it took only a couple of days for me to cover the squirrel's launch sites.

I could relax again. My relaxation lasted exactly twenty-four hours.

The squirrel found new launch sites.

So I found new places to put Perrier bottles.

And then the squirrel started knocking the Perrier bottles down. I filled them with tap water to make them too heavy to knock down. Then the squirrel started bowling: he discovered that if you could knock down one Perrier bottle you could cause most of them to fall. That apparently was not only easier from the squirrel's perspective, but more enjoyable as well. My countermove was to encircle the bottles with copper bell wire to create a single Perrier superstructure that was too heavy for the squirrel to knock over.

Victory at last!

Wrong again. The squirrel decided to ignore the Perrier apparatus altogether and simply hoist himself up to the feeder by grabbing onto the wooden window frame and pulling himself upward as if doing a chin-up. Mr. Squirrel even found that he could use the Perrier bottles as a support to balance his back legs against as he lifted himself into the feeder.

My riposte was to spray the window frame with Teflon, even though I knew it would only last until the next rain. Alas, I also sprayed the window with Teflon, which made it difficult to see through.

Maybe I'm going about this all wrong, I figured. Perhaps the solution lies not in preventing access to the feeder, but in the type of feeder I have. Looking at the feeder, with its wide entry area and well-defined edges—great for holding on to—I understood that I'd been making things too easy for Mr. Squirrel. It was time to play hardball.

I bought a new feeder—a chalet-style apparatus made of pine, with Plexiglas windows along the sides. The seed was dispensed from a gap between the Plexiglas sides and wooden base of the feeder. In order to eat the feed, a bird (hopefully, *only* a bird) had to reach that narrow opening. By putting the feeder on top of the Perrier bottles there would be no way for the squirrel to get its furry little face into that opening; the space was simply too high and far away.

Again, I was wrong. I learned something new about squirrels' capabilities: they can, and will, eat through anything to get to food. In a few days the squirrel had eaten through the feeder to create a reasonably sized hole through which he could munch to his stomach's content.

Enough! It had to be possible for a human to outwit a squirrel! Feeding birds was important, certainly; being surrounded by cardinals and titmice all day long is rather pleasant. "No squirrel is going to stand in my way," I growled through gritted teeth. This was becoming more than a matter of being close to birds. Pride and intelligence were involved and I wasn't about to let a mere rodent get the better of me.

It's at this point in the story about my war with the squirrels that I'd like to digress. My squirrel war was causing personal problems. Frequently while talking on the telephone, I would shout in the squirrel's direction, "Get out of here!" followed by certain epithets. My friends, of course, thought it rather rude that I would hurl insults at them without provocation. When I told them about the squirrel, it increased their concern for my mental health. So be it—I was not going to succumb to the squirrel's strategy.

I bought yet another feeder—a clear Swiss chalet-style feeder that attaches with suction cups to the window and has a wide opening in front. Buying new feeders was to be a recurring phenomenon and part of the squirrel's strategy, I was certain. (If he couldn't win by being more patient and persistent than me, he was going to make me very, very poor. Of course, he probably didn't realize that if I could no longer afford new feeders, I couldn't afford more feed.) Attaching a feeder directly to the window was a return to the old, unsuccessful geometry, I knew, but the height of the feeder on the windowpane was an advantage and I intended to take that advantage. This feeder had an opening in the front and suction cups on the back. The opening of this feeder was arranged so that the squirrel couldn't leap directly in. But I knew that if I simply attached the feeder to the window, the squirrel would be able to leap on top of it and crawl inside. The Swiss chalet had a very steep roof, and it was this characteristic that I intended to exploit. Because of its steepness and Lucite construction, the squirrel would have a difficult time securing himself to the top so as not to fall. (I had discovered by this time that squirrels aren't afraid of heights, falling, losing their balance, or anything like that at all; but they *can* fall.) When on the chalet the squirrel would have to devote some of his claws to supporting himself while he climbed over the top into the feeder which was the only way to the food. Knowledge is the most powerful tool of the human species. By pressing this knowledge to its outer limits I was certain I could win. Carefully, I drilled holes spaced about one-quarter of an inch apart in the feeder's roof, near the front edge. I then placed three-inch nails, pointing upward, in these holes, creating a barrier to prevent the squirrel from leaning over the edge of the roof and climbing into the feeder from the top. I also placed a couple of upward-pointing nails on the feeder to make it more difficult for the squirrel to meander around the top. These nails were positioned more or less in the center of the upside down V-shaped rooftop. The feeder looked intimidating, kind of medieval, and frightful. Sometimes I could see the sun reflect off the nails' points, and suddenly I felt as if my feeder-fortress had a consciousness—it knew its purpose. In a strange way, it was an evil creation designed to inflict good.

And here's what happened. First, the squirrel used the nails as handholds by wrapping one claw around a nail. Second, by some ability I am at a loss to describe, Mr. Squirrel simply passed through my wall of nails as if they weren't there. Because the nails were pointing up along a triangular surface, geometry forced the space between the nails to get larger the farther the nail was from the surface of the feeder. Yet somehow the squirrel lifted himself into the air and pushed through the open part. I countered by weaving copper wire between the nails to fill that space; it looked like a fence. Now the squirrel had to scale the fence, and flip upside down to get inside the feeder. He did.

It was time for heavy artillery. I bought a squirt gun and blasted the squirrel every time he came near the feeder. Naturally, this meant that I didn't get much work accomplished, but so what? War requires sacrifice. Although Mr. Squirrel wasn't too crazy about me, after a while he didn't seem to care about being sprayed with water. It didn't take long for the squirrel to figure out that what I was squirting him with was the same stuff that falls from the sky. So I escalated and bought a dart gun—the kind with the red, rubber tips so I wouldn't actually harm the squirrel. (While bird feeders may *hate* squirrels, we are, deep down, nature lovers.) And I got pretty good—I could hit a moving squirrel at twenty feet. My objective with the dart gun was to annoy the squirrel enough so that he'd move elsewhere—to somebody else's feeder. While I did annoy him (though when the dart hit the squirrel at its maximum range the impact was so soft that the squirrel just shook itself and went back to whatever he was doing), the squirrel developed a countertactic: eat while I wasn't watching. He knew that by the time I grabbed my gun, reached the window and opened the screen, he could be well out of range. In response I would sometimes lie in wait with dart gun in hand—ambush style—beneath my window and spring to fire while the squirrel wasn't looking. Ultimately, however, I tired of this faster than the squirrel did.

It was then that I read about Nixalite in an article in *The New York Times*. Nixalite's another product of miraculous 1980s technology— like Teflon, I guess, only better. The article discussed how effective Nixalite was at keeping pigeons from roosting on building ledges. It was particularly helpful to owners of historical properties, who prefer

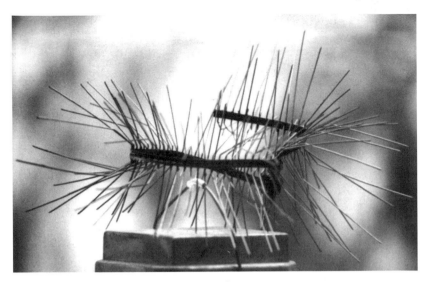

If you were a squirrel, would you get close to Nixalite?

not to have their architectural masterpieces covered with pigeon drop-pings. (I guess it's fair to malign pigeons in a book that's pro-bird, because they're not really birds but are more akin to, as Woody Allen once said, "rats with wings.") Nixalite is a prickly, barbed wire-type of material. It comes in twelve-inch strips, with sharp, three-inch spines protruding out of the strip. The spines all extend in the same direc-tion, but at varying angles, making it impossible for a pigeon to alight on them. Nixalite can be handled from the bottom, but you definitely wouldn't want to grab it from the sharp side. Presumably, a squirrel wouldn't want to leap onto that side, either.

I bought yet another feeder—a new wood-and-Plexiglas chalet feeder (the same kind I had before). I placed the Nixalite around the tops of the Perrier bottles so that the squirrel couldn't chomp away at my feeder. This time I was certain that the squirrel wouldn't be able to get into the feed and that soon he would become frustrated and go away. My feeder was surreal and scary. There it was, with sharp spines pro-truding dangerously in all directions. H.P. Lovecraft would have been proud. I wouldn't want to try to get into the feeder.

But I'm not a squirrel. Mr. Squirrel was undaunted by the Nixalite. At first he tried to eat it. (I've discovered that metal is just about the only thing squirrels can't gnaw through). Instead of giving up (something I've also discovered isn't a squirrel instinct), he just leapt to the top of my alpine-shaped feeder and fed himself upside down.

Attack, retreat, then counterattack. This was truly war and I was not about to lose.

By this time, Nixalite covered the feeder. It was impenetrable, with openings available only to creatures that fly. But again, I underestimated the depth of Mr. Squirrel's determination. At first he began to eat through the sides of the wooden feeder; as he was close to achieving success, he abruptly changed his strategy and decided simply to push the Nixalite away with his claws, risking a bit of discomfort perhaps, but creating a large area from which he could hang upside down and feed.

So I decided to obtain yet another feeder—and this time I placed it entirely out of reach of the squirrel by attaching it to the end of a long pole which I secured to the molding on the side of the window. The pole, made of steel and aluminum, extended up at a forty-five degree angle. My feeder was now about ten inches from the apartment building's wall; only if the squirrel could fly could he get to the feeder.

Wrong again. The squirrel now had a choice between leaping from the side of the building to the top of the feeder or shimmying up the pole to the feeder. "Great," I thought, "I've made things even easier for the little rodent." Well, if the squirrel could discover a simple solution, so could I: Nixalite on the top of the feeder would keep the squirrel off. And it did! Hurrah! I watched with glee as Mr. Squirrel climbed the pole, extended his paw to test the consistency of the feeder's roof, and determined that it was just too pointy and too risky to sit on.

Needless to say, I was very surprised and upset when I walked into my apartment the next afternoon and found a very elongated squirrel connected like a bridge between the building's wall and the feeder. With back claws on the wall and front claws on the feeder, Mr. Squirrel's mouth was happily munching away.

By now I had disposed of my dart gun, and ideas came to mind like blasting him with Formula 409, or running an electrical current to the feeder so that when the squirrel made his bridge, he would complete the circuit.

Instead, I rotated the feeder so that the long ends—the sides with the seed—were unreachable from the wall. To prevent the wind, or the squirrel, from rotating the feeder for easy access, I secured it with a copper wire attached to the feeder and the brick wall—another of the many uses of copper bell wire, which is one of the few things squirrels can't chew through, though not from the lack of trying. Although this meant that I couldn't see the birds that were eating on the far side of the feeder away from the window, neither could the squirrel reach the food. Still, I could watch the birds fly around and perch on the pole. And the squirrel was absolutely frustrated by this—until he figured out that he could just as easily stretch from the window screen to the feeder as he could from the wall to the feeder. It appeared to the squirrel—and to me—that the tiny grating that comprises the screen was designed to be a perfect match for squirrel claws. And I wasn't about to go without a screen: as much as I disliked squirrels, I hated mosquitoes even more.

So there we were: a standoff. Yes, I know, it wasn't exactly a standoff. Actually, the squirrel had won. The electric current idea seemed more attractive than ever, and I even went as far as visiting my local Radio Shack to explore the various paraphernalia—capacitors, more bell wire, waterproof batteries—that would make it work. It was tempting, but deep down I knew that even though the squirrel would be only scared, not electrocuted, by such a system, it wasn't right. Besides, despite my best efforts, I might accidentally zap a cardinal.

I was angry! Frustrated! Not since college, when one of my hallmates stole my towel and room keys while I was in the shower, had I been outwitted by a creature with a brain the size of a walnut.

I ransacked my apartment for devices that could be used to battle the squirrel. I tried the strobe flash from my camera. I figured if people don't like being momentarily blinded with a flash, squirrels probably don't either. Well, you know all those photographs of cute squirrels you see in newspapers, magazines, and slide shows you're forced to watch? All those pictures are there because squirrels enjoy having their photos taken. Shoot a squirrel with a flash, and he puts on a squirrel smile and stares at the camera, ready for another.

Once again, the only solution I could think of was buying a much more expensive feeder. This time I chose the GSP feeder, manufactured by the Clarke Products Company. The GSP is the king of feeders: very sleek, even "high-tech" looking. The feeder is a Lucite dome; birdseed fills a clear, hollow cavity within the walls of the dome. On top of the dome is an aluminum cover that slides up to reveal an opening through which the birdseed is replenished. Because the feeder hangs in the air and because the only way in is through the space at the GSP's bottom, the only creatures that can enter the feeder are those with wings. So I shelled out my sixty dollars and then set up the GSP feeder.

And my theory about squirrels not being able to fly was proved correct. The squirrel was very frustrated by this change of events: all his life he had succeeded in foiling humans, and now, at last, a human had won.

But the victory was short-lived. Somehow, the squirrel figured out a way to lift the aluminum top while standing on a smooth, downward sloping surface, and stick his head inside the opening that was intended for replenishing the feeder.

Well, here I was in possession of a sixty dollar so-called squirrelproof feeder whose only purpose, best I could tell, was to serve as a coordination test for squirrels. I wrote to the Clarke Products company and received a pleasant letter informing me that my squirrel was one of three that had learned how to remove the top cover to the feeder. The others were in Connecticut and Illinois. Fortunately there was a solution, the letter said. Clarke Products sent me a latch that goes above the top, requiring any creature that wants to lift the top to use two hands. And we all know that squirrels can't do that.

But what they can do is stretch from the screen on my window, pull the feeder toward them, and hoist themselves into the feeder. They're pretty adept at that.

I countered by putting the feeder on an even longer pole, extending horizontally from the wall of my building. Now there was no way—repeat *no way*—the squirrel could enter the feeder.

And this time I was right. He tried for days. For weeks. He even tried into the evening hours, when the fragile light was flittering away quickly into dangerous darkness, when squirrels want only to be safe in their nests. But he never could do it. My feeder was perfectly safe from Mr. Squirrel and his friends.

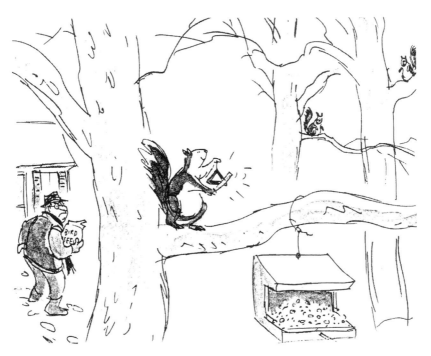

Drawing by Stevenson; © 1988 The New Yorker Magazine, Incorporated.

A few weeks later I read in one of those bird books that it's a good idea to have two feeders with different food in each because you attract more birds that way. So I attached another feeder to my window . . . .

(The GSP feeder and others are reviewed in chapter 5.)

TWO

Attracting Birds and Bird Personalities

Compared to outwitting squirrels, attracting birds to your feeder is virtually effortless. All you have to do is put out some seed, peanut butter, nuts, bread crumbs, or fruit, and birds will flock your way like people to a "50 percent off" sale. Leave the food on your porch, put it in a bowl, or tack it to a tree—that's all you need to do if you want birds in your backyard. This is called the minimalist approach. You don't even need a feeder. However, buying a feeder helps keep the birdfeeder companies in business, and without those companies there would be no wonderful color catalogs of birds and birding supplies. For this if for no other reason, feeders are essential.

Besides encouraging the proliferation of catalogs, there are several advantages to using a feeder instead of throwing seed on the ground. Seed on the ground gets eaten by anything that crawls; feeders provide a modicum of protection from squirrels. Also, many birds don't like to feed on the ground, preferring to eat above ground, plus feeders protect seed from rain, snow, and wind, and keep seed from getting all over the place.

Feeders and Food

Beyond the minimalist, throw-seed-and-watch approach, there are many ways you can coax your favorite species to your feeder and increase the number of birds that visit your yard. The first step, of course, is a feeder. The second step is the right feeder. Chapter 5, "Rating the Feeders," contains the most comprehensive discussion of feeders available anywhere and reveals which feeders are best for attracting which birds. Some important points to keep in mind regarding feeders follow.

First of all, keep your feeder full all year long. If you periodically let your feeder run out of feed, birds are going to seek their meals elsewhere. Birds—especially "desirable" ones such as cardinals and woodpeckers—develop loyalties to a particular area. They like to get to know an area where they feel safe. Birds build their nests where they are accustomed to the surroundings, where they know how to find emergency shelter if a cat or man wearing bright orange approaches. If you feed birds year round you will encourage them to nest near you. Also, some birds, such as red-bellied woodpeckers, appear so infrequently that if you want to attract them you'll have to provide chow all the time. Despite what you may have heard from your nonbirding friends, it's OK to feed birds throughout the year. If you've heard that you shouldn't feed birds in the summer because they'll become dependent on you, regard such utterances as nonsense. You'll bring no harm to birds by offering them seed year round. The truth is that birds do much better because people feed them. In a sense, they do depend on feeders.

But the most important reason to feed birds all year long is that as we turn more and more woodlands into shopping malls and highways, birds' natural sources of food disappear. Bird feeders like yourself are taking on nature's responsibility: you are helping birds survive and prosper. So feed all year long and enjoy.

As the seasons change, your feeding habits should change, too. Suet (hardened fat) is a terrific winter food that's enjoyed by just about every bird and adored by woodpeckers, but it doesn't hold up too well in summer. Suet, especially the home brewed kind, can turn rancid in warm weather, so check it periodically if you use it in summer. You may have to replace the suet before it gets eaten. (Alternatively, you can use suet as a squirrel diverter; it will be quickly consumed that way. See chapter 7 for more information about diverting squirrels.) Sometime in April or May, depending on where you live, hummingbirds appear. They follow the flowers north. As soon as red flowers come up you should put out a hummingbird feeder—these are wonderful birds to watch.

You should also clean your feeder frequently. Mold and fungi can grow in a feeder, especially after a rain, and turn yummy birdseed into deadly birdseed. Cleaning your feeder has another advantage: it gets the dirt and bird dropping off and lets you see the birds more easily.

There are three categories of feeders: window, hanging, and pole feeders. Window feeders attach to windows with suction cups. They can be filled with a variety of seeds and offer the closest view of birds. Birding stores and mail order houses sell one-way transparent film you can place over your window so that you can see the birds, but they can't see you. Window feeders are squirrel-resistant only if one of two conditions are met: a) there are no squirrels around or b) the feeder is surrounded by a sufficiently large area of glass. Squirrels can't climb glass. Hanging feeders come in dozens of different shapes, and in a range of squirrelproofness. They can be suspended from trees, specially designed poles, brackets that extend from houses or fences, or from wires strung between trees. Never hang a feeder from an electrical or telephone wire, as squirrels sometimes chew through the wires that support feeders (unless you like the taste of grilled squirrel). Pole-mounted feeders are designed to be placed on a pole or post. When properly baffled they can be very squirrelproof. These three feeder types enable you to place feeders just about anywhere you want. Chapter 5 discusses the placement of feeders in more detail.

George Petrides of the Wild Bird Center in Cabin John, Maryland, says that if you want to triple the number of birds you attract, "double the number of feeders." He also pointed out that if you put different food in each of the feeders, you'll do even better.

What should you fill your feeder with? There are over a dozen foods that birds like which are easy to purchase. Sunflower seeds, fruit, peanuts, and suet are among birds' favorites. What you put in your feeders will affect the species of birds you attract, and birds' tastes vary from season to season. A wren, for example, may eat hulled sunflower seed in the winter, but shun it in the summer.

I've divided birdseed into three categories: Universal, Specialty, and Gourmet.

Universal

Universal birdseed attracts just about every variety of bird, and every bird will eat it if hungry enough. Types of universal seed include perodovic sunflower seed, sunflower hearts, and peanut hearts. Mix them together and it'll look like a scene from Alfred Hitchcock's *The Birds* around your feeder.

Specialty

Specialty seed attracts only a handful of specific birds, and, perhaps more significantly, is disliked by certain birds. Safflower seed, for example, gets gobbled down by chickadees and finches, but starlings and grackles hate it. Chickadees, nuthatches, and titmice love shelled peanuts, but finches aren't too crazy about them. Most ground-feeding birds like millet, while birds that feed from hanging feeders will usually toss the millet aside. Other specialty seeds include yellow corn and canary seed.

Gourmet

Gourmet seed attracts only a very small number of birds and is expensive. Thistle seed, which brings in finches and can be used to attract goldfinches in particular, falls into this category. Raspberries and orange slices are other gourmet foods.

Seeds and the Birds They Attract

Sunflower seed

Cardinals	Chickadees	Crossbills
Finches	Grosbeaks	Mourning doves
Nuthatches	Sparrows	Starlings
Titmice		

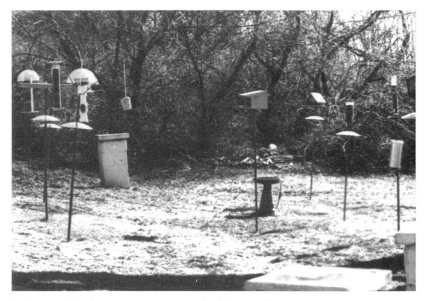

Inside the Wild Bird Center in Potomac, Maryland: there's a feeder for every fancy.

Sunflower hearts

Blackbirds	Cardinals	Chickadees
Goldfinches	House finches	Juncos
Mourning doves	Nuthatches	Redpolls
Sparrows	Wrens	

Fruit

Mockingbirds   Orioles

Suet

Red-bellied woodpeckers	Chickadees
Red-headed woodpeckers	Nuthatches
Downy woodpeckers	Titmice

Safflower seed

(Starlings and grackles don't like safflower seeds)

Cardinals	Chickadees	Purple finches
Titmice		

Thistle seed

Goldfinches	House finches	Indigo buntings
Juncos	Pine siskins	Purple finches
Redpolls		

Shelled peanuts

Blue jays	Cardinals	Chickadees
Grosbeaks	Nuthatches	Titmice
Towhees	Woodpeckers	

Whole peanuts

Blue jays	Titmice

White proso millet

Juncos	Mourning doves	Pine siskins
Purple finches		

Avoid commercial seed mixes sold in supermarkets and hardware stores that contain large amounts of millet and other less desirable seed. When a bird encounters a seed it doesn't want, it flicks that seed aside. People who fill their feeders with mixed seed containing millet usually find the ground beneath their feeder covered with millet. A much better idea is to erect two or three feeders, each with one kind of seed.

Water

Birds must have water to drink and to bathe. Water is so important that you can attract birds to your yard with a water station alone.

Plenty of commercial birdbaths are available, but you can just as easily construct your own. A clay plant dish makes an excellent bird-bath, as does a window birdfeeder or an aluminum trashcan lid turned upside down. Make sure your water station isn't too deep—three inches is the maximum. If the water is too deep, birds may have trouble escaping in an emergency, such as a cat attack. Be sure to locate your water station away from any place cats could hide. If you can put the birdbath on top of a baffled pole, that's even better. Give the bath a gradual slope by putting stones and pebbles along the outer rim.

Birds need water all year long, so don't neglect the birdbath in winter. Some catalogs and stores such as Duncraft and The Audubon Workshop (see Resources) sell heated birdbaths.

You're going to have to clean your birdbath from time to time unless it rains enough to wash the bath out. Bacteria and algae can grow rapidly in a birdbath.

Finally, squirrels like to drink from birdbaths, too. You can try to prevent squirrels from getting to your water station if you want, but water's inexpensive enough that this probably isn't worth the effort.

Nests and Boxes

You've probably noticed that birds like to rise early, sometimes causing you to awaken before your gray cells are ready. But when they're not active, birds do the same thing that you do. They sleep. This they do in nests, and the more nesting areas you have around your house, the more birds there will be.

You've already enticed birds to your yard by feeding them, so they're predisposed to set up home. You can encourage them to homestead by either providing them with nesting material or putting up birdhouses. Duncraft and The Wild Bird Center sell nesting material you can hang from a tree. Commercial nesting material consists of twine, cotton, sisal, hemp, and yarn—for birds these materials are a good adjunct to what they find in nature. You can also leave out thread and twigs for birds to build nests from. Most birds use this material, including chickadees, goldfinches, robins, and orioles.

Commercial birdhouses are available in a variety of shapes. Different species prefer different kind of houses based on entrance size, inside space, and appearance. Chickadees, downy woodpeckers, nuthatches, wrens, barn owls, bluebirds, and purple martins love to live in manmade houses. The Audubon Workshop, Duncraft, and Wild Bird Center all offer a wide variety of birdhouses. If you're looking for a birdhouse that will impress the neighbors, Richard Clark, owner of The Bird House, makes very artistic birdhouses by hand.

You can also build your own birdhouses. Milk cartons with one-inch holes near the top make excellent temporary nesting sites. If you're going to construct a birdhouse, make sure the wood is three-quarters to one inch thick and that it is treated with a wood preservative or, at the very least, paint.

Whichever birdhouse you buy, be sure to protect it from predators. Squirrels eat baby birds and eggs. Cats like to patrol around birdhouses, so make certain that all they can do is watch. Putting the birdhouse on top of a baffled pole is a good idea; Nixalite can also help keep cats and other predators away. Birdhouses must be securely mounted because when they fall baby birds die. If the birdhouse tenants leave for summer or winter vacation, take that opportunity to clean the birdhouse. Make sure that rain can't spill inside, or drill drainage holes if it does. Ventilation should be adequate, and the birdhouse shouldn't be placed in a place where it receives direct sun during the hottest part of the summer day.

The chart below shows the size of birdhouses that various birds prefer. Use this guide when building or buying a birdhouse. For all these birds, the entrance should be about six to eight inches above the birdhouse floor.

Birdhouse preferences
(in inches)

	Floor space	Depth	Entrance hole diameter
Bluebird	5 x 5	8	1½
Chickadee	4 x 4	8–10	1⅛
Crested flycatcher	6 x 6	8–10	2
Downy woodpecker	4 x 4	8–10	1¼
Nuthatch	4 x 4	8–10	1¼
Wren	4 x 4	6–8	1–1¼

Your Backyard

Have you ever wondered why New York has few birds and why those that are there are congregated in Central Park? There's a clear relationship between the number of plants and flowers and the number of birds. The ideal backyard for attracting birds is surrounded by trees and filled with shrubs and flowering plants. Dead trees help, too: if you have dead trees around don't cut them down. Of course, if a dead tree is threatening your house, the house takes priority. If you must cut down dead trees, make sure that there aren't any nests in the cavities and plant new trees to replace the dead ones. Dead trees are excellent sources of food and shelter for many species of birds.

Personality Profiles of Some Common Birds

Now that you know how easy it is to attract birds of different species to your yard, it's worth knowing a little about how these birds behave and what they expect of you. As you spend more and more time at your feeder (and you will, it's an addicting hobby), you'll notice that each species not only looks different but has its own personality, preferred feeding time, and way of eating. The sketches below are intended only to introduce you to these birds as birders know them. For more detailed information, consult the bird books listed in Resources.

Chickadee

Of the various kinds of chickadees, the black-capped is the most familiar. It is one of the smallest and friendliest birds to visit feeders—a chickadee will eat out of your hand if you're patient. Chickadees weigh about one-third of an ounce, the same as four pennies. They are predominantly black with a black cap, white cheeks, and a white-yellow underbelly.

Chickadees are fun to watch. They zip over to your feeder, grab a nut or sunflower seed, then zip to a tree to eat; as soon as they're finished they fly right back. They are constantly active, hopping from tree to feeder to branch; if they were people, they'd probably be offered a sedative. Chickadees will eat whole nuts, sunflower and safflower seeds, suet—pretty much anything. They will eat from platform feeders, hanging feeders, and pole-mounted feeders. Because of their size you can frequently adjust feeders to allow chickadees in, but prevent larger birds from getting the seed.

In flight, chickadees are acrobats. They can change directions in mid-air in three one-hundredths of a second. You'll never get bored watching them. Naturalist George Harrison in *The Backyard Birdwatcher* writes, "If there is such a thing as reincarnation, I want to come back as a chickadee."

Tufted titmouse

Both the titmouse and chickadee are part of the titmouse family, and their behavior is similar. Like the chickadee, the tufted titmouse has a fun-loving, spirited personality. With its diminutive size, strong-looking face and beak, gray back, white belly and tufted top (its crest), the titmouse is probably the cutest bird that visits feeders. They walk and explore the area around your feeder, turning their heads from side to side, raising and lowering their crest. They do this with a quizzical look, as if they were trying to communicate with you.

Titmice are loyal birds, and will stay near a feeder all year long. They are particularly common during winter. Although not as tame as chickadees, you may be able to get titmice to eat out of your hand.

Like the chickadee, the tufted titmouse usually grabs a seed, then takes it away and eats on a branch. They'll do this with even a whole peanut—it's an amusing sight to watch a bird carry a nut that's about one-fifth its size. Titmice pound the seed against the branch to get it open. A friend of mine watching this action and noting the titmice's unusual crest dubbed these birds, "hammerhead birds."

Cardinal

The cardinal is a bird that many high school, college, and some professional sports teams make their mascot, which surprises most birders. Although the cardinal is among the most beautiful birds attracted to feeders, it is timid and aloof. However, cardinals are territorial, and during mating season they will bully their rivals to drive them off. Their mating-season agressiveness may be the link between the coy cardinal and sports teams.

Male cardinals are brilliant red and have a crest. Female cardinals have the same crest, but are rose-colored. In winter cardinals travel in flocks, so if you have one at your feeder you're likely to have several. During the midspring to summer breeding season you'll see cardinals either alone or in pairs. Cardinals don't migrate.

Cardinals are ground-feeders, so you're not likely to find them on a perch at a hanging feeder. Platform feeders filled with sunflower seed (their favorite food) or seed that spills from other feeders will attract cardinals. Nuts, safflower seed, and cracked corn may also appeal to cardinals. These birds prefer to snack early in the morning or just before dark. However, during bad weather and winter they will appear at feeders throughout the day. If cardinals survive childhood, they can live three years in the wild.

Downy woodpecker

The downy woodpecker is the smallest and tamest American woodpecker, and is a frequent visitor to feeders. When not hammering small holes in your house early in the morning (and especially on weekend mornings), downy woodpeckers enjoy beef suet but will also eat sunflower seeds and whole peanuts. A regular supply of beef suet may keep them from turning your house into a toothpick factory.

When you hear a downy—or other woodpecker—go tap tap tap it may be doing one of two things. Irregular tapping noises mean the woodpecker is looking for food and you've run out of suet. A regular drumming sound is a signal that usually occurs during breeding season and probably won't damage your house.

The downy is about the size of a house sparrow, with a larger beak and longer tail. It has black and white markings and the male has a red patch on its head.

Downies are found throughout North America. They make their nests between three and fifty feet above the ground on the bottom side of tree limbs. Downy woodpeckers will help clear your garden of undesirable insects, so attract as many as you can. A healthy downy can live over ten years.

House wren

An adorable little brown bird, the house wren doesn't seem to mind being around people and houses. It nests comfortably in store-bought nesting boxes, in homemade boxes fabricated from milk cartons, or in old shoes and discarded couches.

The wren has an assertive, energetic personality. Despite its small size, the house wren has an aggressive nature when it comes to nests. The males will often fly from nesting box to nesting box in their territory, decorating the interior so that other birds think the box is full. A wren will also follow a downy woodpecker to its nest and may even chase away a pair of downies it finds there. When a wren decides that it wants to nest somewhere, nothing will drive it away.

Wrens eat mostly insects, but are drawn by suet, cornbread, and hulled sunflower seed in the colder months. Once in your yard, they're likely to remain there (and help keep the insect population down).

House finch

One day my friend decides that "the finches are OK because it's nice to have any kind of bird at the feeder," and the next day she declares, "I wish all those noisy finches would go away." But she also adds, "My cat Travis thinks they are great. For any cat, finches are kitty TV." If there's one thing about finches, its that there's no such thing as one finch. They arrive in groups so large that you have to use all your fingers and toes to count them. Finches will crowd closely together at a feeder as they eat—I once saw seven side by side at the feeder in my yard.

House finches are lively, aggressive birds. They will scream and poke at each other for space at the feeder, and sometimes carry on this quarrel in midflight. I've seen house finches successfully challenge downy woodpeckers and chickadees for a position at the feeder.

Still, they are vivacious and spectacular birds, and a flock of them can empty a feeder faster than a squirrel. They're constantly in motion, constantly sounding off, and while they are far from charming to the eye, the males sport a bright red breast that puts house finches in the category of fairly attractive birds. Females, alas, are nondescript.

House finches were originally native only to the western United States. In the 1940s pet dealers in California captured some of these birds and sold them in New York as "Hollywood birds." It didn't take long for U.S. Fish and Wildlife officials to catch up with these dealers—selling wild birds was illegal. Rather than be caught selling wild birds, some dealers released their house finches, and the birds survived and prospered.

House finches will nest almost anywhere. Likewise they will eat almost anything, although they aren't terribly fond of cracked corn, millet, and hulled oats. Unfortunately finches rarely eat insects, so they won't do anything to reduce the number of mosquito bites you receive each year.

One of the most interesting features of house finches is the way they move together. A flock will be eating at a feeder and then suddenly—seemingly without reason—fly away. And then just as suddenly they will return.

The best time to observe house finches is in late March and early April during mating season. To entice females, males do a bit of a song and dance and then feed the females. At feeders you can watch females crane their necks back, open their mouths and wait for males to put seed in it. It's a wonderful sight.

Mourning dove

Oh-cooo oh-cooo oh-cooo. The mourning dove is a cousin of the—dare I use the word—pigeon, but fortunately there's little significant family resemblance. (A closer cousin is the extinct passenger pigeon.) Mourning doves make one of the most satisfying sounds—the dove's soft melody is like a natural Valium. In the winter mourning doves travel in flocks of about twenty, but they nest as pairs.

Mourning doves are twelve inches long, sleeker than pigeons, and have pointed tails. They have a rust-beige head and breast, and gray tailfeathers specked with white and black.

Mourning doves are ground-feeding birds (their favorite food is cracked corn but they like millet and black sunflower, too) so that is where you will usually see them. They are exceptional fliers, and have been clocked at up to sixty miles per hour. Although they are widely hunted as a game bird, mourning doves are a successful species, with an estimated 500 million throughout the United States. Their range extends north into Alaska and south to Panama.

Doves will defend their territory against other birds while nesting, but they are usually shy birds. They quickly launch into the air at the earliest sign of danger.

Starling

People who like starlings are also squirrel lovers. That statement isn't based on a formal study, but it seems to make sense. I'm sure you'll agree.

Starlings are a regular pain at feeders. Most likely a comment like that won't win me any points with the die-hard birding community, which treats all feathered creatures with the utmost adoration, but 99 percent of birdfeeder owners would rather not have them. Starlings are noisy, aggressive, and not terribly pleasant to look at. They chase away other birds, eat plenty of birdseed, and make a big mess at feeders, attracting squirrels to mop the spilled seed from the ground.

Starlings are not native to America, as you probably guessed by the way they respond to our hospitality. They were brought over from Europe in 1890 by birders who thought starlings would make a welcome addition—like perfume or something. Sixty pairs were released in Central Park. As soon as they could they left New York and within fifty years had spread across the country.

Starlings are one of the few birds that dramatically change appearance over the year. In the winter their black feathers are covered with specks of white that look like Vs. In summer they are mostly black and iridescent green. Starlings roost in large numbers—dozens of birds. They're awkward fliers and dislike wooded areas. They will invade nesting boxes with holes larger than two inches. Starlings love suet, peanut hearts, bakery goods, and cracked corn. They shun thistle, whole peanuts, and sunflower seeds.

One fascinating aspect of starling behavior, however, is the way they gather in flocks. Sometimes you can see hundreds of starlings circling a small area, flying 'round and 'round for an hour. It's a fascinating sight.

Starlings are smart. It's rumored that you can even teach a starling to talk like a parrot.

Pigeon

Not a bird. Put here by mistake.

Goldfinch

If   int to know how arbitrary humans can be, just measure their
re   n to the goldfinch versus the house finch. The major difference
h   en goldfinches and house finches is color. The goldfinch's bright
        d feathers (which become grayish-yellow in winter after molting)
        e a stark contrast to the house finch's drab looks. They are both
        around the same size, have many similar behavior traits, eat the same
seed, and eat in the same manner—they gorge themselves.

Entire chapters in bird books are devoted to goldfinches, but house
and purple finches usually get grouped under the heading of "other
birds." I'm not trying to defend house finches—I'm wooed by goldies'
looks like every other feeder—and I certainly think that house finches
eat far more seed than they deserve. I just want to be honest.

Goldfinches are sometimes mistakenly called "wild canaries" because of their color and their song. If you want to draw goldfinches
put out niger (thistle) seed; although goldfinches like black sunflower
seed, they will travel anywhere for thistle. So much do they love it,
you could probably attract them into your house with a trail of thistle.
Goldfinches prefer to eat at perches. If you want to deter house finches,
cut the perches on your hanging feeder to about one-third of an inch;
the goldfinches can grab on, but house finches can't maintain their
balance and eat.

Goldfinches like to live in open areas such as orchards beside roads
and in swamps. Man's clearing of woodlands has encouraged their
spread. In the wild they thrive on thistle and insects. In September the
goldfinch's feathers molt, changing from gold to a dark olive color.
Goldfinches are not territorial. Instead they are tolerant of other species of birds, even during breeding season.

The goldfinch is the state bird of Iowa, New Jersey, and Washington.

Nuthatch

Small children and adults from New York call the nuthatch "the upside-down bird," because it can often be seen climbing down trees
upside down. It's unusually designed feet enable it to walk down trees
head first. Most birds have four toes; three in the front and one in the

back. But the nuthatch has two on either side. This feature also enables nuthatches to capture many insects that other birds miss on trees.

The nuthatch is bluish-gray—a pretty bird, though not spectacular like the cardinal or blue jay. Its call, *ank ank ank*, is distinctive. The white-breasted nuthatch is the largest and most common nuthatch in North America. The red-breasted nuthatch is usually found in the forests of the West and north of the Great Lakes.

Nuthatches live in cavities or in abandoned woodpecker holes in trees. They eat plenty of insects in summer, and in the winter are frequent visitors to feeding stations, where they consume sunflower seeds, sunflower hearts, suet, and shelled peanuts.

Nuthatches' ranges extend up to fifty acres. Like chickadees and titmice, nuthatches aren't bothered by human company—they can be tamed to eat sunflower seed out of your hand. Some people even claim that nuthatches can be trained to get used to particular individuals so that they come when called by that person.

Blue jay

I have to admit a bias. I'm partial to the blue jay. Like its western cousin, the striking Steller's jay, the blue is one of the most beautiful birds that visits feeders. Within the birding community there's a debate over which is more beautiful, the cardinal or blue jay. The verdict is not in.

Blue jays are about twelve inches long, and are covered mostly with blue feathers. Around their neck is a "bright" band of black. The blue jay's iridescent color isn't entirely intrinsic to the bird's feathers; in certain lights blue jays appear almost colorless.

Blue jays receive a lot of bad press. They're blamed for scaring other birds away from feeders with their aggressive approach. Jays can imitate the sound of hawks. There's another myth that a blue jay will give a fake warning call when it arrives at a feeder to give the impression that danger abounds. Both assertions are only marginally true. Jays sometimes frighten other birds, but are no more aggressive than house finches, and given their relative size, blue jays can even be considered

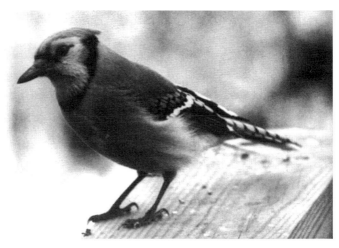

The striking blue jay.

docile. Jays don't hang around feeders for long periods of time, either. If blue jays are disrupting your feeder, put a separate feeder aside for jays and fill it with peanuts. As for the "false alarm" myth, sometimes jays will squawk as they approach a feeding station, but other birds either learn to ignore this or simply wait a couple of minutes before returning to the feeder.

There are those who claim that blue jays raid nests, eat eggs, and occasionally eat young birds. These claims come from the same people who have explored the interiors of UFOs. Blue jays are protective parents. They will attack any creature that approaches their nest. Some jays migrate south during the winter, others prefer to stay put.

To entice blue jays, it helps to have acorns in abundance. (Blue jays compete with squirrels for the acorn crop. The more jays the merrier.) Shelled or whole peanuts are their second favorite dish, followed by black sunflower seed and suet. Jays nest in shrubs and small, wide trees—the more plant cover, the better. Jays are fond of birdbaths, too.

Jays store food by burying nuts. You can also see them carrying several shelled nuts in their mouths at a time. The number of jays in any given year depends in large measure on the number of acorns during the previous season.

Junco

The junco is one of people's favorites. It's handsome (though not spectacular), doesn't make much noise, doesn't bother other birds, doesn't eat too much, doesn't spill seed around, and doesn't come in large flocks. In spring and summer juncos gorge themselves on insects and enjoy eating seeds that other birds shun such as red proso millet (their favorite), cracked corn, and canary seed. They also eat black sunflower seed and suet. Juncos are primarily ground-feeding birds.

The junco also goes by the name "snowbird" because it usually appears at feeders at the first snow. It lives in the northern, western, and eastern parts of the United States, journeying south during winter. The junco is not only well behaved, but has a sense of loyalty, too, and will return to the same feeder year after year. The junco likes to get up early.

In 1984, Lafayette Park, across the street from the White House, once had more squirrels than any other place in the world. "The density of squirrels in that park is the highest ever recorded in the scientific literature," said David Manski, an urban wildlife biologist. There were an estimated 120 squirrels in the eight-acre park, thanks in large part to tourists and residents who feed them every day. One Washington resident confessed to spending between $60 and $90 a week on nuts for squirrels. These "volunteer feeders" provide 75 percent of park squirrels' diets in winter. U.S. Park officials resorted to squirrelnapping and moved squirrels to other Washington parks to reduce the number of squirrels in Lafayette Park.

THREE

Know the Enemy

Everything a Bird Feeder Needs to Know About Squirrels

Who does not know and like squirrels?

—*Animals of the World*

The large gray squirrel (*Sciurus carolinensis*) I do not find as plentiful in Campton, Massachusetts, as the other two species; for several seasons past, very few have appeared in the wood or on the roadside. In Roxbury, a part of Boston, they are quite common among the trees on some of the old estates, and they are often seen in the hemlock grove in the Arnold arboretum. Nothing can be more graceful than their scalloped lines of flight along a tree bough.

The gray squirrel is a sociable little animal who likes the company of a man with a few nuts in his pocket. One cannot walk across the square in Richmond, Virginia, without encountering two or three tame individuals who regard a man as a species of aniated nut tree created for his especial benefit!

If we will watch a squirrel closely we may observe him tuck away two or three small nuts in his cheeks and carry another in his teeth. Last summer one of my friendly chipmunks made six journeys within two hours from a certain corner of the house to his nest beneath a fence post by the road, for the purpose of transferring his summer stores. One would suppose upon beholding his bulgy cheeks that he was afflicted with a severe form of mumps.

—F. Schuyler Mathews, *Familiar Features of the Roadside*

If you're going to do battle with squirrels, you're going to lose every time—unless you know as much about them as you possibly can. Intelligence is frequently 90 percent of any war—and the war against squirrels is no exception. The Japanese knew all about Pearl Harbor in 1941. Israel's victory in 1967 was due in large measure to superior Israeli intelligence. The Soviet bugging of the U.S. Embassy in Moscow rendered our embassy virtually useless for confidential work. Mata Hari was famous only because she gathered facts. Regular soldiers may be interned in prisoner of war camps during wartime, but spies are shot because one scrap of useful information about the enemy can be worth a thousand soldiers.

I repeat: you have to know everything about squirrels. Because they know everything about you.

Squirrels know that when you fill a feeder, you're ringing the dinner bell for them. Squirrels know that you're going to put baffles on top of feeders, so in the meanwhile they practice their jumping skills. Squirrels know that you may occasionally scream and flail your arms at them, but that in a few minutes you'll go away. Squirrels know that if they gnaw through one feeder, you'll buy another for them to sharpen their teeth on. Squirrels know that if you string a feeder between two trees on a thin wire, they've rehearsed their tightrope-walking skills. Squirrels know that if they eat the feed you've put out for birds, you'll just put out more. Squirrels know not to attack your spouse, children, and pets, because that might cause you to react violently. Squirrels know that no matter what, there's going to be delicious seed in your yard. Yes, indeed, squirrels know humans pretty well.

The gray squirrel is called *Sciurus carolinensis* by those who study them for a living. There are dozens of species of squirrels, some of

Gray Squirrel Fact Sheet

(Remember, you can't tell the players without a scorecard.)

Latin name:
Sciurus carolinensis

Adult female weight:
16–24 ounces

Adult male weight:
16–24 ounces

Length:
8–11 inches with a tail that measures 8–10 inches

Home range size:
1–7 acres (some biologists report that squirrel ranges
extend to 20 acres)

Number of plant species eaten (most are eaten rarely;
however, gardeners beware):
30–60

Foods:
Tree nuts, plant seeds, fruit, flowers, mushrooms,
buds, birdseed, peanut butter (preferably Skippy
Super Chunk)

Percentage of food from animal matter (including bird eggs):
2–11 percent

Mean annual survival rate in the wild:
52 percent

Life span:
About one year in the wild; up to twelve years as pets
(which is far longer than the furniture survives)

Reproduction:
Usually two litters a year

them very cute. (There are thirty-six species of flying squirrels in Europe, Asia, North America, and Central America.) The cute squirrels stay in forests and eat only acorns, wild berries, hickory nuts, and other foods that squirrels were originally supposed to eat. Squirrels are generally classified into two groups: those that dwell in trees, such as the gray squirrel, the flying squirrel (*Glaucomys volans*), the tassel-eared squirrel (*Sciurus aberti*), and the eastern fox squirrel (*Sciurus niger*) are called tree squirrels. The second group are ground squirrels—squirrels that think it isn't wise for a ten-inch-long animal to climb a sixty-foot-tall tree, and consequently never venture up. These include the beautiful golden mantle squirrel.

Squirrels are members of the rodent family, sometimes called by zoologists the "order of gnawing animals." The word "rodent" comes from the Latin *rodere*, meaning to gnaw—and there are over 1,600 species of rodents. But there's a forest-wide difference between the various members of the rodent family, which include squirrels, beavers, rabbits, mice, and rats. Rodents behave differently, eat different foods, and look different, which is a real blessing. Could you imagine how much more awful the squirrel problem would be if squirrels not only pilfered birdseed, but also looked like their distant relatives, rats?

Squirrels evolved between fifty-four to thirty-seven million years ago in North America during the Eocene epoch. Using the land bridges that existed between continents, squirrels may have spread to Africa during the Miocene era, some twenty-five to five million years ago, and into South America after the Panama land bridge formed about three million years ago. Near the end of the Oligocene era, roughly thirty to twenty-five million years ago, squirrels diversified into true tree- and ground-dwelling squirrels, a metamorphosis that apparently came about because of changes in climate and vegetation. The origins of *Sciurus carolinensis*, the gray squirrel, are unknown.

Squirrels have only one thing to do all day long: eat. Practically every activity they're involved in concerns food. Their physical make-up enables them to be perpetual eating machines. A mere 2 percent of a squirrel's energy goes into making babies. (No Dr. Ruths in the squirrel world.) Just about all of the remaining 98 percent focuses on food. Your food. Squirrels are land sharks, living eating machines.

Squirrels and Food

Squirrels eat a lot. You don't need a zoologist to tell you that. Adult gray squirrels consume roughly one and a half pounds of nuts or seed a week. That may not sound like a lot, but squirrels eat as much as or more than their entire body weight each week. (You try that and see what happens.) A mere four squirrels will polish off six pounds of birdseed in a week. Squirrels can demolish about three ounces of food in one sitting, which means that four of them will empty a small one-pound feeder in the time it takes you to mail order more birdseed.

Crammed into the tiny squirrel is a seven-foot-long digestive tract, capable of handling a variety of foods. Squirrels' favorite fares, more or less in order of preference, are hickory nuts, pecans, black walnuts, and acorns. They enjoy just about every kind of nut and berry that forests provide, including pine seed, corn, black gum fruits, sugar maple seeds, dogwood fruits, wild cherries, and beechnuts. Although acorns provide more nutrients for squirrels than hickory nuts, they prefer the latter hands down. One of the reasons may be that the hickory nut's hard shell helps squirrels sharpen their teeth. Another may be because hickory nuts taste terrific. But most likely the reason is that hickory nuts have a very high fat content, 29 percent, and fat is essential to a squirrel's nutrition. According to naturalist and writer Ernest Thompson Seton, a squirrel's love for hickory nuts "amounts almost to a passion." Seton elaborates:

> A squirrel will pass by all other foods, and brave innumerable dangers for a feast of his favorites. So eager is he for the annual bounty of his mother tree, that he cannot await the decent time of ripening, but cuts them while they are green. He is like an overeager, greedy small boy who is too impatient to wait for the thorough baking of his cake, so he nibbles and nibbles at the unsatisfactory, unwholesome dough (*Life Histories of Northern Animals*, Charles Scribner's Sons, 1909).

In all, there are over seven major squirrel foods. Gray squirrels will eat between thirty to sixty different plants. (Compare that to the average American, whose major sustenance consists of a Big Mac, fries, and a Coke, with occasional experiments with exotic dishes such as chili dogs or onion dip.)

Acorns, however, are among the most important food for gray squirrels, both the city and forest varieties. Oak trees go through five-year cycles of acorn production, and as a result squirrel populations go through five-year cycles. You can predict how many baby squirrels there are going to be by the acorn crop.

Which birdseed do squirrels like best? An experiment was conducted at the Schlitz Audubon Center in Milwaukee, Wisconsin, to test birds' preferences for seed. Twelve Droll Yankee feeders were strung along a wire, each filled with a different seed. The entire apparatus was protected by various baffles. The birds never had a chance. Within minutes several gray squirrels attacked the feeders. The researchers discovered that squirrels prefer black sunflower seeds; once sunflower seeds are gone, squirrels begin on other seed. Squirrels are not too fond of thistle but will eat it when they're hungry enough. Gray squirrels prefer white acorns to red and black acorns when given a choice, possibly because of the relatively high tannin content of red and black acorns. Tannin may make acorns less tasty and less digestible.

Gray squirrels are omnivorous. In addition to vegetable matter, such as berries and nuts, they also eat minerals and animals. Squirrels also strip bark on trees, possibly for several reasons: to sharpen their teeth, to obtain some of the nutrients in the sappy tissue beneath the bark, to gather material to line their nests, and as a behavioral characteristic.

Gray squirrels have earned the term "tree rat" because of the damage they do to hardwood trees by stripping bark. They gnaw at the bark until they make a hole, then use this notch to strip the bark off by pulling on it. Occasionally squirrels will kill a tree by stripping the bark around a tree's entire circumference. Other times, bark stripping makes trees susceptible to a variety of fungal diseases. The problem of bark stripping is particularly prevalent in England, where the European sycamore and beech trees have been severely damaged in tree plantations. Squirrels also eat buds and shoots on trees, damaging new growth.

Squirrels also eat mushrooms, including the deadly amanita, apparently for the nutrients they offer. They have no problem with nontraditional foods, either. Apples, peanut butter, peanut M&Ms (they don't seem to like red ones), and corn on the cob, buttered or unbuttered, meet their requirements for taste.

Squirrels will also eat bird eggs, baby birds, and the bones of dead mammals. Approximately 10 percent of their diet comes from animal matter, which also includes insects. Apparently squirrels derive some nutrients, probably calcium, from these meats.

Although squirrels obtain some of the water they need from non-nut foods such as berries, fruits, and grasses, squirrels must drink water twice a day. You'll notice that squirrels visit your birdbath as often as birds do. In winter squirrels will eat snow for water.

A squirrel's teeth are its most important tool. Two pairs of surgically sharp incisors enable squirrels to gnaw through the outside of any nut, and practically any substance. Wood and plastic pose no problem for squirrels; squirrels can even make holes in certain kinds of metal. One of my friends swears that a squirrel gnawed through the telephone wire that her feeder was hanging from. Flesh, as I unfortunately discovered while examining a squirrel closely, is the easiest material for squirrels to bite through. A squirrel's incisors grow about six inches a year, and must constantly be worn down by eating or chewing on various objects like fence posts and fingers. If a squirrel looses its teeth, or if it suffers a malocclusion, that's the equivalent of a death sentence.

After the squirrel uses its incisors to cut and strip the food, it passes it to four pairs of premolars, which look like pegs, where it is ground into fine fragments. Peeling is an important part of the eating process. If you watch a squirrel eat a raw peanut or acorn, you'll see how it carefully strips away the undesirable parts. Squirrel jaws make two motions. First, the lower jaw is pulled forward so that the bottom and top incisors can gnaw the food, then the lower jaw pulls back so the cheek teeth can grind the food.

Gray squirrels prefer to dine while sitting on their back legs, but can eat from any position, including upside down. A squirrel hanging from its back legs, its paws wrapped around a chain with a sunflower seed in its front paws, is a common sight among birders. Squirrels can even eat when their bodies are stretched out between a tree and a feeder. Squirrels bury nuts to store for the winter, when there's little natural food. That's not news. What is interesting is that despite squirrels' intense interest in food, squirrels cannot remember where they've buried a nut for more than twenty minutes. Not very smart animals, after all, it seems. Or are they? Although squirrels don't know where their nuts are buried, they have no problem locating nuts that they or other squirrels have buried. Squirrels locate buried nuts using their sense of smell, and can find nuts buried under several inches of snow. In fact, most of the nuts a squirrel recovers will not be the ones it buried. Caching nuts is one of their most important survival instincts. Squirrels bury nuts communally so that all members of the species in the area benefit. Almost as soon as they leave the nest, young squirrels start burying nuts, although at first they don't completely cover the nut.

Squirrels can bury up to twenty-five nuts an hour. They bury nuts over a widely scattered area, which is called scatterhoarding.

There's another advantage to scatterhoarding besides providing nuts for other squirrels. There are many other species that forage for buried nuts, and if a competing species finds many nuts in a small area it will probably stay there. However, scatterhoarding, with its low density of nuts, prevents competitors from finding a large cache, because there is none.

In semi-urban areas squirrels become desperate for places to bury nuts. According to the *Washington Post*, "an alarming number . . . have chosen to stockpile their nuts in electrical transformers at the top of power poles." The result? "Squirrels are getting zapped and electrical blackouts are increasing." In one day in the Washington area there were seven squirrel-inspired blackouts.

Squirrels' burying instinct is powerful. In the building where I have my writing studio there's a woman who feeds squirrels on her windowsill. She mentioned that squirrels occasionally come into her apartment through the window. They steal peanuts from her kitchen counter and bury them in her avocado plant.

Spring is a crucial season for squirrels, because during the winter they loose a considerable amount of weight. At the end of March, when squirrels are at their lowest weight, they must seek new plant growth—buds, berries, and stalks—and new birdfeeders. A squirrel's weight varies by as much as 25 percent between autumn and spring. That's some diet!

Physical Capabilities

When you read a list describing the prowess of squirrels you might think that they are the supermen of the lower animals. They have immensely powerful hind legs. Squirrels can jump up to six feet. They can leap between trees that are eight feet apart. They can climb up dozens of feet and scale just about every surface except glass. They're swift, too. Squirrels have been clocked at nineteen miles per hour—definitely not faster than a speeding locomotive, but a heck of a lot swifter than many people. Squirrels can swim. Yes, swim. Up to a mile. To swim, squirrels manage a variation of the dog paddle, keeping their heads above water and their tails either just above or on the surface. Squirrels can dig up earth and burrow through snow to create tunnels.

Squirrels have acute senses. Their sense of smell is uncanny. Their hearing enables them to be aware of any changes in the flow of sounds in the woods. They can hear doors opening, a predator walking, or a feeder being filled. A squirrel's vision is also remarkably powerful, and its eyes, which are situated on opposite sides of its head, give the squirrel a wide range of vision without moving its head. It was once thought that gray squirrels had only cone cells in their eyes, but now researchers are sure they have rod cells (sensitive to light) near the center of their retina, and cone cells (for distinguishing colors) around the rods. This gives squirrels the ability to see fine detail including vertical objects, which is a necessity if you're leaping from tree to tree. It's said that one squirrel can distinguish another from a distance of fifty feet. Squirrel eyes also respond quickly to changes in their field of vision; they can see objects moving twice as fast as a human can. Grays possess dichromatic color vision (humans have trichromatic vision). They can't distinguish between red and green, which may help explain why so many never make it across the street.

Squirrels have two peak activity times during the day in the spring, summer, and fall: the first two hours after sunrise and midafternoon. In the winter they are active only around noon. In February they spend 73 percent of their time foraging for food; in August only 31 percent. Dawn is a more important signal for the start of squirrel activity than dusk is for ending it. In cold weather squirrels spend more time in their nests, and have been known to spend several days there during particularly severe weather. Squirrels become lethargic in hot weather, and may take a siesta in the middle of the day. Rain doesn't bother squirrels.

Squirrels mark travel lanes which they journey along, just as we might use a path. These lanes, which are on the ground and among branches in trees, are marked by scent from the squirrels' glands. Because they know these paths, squirrels can swiftly leap from branch to branch, certain of what lies ahead.

Squirrels molt twice a year, in spring and autumn. Molting starts at the nose and eyes and then moves in a fixed pattern across the body.

Squirrels are either right-handed or left-handed.

Squirrel Anatomy and Growth

Although this may come as a surprise to most birders, there are other parts to a squirrel besides its eating and digestive system. Indeed, many lay people who study squirrels divide these mammals into two anatomically distinct systems: the part that eats, and the rest of the squirrel.

Perhaps the most prominent aspect of the squirrel is its tail. A squirrel's tail extends between eight and ten inches, as long as the squirrel is itself. A squirrel's tail is covered with soft, fine fur, and without it you would have a hard time telling the difference between a squirrel's tail and a rat's tail. The name "squirrel" is derived from Greek words meaning "shade" and "tail." Squirrels' tails fulfill many purposes, including providing shade in the hot summer. Squirrels use their tails for balance when leaping and climbing, for warmth in the winter when they wrap their tails around them as they sleep, and to communicate with other squirrels. Because tails are so important, squirrels spend considerable time grooming them. Naturalist Alan Devoe wrote, "The tail is to the squirrel what vision is to the hawk or fleetness to a deer or wariness to a fox. He lives by it" (*Our Animal Neighbors*, McGraw Hill, 1953).

Squirrels use their wide whiskers to determine whether the hole they're climbing into is large enough for them.

Squirrel coats have never faded from fashion. Men and women who own squirrel coats discover that the soft fur is pleasant to touch (assuming there are no live teeth attached to it), and very warm. Squirrels think so, too.

The gray squirrel isn't exclusively gray. The fur is a mixture of brown, gray, and yellow on top, white and gray underneath; a squirrel's coloration changes as the seasons change. The tail is silver, with dots of frosty white on the tips of the hair. There's no discernible difference between the appearance of male and female squirrels. The only way to tell which is which is to turn them upside down. It's not worth the effort.

The squirrel is a miracle of energy efficiency. Because squirrels do not hibernate, they must be prepared to brave the winter chills without the benefit of L.L. Bean. A squirrel's fur provides the first defense against the cold. Beneath the outer layer of fur is an underfur that gives squirrels added insulation and protects the skin. And beneath the skin is a layer of fat.

Squirrels grow rapidly. When they are one day old, squirrels measure about four inches long, and are furless, pink, and blind. They really do look like rats. When squirrels are two weeks old they've grown another one and a half inches, their skin has begun to darken, and—thank goodness—their hair has begun to appear. It is in the following week that a squirrel's incisors start to appear in its lower jaw. At week five squirrels open their eyes. They are now between nine and ten inches long, have developed their lower gnawing teeth and upper teeth, but still have no grinding teeth.

Grinding teeth appear in their sixth week of life. Around their seventh week squirrels have had their first taste of bark, twigs, buds, or leaves, but continue to derive most of their sustenance from their mother's milk. The baby squirrel's teeth make suckling at times uncomfortable for the mother squirrel. It's around this time that squirrels first leave the nest, but many continue to be nursed until they are twelve weeks old. As Professor Vagn Flyger of the University of Maryland points out, "It takes longer to make a squirrel than other mammals."

Squirrels born in forests and New York must forage for their food. Those who live in the suburbs where birdfeeders are plentiful have it made. Throughout the nursing stage, squirrel mothers are not only attentive but extremely protective of their young. People who try to inspect squirrel nests while the mother appears to be away are sometimes attacked by the mother squirrels who run to their children's defense. But once squirrels leave the nest for good, the squirrel family dissolves, and each squirrel is on its own.

Young squirrels are not automatically welcomed into a range. They must establish their own position, and an estimated 10 percent of young squirrels are forced out of a range by more dominant ones. Ranges overlap.

Gray squirrels come in several pigments: gray, silver-gray, black, and albino. In the eastern United States, black squirrels, also familiar in the Northwest, have been increasing in number over the past decade. They seem to prefer cities (being numerous in Washington, D.C.) and do OK in the suburbs, but are rare in rural areas in the East. One theory explains this abundance of black squirrels by suggesting that city dwellers are especially protective of them. But the real reason behind the resurgence of black squirrels in cities remains unknown. Squirrel-watcher Vagn Flyger explains:

> We can only make wild guesses, but there seems to be an advantage to being a black squirrel here [in Washington, D.C.]. In rural areas black squirrels may not do as well because gray is better camouflage. Several hundred years ago black squirrels, which are more timid than grays, were more numerous, but destruction of forests probably gave grays an advantage over the decades—black squirrels were easier for predators to spot.

Squirrels thrive in urban areas, despite automobiles. One reason appears to be the prevalence of "urban islands": parks and other green spaces where squirrels have few predators. There's frequently an abundance of food, a sort of "squirrel grocery" thanks to the carefree attitude of tourists and other do-gooders. The squirrels within these islands mate exclusively with each other, so you're likely to see a preponderance of black, gray, or even white squirrels in a park or similar area.

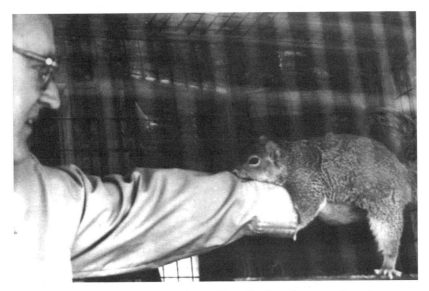

Professor Vagn Flyger and his pet squirrel, Fitzwilliam. (Don't try this stunt at home.)

The Sex Life of Squirrels

Female squirrels usually have two litters a year, each consisting of three or four infants. Once they've mated, the father squirrels usually desert their families and go off in search of food, other female squirrels, and birdfeeder owners to harass, generally having a good time. Squirrels do not mate for life. You may think this is rather rotten, and that the male squirrels are sexist, but actually it's a good idea. Mating among different squirrels prevents inbreeding, ensures a stronger genetic pool, and helps the species survive. As another benefit to the species, females usually mate with older, more dominant males. The older males are better equipped to survive, and pass along those genes. After copulation, the male squirrel fills the female's vagina with a kind of waxy plug that prevents other males from copulating with her and locks the semen in.

Even though female squirrels bear the responsibility for rearing their young, life isn't so bad for females. First, they still get to raid birdfeeders. Second, females do invite and receive sex from younger males. Third, females control the sex act. Finally, they live longer than the males.

Smell plays a major role in mating among squirrels, as males use it to locate females. Copulation can take place only when the female is in heat, called oestrus, which lasts for one day only. Five days before oestrus occurs males begin to follow females. As many as twelve males will follow a female in a *mating bout* or *chase*, during which the males will scream at and chase each other. One by one the less dominant males will go away in search of other partners. Dominant males expend considerable energy during this process. The winning male will follow the female through her home range, until she allows copulation.

Litters are spaced about thirteen to fourteen weeks apart, allowing females time to wean the babies. The gestation period is approximately forty days. Peak birth times—during which 75 percent of the young are born—occur between the end of July and early August, and again in winter between late December and early January. This timetable is not fixed, but varies as weather and food conditions change.

You can use your knowledge about breeding to predict when the next crop of hungry squirrels will appear from their nest. Soon after young squirrels leave their nest you might want to temporarily cease feeding birds, or switch to thistle seed to encourage the squirrels to travel elsewhere.

Enemies of Squirrels

The life of a squirrel in the wild is brief. Ten to twelve months, just long enough to see each season, is typical. In captivity they may live as long as ten to fifteen years; one such squirrel lived long enough to die of prostate cancer.

Squirrels have several enemies, but birders aren't among them. Squirrels may run away from you when you come at them flailing your arms and screaming, but they learn that you aren't going to hurt them because they know you don't want a dead squirrel in your yard. At window feeders squirrels discover that glass is a perfect protection and no matter how loudly you pound the glass you're not going to stick your arm through it.

Some squirrel "enemies" such as woodpeckers merely annoy squirrels. According to *Animals of the World*,

> . . . the gray squirrel is not the only claimant for the nuts; the red squirrel and the red-headed woodpeckers demand the lion's share.

The birds seem to think that these nuts are exclusively their property, and vigorously do they protest if a squirrel appears. One
determined woodpecker will sometimes send a gray squirrel scampering after a few moments, for the blows from that long sharp
bill of his are severe. The squirrels, being the earlier risers, are
often feasting when the birds appear, but they beat a hasty retreat before these tri-colored warriors.

Crows, blue jays, and mockingbirds are other feathered friends who
will harass squirrels.

But squirrels have many deadly enemies in urban, rural, and sub-
urban areas. Hunters kill roughly forty million squirrels each year in
the eastern part of the United States. And although that doesn't make
a significant dent in the American squirrel population, it's something
squirrels aren't crazy about. A greater danger to squirrels is the auto-
mobile. A familiar scene: a squirrel runs exactly halfway across a road
as a car approaches. The driver accelerates. The squirrel turns around
and runs back. Bam! Flattened fauna. It's not entirely clear why squirrels do this, and none of America's leading squirrel experts can
satisfactorily explain the phenomenon. However, the *Dick E. Bird News*
offers this reasoning:

> Their tail scurries across the ground at around ten miles per
> hour and jumps from tree branch to tree branch pushing their
> bodies ahead of it. Talk about being pushed around all the time.
> One big problem is that quite often a squirrel will get out into
> the middle of the road when a car is coming. When this happens
> the tail usually wants to go one way and the body wants to go
> another. But the time they get their differences worked out, it's
> often too late.

The worst kind of streets for squirrels are those with median dividers. In those cities with concrete dividers, such as Boston, life is even
harder. "You make it across the first four lanes of traffic, and you're
still stuck," said Dr. Thomas French, a zoologist at the Massachusetts
Division of Fisheries and Wildlife.

Predators are a problem for squirrels. These predators include cats, dogs, snakes, weasels, ferrets, red-tailed hawks, barred owls, foxes, raccoons, boys with BB guns, and even largemouth bass (one was found with squirrel remains inside). Predators pose different threats to squirrels, causing squirrels to react differently in each case. Dogs, cats, barred owls, and hawks will attack and dine on squirrels of all ages. A squirrel that is out in the open—in a field not near a tree—is essentially squirrel meat when chased by one of these. Sharp as a squirrel's claws are, squirrels are no match for these creatures. A squirrel's best, and sometimes its only, defense is hiding in trees. Just about everyone who has watched squirrels has noticed their ability to hide from their enemies by lying flat against the opposite side of a tree. As the enemy moves, the squirrel moves.

Snakes and raccoons enjoy the taste of young squirrels, but tend to leave the larger ones alone. These predators can enter squirrels' burrows.

When confronted by a dog, cat, or predatory bird, squirrels will run as quickly as they can to the nearest burrow or tree, observe the predator, and retreat only when approached. Squirrels will often stand their ground against weasels, ferrets, and snakes—squirrels will confront them and even harass them.

When threatened, squirrels often chatter, scold, and try to warn other squirrels.

Becoming dinner isn't the only danger that squirrels face. By far their greatest enemy is malnutrition. Not enough food kills the majority of squirrels in the wild, either directly or by making them susceptible to disease. Squirrels live in a harsh environment. Babies born in the summer may face their first winter storm when they are only fifteen weeks old and it's hard to gather food in that kind of weather.

Sarcoptic mange claims a large percentage of squirrels in winter. Caused by mites, this disease strikes underfed squirrels causing them to lose their fur. In the summer mites are only a nuisance for squirrels—all they have to do is scratch—but in the winter fur loss is deadly.

The warble fly begins to bug squirrels in August and September, causing swellings behind the forelegs and on the shoulders. These lumps occur where the warble fly has deposited its larvae. Squirrels infested with the warble fly often have blood oozing from lumps on their skin.

Various nematode worms and cysts plague squirrels as well. Some squirrels have been found with over one hundred worms in them, a condition squirrels aren't enthusiastic about.

Social Activities

For all their running around, squirrels don't go very far. (Why should they with people like you who graciously feed them?) A squirrel's range is between one and seven acres. The home range of males is twice as large as the range of females, possibly because males are more persnickety than females about what they eat. Females are happier with leaves and berries, while males really want nuts. The range of males increases during breeding seasons, which enhances their chances of getting a mate.

Territoriality doesn't seem to be a trait of gray squirrels. They roam freely within their home range, pretty much ignoring other squirrels except under certain circumstances. Female squirrels will defend their nests. When males vie for dominance over females they yell and harass each other. At birdfeeders both male and female grays will argue over who has rights to the feeder first. Arguing squirrels rarely come into contact—their chisel-sharp teeth are reserved for you. Instead squirrels like to scream and shake their tails at one another. (A few species of squirrels do exercise territoriality. Fortunately none of these species is interested in birdseed. Could you imagine one squirrel defending a feeder from all other squirrels?) While home ranges overlap, newcomers to a particular range may be met with aggression.

Some mornings you may be awakened by the sweet songs of birds. Other times you may bolt upright after hearing the shrill, piercing sound that goes something like *cheeoo eeeeoooo*. That's squirrel talk. What are they saying? They must be doing something other than deliberately trying to deprive you of sleep. Squirrels are unusually vocal animals and actually use their voices to communicate. There are no direct relationships between particular sounds and what squirrels are trying to say; in other words, squirrels have no vocabulary or language as we understand it. As Donald H. Owings and David Hennessy put it in their scholarly article, "The Importance of Variation in Sciurid Visual and Vocal Communication," squirrel calling "is not structurally unitary but varies at multiple levels and correlates with variation in calling situations" (*The Biology of Ground-Dwelling Squirrels*, Jan O. Murie and Gail Michener, eds, University of Nebraska Press, 1984).

In other words, squirrel sounds do not have meaning in isolation from the conditions they are in. Even calls under the same circumstance may mean different things to different squirrels. For example, when a snake is in the vicinity, adult squirrels may be warning other squirrels with their call, while young squirrels may be recruiting help. Squirrels use their calls and tail signals to alert other squirrels and to intimidate their adversaries, including other squirrels. Squirrels continue to call after the danger appears to have passed, possibly because they know that the danger may persist beyond their line of sight and other squirrels may be in jeopardy. Through their calls squirrels exhibit a strong determination to preserve their species.

How the squirrel uses its tail is not entirely understood. Unlike a squirrel's call, tail movements are not restricted by the amount of air a squirrel can manipulate. Tail movements can be held for a long time and varied within that time, and a squirrel uses this motion for many of the same purposes as their calls. However, tail motion also helps a squirrel balance, and at times may be used simultaneously for balance and signaling.

Squirrels also use smell to communicate. Marking the underside of branches with urine so that the smell isn't washed off by rain, and anal dragging are two common forms of scent marking.

Although you may see gray squirrels chase each other, especially the males around mating times, squirrels are cordial animals. This trait is particularly noticeable in their nests. According to Vagn Flyger, "Males and immature females will sleep together. I've seen as many as six or seven squirrels in one nest." Mature females are not included in this crowd: it would become sexually confusing if they slept in the same nest as several males. "Mature females become loners," says Vagn Flyger.

There are four kinds of squirrel nests. Both males and females help build nests. The one most commonly seen by humans is the drey, or winter nest. They are roughly twelve to sixteen inches in diameter, waterproof, and made of twigs on the outside, and moss, bark, fur, feathers, lichen, and leaves on the inside. Winter dreys take one to three days to construct and are strong enough to withstand harsh

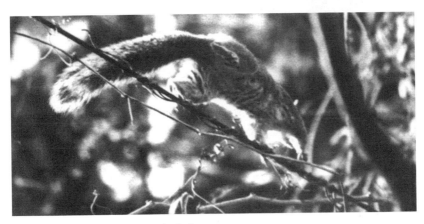

Mr. Squirrel trying out for a part in the high-wire act.

winds. They are never built too low where predators can reach them, nor too high where the winds are more severe. Summer dreys are smaller and more fragile, consisting of twigs and leaves.

Squirrels also live in cavities of trees, called tree dens. These cavities are created by woodpeckers or branches that have fallen away. Finally, squirrels sometimes build their nests in holes in the ground, which can provide considerable insulation against the cold.

The hierarchy that is manifest in squirrel mating behavior is also apparent in day-to-day life, and is strictly adhered to. Less dominant squirrels defer to the older, larger, and more assertive males, not only during mating but at food sources. Dominant squirrels eat first. Squirrels yell, wave their tails, and chase each other, but as I mentioned earlier, there is very little physical contact between them. They know who is dominant and who is subordinate. This hierarchy, Professor Flyger speculates, helps keep squirrels from fighting one another.

Several times in this chapter I've made references to squirrel behavior that helps preserve the species, behavior that can sometimes be described as altruistic. This behavior includes:

1. Burying nuts for all squirrels in the range

2. Males mating with various females to prevent genetic inbreeding

3. Sleeping together to preserve body heat

4. Warning other squirrels of danger

The Expert Squirrel Watcher

There was one name that continued to crop up in my reading and interviews about squirrels: Dr. Vagn Flyger. In *The World of the Gray Squirrel* there was Vagn Flyger and his studies of squirrels. In an article entitled "Climactic Influences on Life-History Tactics and Behavior [of Squirrels]," Vagn Flyger appeared again. He wrote a seminal article entitled "Movement and Home Range of the Gray Squirrel." Who is Vagn Flyger? He has written extensively on the nesting behavior of squirrels and their population dynamics. How did he become one of the foremost experts on gray squirrels? What is a squirrel expert like? I decided to visit Vagn Flyger to find out.

Vagn Flyger looks the way you'd expect the movie character Indiana Jones, played by Harrison Ford, to look in twenty years or so. A little thicker around the middle than he once was, a little less hair, and a walk that is less speedy than it once was, but still strong. He has a definite outdoors look to him: thick hands, weathered skin, a pleasantly rough face—the marks of a man who has spent much of his time outdoors and does plenty of physical work. His eyes appear sharp, as if they are practiced in spotting objects that most people wouldn't see. He appears jovial and confident, an enviable combination.

Vagn Flyger lives in Silver Spring, Maryland, a suburb of Washington, D.C. (squirrel capital of America) which is near the University of Maryland, where he teaches about mammals. The drive takes about forty-five minutes from downtown Washington, passing mostly highway and convenience stores, until you near Vagn Flyger's house. As you turn into the semi-paved road that leads to his home, you begin to think that not too far from here is the perfect location for someone who has made his career the study of mammals.

Professor Flyger seated me in one of the many comfortable, oversized chairs in his house and began to tell me about squirrels. I didn't need to ask many questions; a simple mention of the word squirrel and he was off talking.

Vagn Flyger's first academic encounter with squirrels came when he was asked to do a study in Maryland on whether the length of the hunting season affected the squirrel population. At the time Maryland had a short hunting season. Flyger recommended that the season's length be extended. Although forty to fifty million squirrels are killed by hunters in the Eastern part of the United States each year (one-half million in Maryland alone), "no one has been able to demonstrate that hunting has reduced the population at all." One of the reasons for that is "a hunter sees only one-sixth of the squirrels that are out there. We know this because we put radio transmitters on squirrels." During this project, Professor Flyger found that "squirrels were convenient animals to study."

It was at this point that I asked Dr. Flyger, "Have you ever been bitten?" That's kind of a rhetorical question, of course, for a man who studies squirrels, but I had to ask. Flyger responded. "Oh yes. But it's not too bad. It's a relative thing. After all, I used to work with polar bears."

This question prompted Vagn Flyger to begin talking about the kinds of things that squirrels eat. "They eat many different things," he said. "Most people don't realize that squirrels eat fungi and tree bark, which are just about as important to squirrels as nuts. Squirrels dig for truffle-like mushrooms." Now you know who's to blame for the outrageous price of truffles, I thought, as Flyger continued. "Nineteen eighty-eight's going to be a bad year for squirrels, because we had a bad acorn crop last fall," he said, sounding slightly solemn. "The fall of 1985 was a great acorn crop for squirrels. But this last fall there was the seventeen-year locust and squirrels were filling up on cicadas. Breeding reflects the amount of food there is for squirrels, so there was a bumper crop of young. We came into the fall of 1987 with a lot more squirrels than we should have." Flyger's silence said the rest: a lot of squirrels died over the winter. But this was not the worst loss because of an acorn shortage. "Between 1953 and 1954, 95 percent of the squirrels disappeared."

The squirrel's day is not as hectic as it may appear from watching them attack feeders and run up and down trees. "A squirrel spends a large part of its day just snoozing," Vagn Flyger said, changing the subject. "When the weather is warm, he just stretches out on the branches and sleeps. On a typical August or September day a squirrel will spend a lot of the day eating and building up fat." Listening to Professor Flyger, I began to feel that squirrels were a lot more like people than I had ever thought. He continued, "In winter they don't eat as much. They're not as active—they get up later and go to sleep earlier."

Professor Flyger reinforced the notion that squirrels are a disciplined lot. "*Chuck chuck chuck* is the alarm call of squirrels. When they do that and start waving their tails, they're excited about something. It tells other squirrels that they should be on the alert. Other squirrels take notice and run half way up a tree, watch, and wait."

By making this alarm call, a squirrel may be drawing the attention of predators away from other squirrels, toward itself. If this is true, then this is an example of highly altruistic behavior.

Vagn Flyger has also spent considerable time studying the red squirrel, which "sings like a bird." He mentioned this because the interaction between grays and reds shows that gray squirrels are not so omnipotent after all. Smaller than the gray squirrel, the red is territorial. Although grays bury their nuts communally, red squirrels defend their nuts. So what happens when the two subspecies come into contact? "The red treats grays like a red and will chase them. Even though the grays are larger, they usually defer to the reds." (But if you're thinking about importing red squirrels to your yard, be forewarned, reds like feeder foods, too.)

I asked Vagn Flyger about protecting birdfeeders from squirrels. I asked which is the most squirrelproof feeder. He mentioned a couple of feeders but then pointed out perhaps the best way to outwit them: "The best way to cure the problem is to treat a squirrel like a chicken." "Like a chicken?" I asked. "Yes," he continued. "Any recipe that works for chicken will work for squirrel. And they're low in cholesterol."

Vagn Flyger explained further. The ability of any particular area to support squirrels is limited. That's called the "carrying capacity." "When you move a squirrel to a new area"—many birders trap squirrels and ship their problem elsewhere—"it increases the amount of stress on the carrying capacity in that range because the squirrels that moved there increase the number of squirrels in the range. Either the new squirrels or the less dominant squirrels have to leave or die. I discovered this by dyeing transported squirrels purple." That's why "it's better to trap and eat squirrels than move them." Then he added, "depending on the game laws."

After we talked for a while at Professor Flyger's house, he gave me a tour of the grounds. It's difficult not to feel uplifted by the surrounding acres of unspoiled woods, especially when you were on a highway only minutes before. But the woods aren't entirely untouched; there were about a dozen feeders, nesting boxes, and other contraptions. The first place Flyger brought me to was a large cage about a hundred feet behind his house. The cage was big enough to hold several people. There he introduced me to Fitzwilliam, Flyger's pet squirrel. Fitzwilliam is a fox squirrel, which at first glance looks like a gray, but is actually a little larger, has a rounder face, sort of like a fox, and a reddish-brown hue. I'd never seen a squirrel as a pet before, although I'd heard stories about people who kept them inside in order to lower the value of their house to keep their tax assessment down. Fitzwilliam, adopted from one of Vagn Flyger's former students who had been studying him, stays in his cage all the time, but this doesn't dampen the squirrel's spirits. Without hesitating, Flyger opened Fitzwilliam's cage and stepped inside. I had a different reaction: I adjusted my telephoto lens and stepped back. But as soon as Professor Flyger was inside, Fitzwilliam jumped on his arm and ran over his shoulders, just like a kitten. Later when the squirrel expert played with Fitzwilliam by rubbing his nose, Fitzwilliam played back by batting Flyger with his paw—playfully. Vagn Flyger discovered how good a squirrel's memory can be by watching Fitzwilliam: when Flyger returns from a trip Fitzwilliam runs and jumps because he's glad to see his friend.

Flyger then showed me an L-shaped apparatus he uses to feed squirrels that was originally designed in Great Britain to poison squirrels. He fills the L-tube with corn. "The squirrels eat the germ of the corn and the birds eat the rest." More than anything else I saw that morning, this squirrel feeder satisfies Vagn Flyger's sense of total ecological utility. While we were standing by the squirrel feeder a squirrel yelled at us from a nearby tree. "He's mad because we're at his feeder," Flyger pointed out.

But lest you think that Vagn Flyger is in the other camp (you know, the prosquirrel side), I should add that his birdfeeders are prominent and popular. The best way to describe Professor Flyger is to say that he is an unbiased observer.

The size of a squirrel's litter is positively correlated with latitude. The warmer the climate the greater the number of litters produced each year by squirrels.

Despite their "tameness" squirrels are difficult to breed in captivity. Their elaborate courtship ritual involving several males chasing a female is an essential prerequisite to mating.

FOUR

The Unbearable Persistence of Squirrel Appetites

Squirrels consider birdfeeders as special challenges.
— *The New York Times*

It was during that indefinite time between late winter and early spring when flowers appear despite the fickleness of the weather that my friend Randy Rieland discovered I was writing a book about outwitting squirrels. Randy said he watched the crocuses pop up in his yard one afternoon and disappear the following afternoon. Randy suspected a culprit. "Do squirrels eat crocuses?" he asked.

"They do," I replied. "They eat the buds and bulbs from many flowers. It's something they look forward to all winter long. They also like tulips."

Squirrels have a way of creating maximum annoyance in gardens. You never know what they're going to do. Henry Mitchell, a writer for the *Washington Post*, reported that for two years squirrels "made surgical slanting cuts on some Ilam and Exbury azaleas as the buds began to swell, just before blooming season. I had heard squirrels sometimes like to eat the resinous buds, so I covered them with nylon stocking. It was then that the squirrels cut the stems and carried off the buds in their stockings."

While most bird feeders worry about pilferage of seed, other outdoor hobbyists are devastated by squirrels, too. The squirrel is the nemesis of the gardener. A hungry squirrel—is there any other kind?—will devour any flower-like growth in sight. They're particularly tempted by buds, but they will eat everything save the stem. Having squirrels in your yard when the first flowers come up is like having a lawnmower run amok. Mary McGrory pointed out that if you feed birds and have a garden, you're in lots of trouble. "They do vindictive landscaping."

Squirrel appetites extend into our National Parks. In 1983 the National Park Service conducted a census of squirrels in Lafayette Park, across the street from the White House. Park spokesman Duncan Morrow suspected that many squirrels were subsidized by White House staffers. "There are a number of White House staff people who show up pretty regularly with stuff they feed the squirrels."

The park is the nation's most popular spot for demonstrations. Still, a park service spokesman said, "There is not much damage to the park from demonstrators. The biggest damage we get is from squirrels eating the bulbs of plants."

Bird, squirrel, and garden lover Heather Perram has a solution for vindictive gardeners. She said that if you plant mothballs around your flowers the squirrels will leave them alone.

Biologist Roger Swain, science editor of *Horticulture Magazine*, is keenly aware of the squirrel problem. Swain, who wrote his doctoral dissertation about tropical ants, has spent countless hours trying to figure out ways to outwit squirrels from a gardener's point of view. (The shift from studying ants to what he now does was natural, he said: "I just added a 'p' and an 'l'.") His opinions are blunt. "The best thing to do is to get rid of squirrels. They're terrible for plants. Squirrels eat fruit and buds just as they're coming out.

"I was once giving a lecture in which I said you should get rid of them. Unfortunately there was an officer from the humane society in

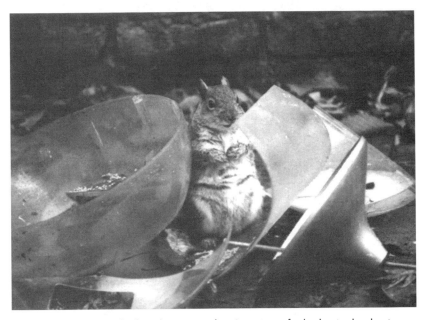

This could happen to any feeder: when a squirrel can't get into a feeder, he simply takes it down. Notice how fat the squirrel in this photograph is.

the audience who said he just gave a $250 ticket to someone for killing a squirrel. I'd gladly pay the bail of that person."

I suggested that perhaps birders and gardeners should join forces to outwit squirrels. Horticulturalists have discovered how hard it is to thwart squirrels, especially because you can't hang plants in the air as you can with feeders. "The one thing you can't do is educate a squirrel through terror." said Swain. "People, who are higher up on the food chain, remember terror. But when you are squirrel size you're scared witless many times a day. Their whole day involves fear. To survive as a squirrel you must be able to forget the last time you were scared." Fear is not imprinted into a squirrel's memory. "If a squirrel or woodchuck remembered fear it would die of fright: it's scared too many times." Swain offered this analogy: "A short order cook can only succeed by forgetting the last thing he cooked."

In the following essay, Roger Swain elaborates another side of the squirrel problem.

The Squirrel and the Fruitcake

Pecans are a choice ingredient of both fruitcake and squirrels. Some ten million pounds are incorporated annually into each. In fruitcake, pecans improve the color, texture, and taste, for the nuts offset the darkness, gumminess, and molasses flavor of the candied fruit. In squirrels, the nuts are vital. A diet of pecans, with their 70 percent oil content, is responsible for a higher birthrate, increased survival of the young, reduced emigration, and longer life for adults. In short, more squirrels.

With the quality of both squirrels and fruitcakes dependent on the seeds of *Carya illinoensis*, there has always been competition for the nuts.

From the point of view of the nut grower, squirrels make off with far too many pecans. Climbing into the trees, the squirrels begin to feed on the nuts even before they are ripe and later remove the largest and finest nuts from the opening shucks. Nuts that have fallen are picked up off the ground. In all, a single squirrel may make off with fifty pounds of pecans in a four-month period. Some of these nuts are eaten on the spot; others are carried up to a hundred feet away and cached singly in shallow holes dug in the ground.

From the squirrel's point of view, the human is far too successful at usurping the harvest. Nut trees that have been planted far away from adjoining forests are often surrounded by a dangerous expanse of closely mown ground; crossing this open ground means exposure to hawks, foxes, dogs, and other squirrel eaters. Reaching the grove may provide little sanctuary: guns and traps baited with pecans constitute another, greater hazard. If someone has protected the trees with eighteen-inch-wide bands of aluminum flashing tied around the trunks, the trees are unclimbable anyway. Scarcely any nuts are on the ground until they are knocked or shaken from the trees by the harvesters, and when that happens the grove is filled with people. For a squirrel whose ancestors harvested pecans long before humans appeared on this continent, this is an unpleasant development.

"The Squirrel and the Fruitcake," copyright Roger B. Swain, first appeared in *Horticulture Magazine*. This essay was reprinted in Swain's book *Earthly Pleasures*, published by Penguin Books, 1981. It is reproduced here by kind permission of the author.

The displeasure that humans and squirrels may share at having to divide up the pecan crop is compounded by the periodic disappearance of pecans from a tree altogether. The nonproduction of nuts is a periodic occurrence, especially in the year following a heavy harvest. A heavy crop will exhaust the tree's supply of stored carbohydrates, and the ripening of so many nuts prevents the tree from storing enough carbohydrates to bear the following year. Pecan growers refer to this as "alternate bearing" and determinedly try to prevent it through breeding, high fertilization, and careful spacing and pruning of trees to promote additional photosynthesis. As a further strategy, growers often plant four or five pecan cultivars in a single grove so that some of the trees will be bearing each year.

While growers and squirrels may both consider a year without pecans to be a crop failure, from the point of view of the pecan tree itself, such a year is not a failure at all. Pecans are reproductive units intended to increase the population of pecan trees, not squirrels. A given pecan tree might fruit every year, but then there would always be the same number of squirrels, pecan fed and ready to consume all of the crop once again. On the other hand, a pecan tree that saved up its carbohydrates for several years would not be feeding squirrels. There might be fewer squirrels in the absence of pecans, and when the tree did fruit, producing a much larger crop because of its stores of carbohydrates, the reduced squirrel population might be unable to consume all of the nuts. Some pecans would escape to become pecan trees.

For a pecan tree to effectively elude nut predators by concentrating its nut production into one year, all the trees in the vicinity must bear nuts the same year. Otherwise the predators will simply feed on the nuts of one tree one year and the nuts of another the next. This synchronization is not as improbable as it sounds. There already exists remarkable synchronization among nut trees, even in forests containing many species. Measurements on the amount of hickory nuts, acorns, beechnuts, and other seeds in a forest in southeastern Ohio from year to year showed a range of 35 to 220 pounds per acre.

Whether in a forest or a grove, the concentration of nut production into only a few years results in lean years, which to both squirrels and pecan growers are entirely unwelcome. But from the point of view of the pecan tree, nonproduction means that the tree is not losing its nuts to predators. The pecan tree can't give up fruiting altogether, because eventually the tree must reproduce itself. The tree has simply evolved a specific behavior, in the form of irregular fruiting, that serves at least partially to prevent the total destruction of the nut crop by squirrels and other predators.

Ecologists and evolutionary biologists term this behavior "predator satiation." There are some extremely dramatic examples among plants. The bamboo *Phyllostachys bambusoides*, for example, fruits only every 120 years, with all the plants doing so at once. Among nut trees the interval is much less, usually a year or two between seed crops, but the bitternut (*Carya cordiformis*) has a three-to-five-year interval and the white oak (*Quercus alba*) a four-to-ten-year interval. The European beech (*Fagus sylvatica*) accumulates starch in the parenchyma of the sapwood for about eight years. It is then virtually completely incorporated into a single seed crop and then storage is resumed.

While the pecan trees have evolved a way to assure the survival of some of their nuts, they also have become dependent on squirrels to distribute and plant those same nuts. The thickness of the shell of wild pecans is largely a result of selection by squirrels. Pecans whose shells are too thick or too hard to be pierced by squirrel teeth will not be collected, and the trees producing these nuts will remain unpropagated. Pecans whose shells are too thin are likely to be eaten much too readily rather than buried in the ground where a small percentage will remain to germinate.

With the arrival of modern agriculture, the pecan is no longer dependent on the squirrel for propagation. Seedlings are grown in nurseries and transplanted into groves. Careful breeding and improved cultural practices have greatly improved the pecan tree. New cultivars bear early, annually, and prolifically. Nuts are larger, have thinner shells, and are well filled. The only situation that hasn't improved is the problem with squirrels.

The annual loss of pecans to squirrels is difficult to compute. In Georgia alone, an estimated ten million pounds of pecans are eaten by predators, including crows, blackbirds, and jays as well as squirrels. If we assume that squirrels account for one-third of this amount and, further, that Georgia produces roughly one-third of the nation's pecans, then we arrive at an annual nationwide loss to squirrels of ten million pounds of pecans a year.

Boxcar figures are not very useful and indeed they tend to obscure the much greater losses experienced by certain pecan growers. Especially in years of a small harvest, the loss may amount to more than 50 percent. In such "short crop" years, every nut on a tree may be stolen. One expert remarked sardonically that, in some areas of Georgia, pecans are borderline between a cash crop and wildlife feed.

Some people, especially those who have just lost a sizable portion of their pecan crop, would be in favor of exterminating squirrels. Because attempts to exterminate them would almost certainly fail, current efforts are focused on reducing the numbers of squirrels by hunting and trapping or keeping them away with noisemakers, metal barriers around trunks, or fine-wire fences reinforced with electricity.

From what we have learned of the behavior of squirrels and pecan trees, an alternative squirrel control method suggests itself. Since we have undertaken to improve the pecan tree through artificial breeding and selection, why not produce a squirrelproof pecan? Whether or not the effort of selecting for squirrel resistance is economically feasible remains to be determined, but such a cultivar is certainly possible. This hypothetical squirrelproof pecan cultivar would have the following two characteristics, traits the opposite of those being favored by current selection practices.

1. The cultivar would fruit only after long intervals of time, five to ten years if possible, with little or no nut production in intervening years. With all the adjoining trees fruiting at the same time, there would be a single enormous crop that would satiate squirrels and other predators.

2. Nuts of the cultivar would have a very thick shell, too thick for squirrels to gnaw through easily. If the costs in energy of breaking into a nut exceed the nutritive value of the nutmeat therein, the squirrels will turn to other foods. Thicker-shelled pecans would prompt squirrels to seek more accessible nutrition.

Groves of this new pecan should still be isolated from other food sources of squirrels to make it difficult for squirrels to move into a fruiting grove. Home gardeners who might have to plant these trees close to an adjoining squirrel habitat would probably benefit more from the thicker-shelled feature than from the concentrated bearing. On the other hand, concentrated bearing would offer both the home gardener and the commercial grower considerable relief from such insect pests as the pecan weevil and the hickory shuckworm. These pecan pests are much more dependent on pecans for survival and their populations will crash more dramatically than squirrels in the nonbearing years.

A number of objections to squirrelproof pecans come immediately to mind and must be addressed. Will pecan trees that fruit only once a decade mean nine years of nutless fruitcakes? Absolutely not. Different parts of the country could be on different schedules with one grove bearing this year, another the next. It would only be necessary to establish nut-free zones between unsynchronized groves of pecans. A second solution is to store pecans between harvests. Fifty years ago pecan storage had not progressed beyond that achieved by squirrels. Pecans could be kept fresh during the cool winter months, but as soon as spring warmth arrived, the nuts became stale and rancid. Since then, however, it has been shown that in controlled cold storage, pecans can be kept for eight years with no loss in color, flavor, or texture of the shelled pecans. A long hiatus between harvests will deprive only the squirrels, not the fruitcakes.

A second objection will come from fanciers of paper-shelled pecans, those nuts that are easily shelled by hand. However, less than 10 percent of the pecan crop each year is sold to consumers in the shell. The remaining 90 percent is machine shelled. There is no reason why the established cultivars could not continue to provide nuts for the in-shell market. The new thicker-shelled cultivar would simply require a stronger machine.

Finally, conservationists concerned about preserving the squirrel population need not be alarmed. Squirrels have sufficient quantities of food available to them in the form of a host of wild edibles that they face no danger of extinction.

This highly hypothetical proposal for a squirrelproof pecan is illustrative of a different approach to crop plant design. In breeding plants to conform to our commercial needs, we tend to ignore their peculiar characteristics, traits that have evolved during centuries of selective pressure, in this case the fruiting cycles of nut trees. More efforts should be directed at reexamining the biology of wild crop plants for clues to their natural resistance to pests and disease. In some instances we may have overlooked a trait, and in the process of artificial selection, we may have exacerbated a problem rather than alleviated it. Domestication of plants has removed some ecological constraints, such as a need for natural propagation. In seeking means to meet existing pressures, we may be able to select more vigorously for a certain trait than previous ecological constraints would allow. Most trees fruit more often than once a century because there is too much danger of their being blown down or burned up before they reproduce. Having undertaken to propagate pecan trees ourselves, we can select for longer rather than shorter intervals between harvests and for nuts with heavier shells. This may ultimately prove to be an easier way to reduce nut losses than trying to exterminate the predators. With new pecan cultivars, we could have our fruitcake and squirrels, too.

Ground squirrels consume twenty-four ounces of nuts a week. They can eat three ounces at a sitting.

FIVE

Rating the Feeders

Which feeder to buy? Which will attract the most birds? Which will attract the kind of birds you covet? Which are easy to fill, and which are pains in the neck to fill? Which will fend off squirrels? This chapter answers these irksome questions, and gives advice on how to select the best feeder for your needs.

Squirrelproof or Squirrel-Resistant?

Or have you merely created a diner for squirrels? Dozens of different birdfeeders are on the market, and not all of them are going to offer the kind of squirrel resistance you want. Selecting the appropriate feeder is often a matter of trial and error: squirrels first break into your feeder and then you notice your error in buying that feeder.

There's no perfect feeder. Although a couple are highly squirrel-resistant—especially the GSP, Mandarin, and Looker SPF Feeder—and others can be made squirrel-resistant with the use of baffles, grease, and other barriers, there is no feeder that is squirrelproof all the time. These critters are capable seed stealers. Even when they can't leap into a feeder, squirrels can claw a few seeds out, shake seed to the ground, knock the feeder to the ground and feast on the booty, or bite their way through. Squirrel resistance varies, too, depending on how you place your feeder. Certain feeders, for example, are squirrel-resistant when placed on top of a pole, but lose their resistance when hung from a tree. I prefer the expression "squirrel-resistant" to "squirrelproof." Squirrelproof exists only in an idealized state. Peggy Robin, a Washington, D.C. bird feeder, points out that whether a feeder is squirrel-resistant or squirrelproof is a state of mind. If you can't tolerate squirrels at all, there's no such thing as a squirrelproof feeder.

Some Strategies for Making Feeders Squirrel-Resistant

If a feeder isn't as squirrel-resistant as you would like, attempt some home-brewed remedies. Take the initiative! Don't cower to a tiny animal! Show those squirrels who's boss! Turn your anger into a positive force! There are plenty of things you can do besides yelling and throwing Frisbees at the squirrels. For example, if your feeder is hanging from a tree that's not near any other tree, place a sheet metal skirt around the tree to prevent squirrels from climbing up. Maybe the hanging chain the feeder came with isn't long enough—lengthen it with coated, copper wire. Put Vaseline on the wire once a month if that helps. Perhaps the feeder needs a baffle or two, or the baffle the feeder came with isn't large enough. If the feeder is too close to a tree, move it further out on the branch. The cardinal rule is a feeder can't become squirrelproof if it's in a place where squirrels can get to it. (Chapters 6 and 7 discuss antisquirrel devices you can buy and build.)

Certain locations should be avoided, such as tree branches, according to Marlene Couture of the Duncraft Company in Penacook, New Hampshire. "We try to tell people not to hang feeders from a tree. It's the worst place possible, but people put them there because it's the only place they can see them. No matter what you do, no matter what baffles you use, the feeder is right there under the squirrel's nose. It's like hanging lunch in front of them. Eventually they will get to it. And if they can't get to it, they'll knock it down." If you do hang your feeder from a tree, there are certain precautions that may help. Place the feeder as far out on the branch as possible, and use a wire instead of a chain because the wire is slicker. Baffle the feeder. If you can't hang the feeder far out on a limb because the tree limb is too fragile to support a feeder at its end, use a narrow tube feeder that squirrels won't be able to reach from the tree trunk.

Couture recommends poles and brackets instead of hanging feeders from trees—her ideal place is on top of a pole with a squirrel guard baffle beneath. Keep the pole as far away from trees and fences as possible. Failing that, she suggests stringing a heavy fishing line or wire between two trees and hanging the feeder from the line, along with some devices to discourage squirrels from walking along the line.

Be imaginative when it comes to where you put your feeder.

There's More to a Feeder Than Squirrel Resistance

Squirrel resistance isn't the only criteron that you may have for a feeder. Another important consideration is how easily you can view the birds. Bird visibility doesn't depend just on the kind of feeder, either: how you position it is crucial. The GSP feeder, one of the few that could be called squirrelproof, sometimes gives a good view of birds, and sometimes offers a lousy view as it rotates. Wooden hanging feeders only let you view the birds that are on your side of the feeder because wood is opaque. When you're buying a new feeder, think about where you're going to put it and where you're going to watch it from. It's no fun to feed birds you can't watch.

You can improve the visibility of birds by blocking those openings on the opposite side from where you view the feeder, which will encourage birds to flutter around to the side where you want them. You may block particular openings to deter squirrels as well. If the feeder's on a chain that rotates, replace the chain with a metal rod. (Metal rods are easier to grease than chains, too.) After a while baffles can become dirty and scratched; clean them or replace them.

Seed capacity is crucial, too. You don't—repeat *don't*—want to fill your feeder every day, so tiny feeders are out. If your yard sports several feeders or if you're going to be outside frequently, then it's okay to have a small-capacity feeder. But nothing discourages feeding birds more than filling a feeder daily. Window feeders have notoriously small capacities, but they are an exception to this rule because you can usually fill them from inside. I suggest a quart as an absolute minimum for a non-window feeder; the gallon-plus feeders are the smartest buy.

If your feeder is in a hard-to-reach location then seed capacity may be the most important criterion in your choice of feeders.

However, having too large a feeder isn't good either. If the seed in your feeder isn't consumed within a week or two, consider switching to a smaller-capacity feeder. The longer seed sits in a feeder the more likely it is to rot and become disease ridden. There's a trade-off between convenience and serving safe seed. More on this later.

Ease of refilling goes hand in hand with seed capacity. The most annoying feeders are those with tiny seed capacities and those that are difficult to fill. Ideally you just want to pour the seed in, as most window feeders allow; the second best option is to lift a light lid and pour the seed. Many feeders have caps that must be pulled or pried off and are a real pain. Besides, eventually these caps get lost. Beware of feeders that need two hands to hold the seed cavity open, or that require a strong arm to do the trick. The larger the opening, the better, too. The Mandarin, one of the best-designed feeders, has an opening for seed that is so large you could pour a bucket of seed in. Watch out, also, for feeders where you must tilt the seed dispenser at a specific angle in order to get the seed in. Ask yourself: will I be able to fill the feeder easily from where I am going to put it?

Another important question is what the feeder looks like. Every time you peer into your yard you're going to see that feeder, so you had better be certain that you like the way it's designed. A feeder that looks unpleasant in the store will look even worse when you bring it home. Birds couldn't care less about a feeder's construction; a dogfood bowl with sunflower seed in it would make them happy. Most feeders sold in catalogs are fairly ordinary. Others are engineered to resemble Swiss cottages and are usually made of clear, sturdy plastic, which may become muddy-looking over time.

For the most artistically demanding birders, a number of craftspeople are putting art and imagination to the design of birdfeeders. Richard Clarke, who runs The Bird House in Portland, Oregon, handcrafts his feeders. Of the dozens of designs that are available, you should be able to find the one that suits your taste. One word of caution: squirrels will eat through feeders to get at seed, so if you buy a beautiful feeder, make certain that squirrels either can't get to it, or if they can, they can reach the seed without having to make a hole in your feeder.

One last consideration is a feeder's weather resistance. Wet seed quickly becomes covered with dangerous mold. Rain, snow, and wind affect feeders differently. A stiff wind can empty some feeders as quickly as a family of squirrels. One feeder, the GSP, is fantastically weather-proof; for others such as the Cardinal Barn, it depends on the direction of the rain; still others, such as platform feeders, rate a zero in this category. Baldwin's Sheltered Birdfeeder takes advantage of the wind to protect the seed inside. Some feeders, such as the Droll Yankee, have sophisticated drainage systems to help keep the seed dry. But the type of feeder alone doesn't determine how resistant to weather it may be. Where you locate your feeder (is it sheltered by a fence or tree, or out in the open on a pole?) and how you baffle it also plays a role in the ability of the feeder to withstand Mother Nature. If your feeder spills too much seed or gets too wet after a storm you may need to replace that feeder—or you may simply need to move it.

Care of Your Feeders and Your Birds

Squirrels alone don't contribute to the demise of feeders. Although their daily climbing, clawing, and biting regimen can cloud, scar, and weaken feeders, fluctuating temperatures, hail, bird droppings, falling berries, small children, and mildew all take their toll on birdfeeders. Fortunately many birdfeeders are inexpensive enough to replace from time to time, but with a minimum of cleaning a feeder will last years. It's important to clean your feeder periodically for another reason: moisture and seed make mold which may kill birds. Wash your feeder with hot water and soap once every couple of months. That's all. Use only nonabrasive soaps, disinfectants, and cleaning pads because plastic feeders easily scratch, and the more scratches, the less visibility. Dry the feeder thoroughly, refill it, and enjoy. If the seed inside becomes damp after a storm, discard that seed, dry (or clean) the feeder, and refill. I know it goes against the grain to throw away seed, but it's much better to waste some birdseed than to see your favorite titmice in legs-up position. Remember, the birds trust you.

Many feeders collect moisture. Bowl-shaped feeders, some window feeders, and multi-tube feeders can gather considerable moisture. In addition, birds hop around the inside of some feeders and defecate on the seed, which can turn healthy seed into deadly seed overnight. Inspect your feeders regularly for moisture and droppings. Heidi Hughes, proprietor of the Wild Bird Company in Rockville, Maryland, says, "When it rains, discarded sunflower seed shells act as a wick, sopping up water and mold." Hughes says the flatter the feeder the better. Check your feeder regularly for moisture content.

There's a debate over whether a feeder should spill seed onto the ground. When seed spills—or when birds flick away undesirable seed—ground-feeding birds such as mourning doves and cardinals are attracted. However, seed on the ground quickly becomes moldy, especially after a rain. In addition, seed below a feeder gets contaminated with bird droppings. Moldy seed and seed covered with droppings are vectors for disease, including salmonella and deadly avian pox. If you notice any bird looking ill, especially around the eye or beak, switch feeders, remove spilled seed from the ground every day, and consider placing a seed catcher below the feeder. Always keep in mind that bird droppings and moisture poison seed.

You can reduce the amount of seed that spills to the ground by avoiding seed mixes. When a bird encounters a seed it doesn't like, the bird flicks that seed to the ground. Feeders with a single seed inside have much lower spillage. The safest arrangement is to have several feeders, each with its own seed.

It's very hard to find a feeder that doesn't spill any seed to the ground. And it's very hard to curtail the desire for spilled seed because it attracts such wonderful birds. What to do? If you're worried about spillage, buy a feeder that has little spillage, such as Looker Products's SPF (or that hexagonal feeder). In addition, you can buy feeding platforms with drainage.

Feeders can pose another danger to birds. Birds, especially small ones like chickadees, can enter feeders with holes of an inch or more, as well as get inside barn-like feeders. And birds may try to get inside these feeders when they can't reach the seed by just sticking their heads in the opening. Once inside they can't escape. A feeder with a one-inch or larger hole that is low on seed can be a death trap for birds. You must keep these feeders full or have an second feeder to attract birds because a bird may crawl inside and get stuck.

I'd like to mention a couple of miscellaneous—but crucial—points about birdfeeders. First, always, always, *always* wash you hands with hot water and soap after handling your feeder or birdseed. Never handle your feeder when you have an unbandaged cut or other open wound on your hand. This is especially true for small children who are forever putting their fingers in their mouths: keep children away from the feeder. Birds are pretty, their songs sweet, and they are plenty of fun to watch, but they carry dangerous diseases. Their droppings are filled with bacteria that is harmful to birds and to you. If you'd like to know what you can catch from birds, here's the short list:

Hypersensitivity pneumonitis, an allergy, sometimes called pigeon breeder's disease

Psittacosis, a lung infection that gives you many hours of a hacking cough, severe headache, chills, fever, and loss of appetite

Histoplasmosis, a fungal disease whose symptoms resemble tuberculosis

Cryptococcosis, a fungus that causes meningitis

Salmonellosis, a bacterial infection that produces food poisoning

Try not to purchase too much seed in advance because it decays with age, especially hulled and cracked seeds. As a general rule the warmer and more humid it is the shorter the lifetime of the birdseed. Seed won't last longer than one season, unless you refrigerate or freeze it, which may not be the most energy efficient scheme, but it does have several benefits. Besides preserving your seed, freezing kills bugs. Stephanie Faul, a Washington, D.C. birder, passed this tidbit along to me. Whenever she bought seed in bulk, lots of flying critters appeared along with the seed, and Stephanie, who lives in an apartment, wasn't pleased with releasing moths inside, even if her cats adored the situation. Now Stephanie puts the bags of feed in her freezer for a few days and *voila*—no bugs. A few pages ago I mentioned that a feeder's location plays a role in how squirrel-resistant it is and how easily you can fill the feeder. But location matters to what's underneath the feeder as well. Wherever you place your feeder you are going to accumulate lots of bird droppings. Still worse, the shells from sunflower seeds and spillage of hulled sunflowers will kill the lawn beneath. So wherever you put your feeder, consider the ground underneath a dead zone.

Feeders should be put close enough to your house so you can see them, but not too close so that you scare the birds. By the same token, don't put your feeder near the picnic table because every time you eat at the table the birds are going to fly away.

The Mandarin

Type: Hanging feeder
Dimensions: 17" x 17"
Seed Capacity: Over 5 quarts
Attracts: Just about everything except nuthatches. Downy woodpeckers will occasionally feed at the Mandarin; cardinals, juncos, and mourning doves enjoy the seed that spills to the ground. You'll even see blackbirds at this feeder. Starlings love the Mandarin.

The Mandarin is among the most uniquely-shaped feeders. A fat cylindrical tub with four holes and perches in it is covered by something that looks like an upside-down funnel with a skirt. Both the funnel and skirt are steep. The entire feeder is constructed out of rigid, transparent plastic. The skirt angles down over the perches, providing a roof.

The Mandarin is supported by a chain that extends into the center of the feeder. You refill the Mandarin by lifting the funnel skirt, raising this lid, and pouring the seed in. Unlike most feeders, the Mandarin has a huge opening—over six inches in diameter—through which you can pour seed; there's very little spillage during this frequently wasteful process. You have to hold the top while filling the feeder (it doesn't come off) but that doesn't present any problem.

Birds are visible from three sides. Like all four-sided feeders, you can block off the opening that doesn't face your window. The birds won't mind.

This feeder gets covered with bird droppings fairly quickly. Fortunately, it can be cleaned in minutes. The Mandarin is as close to 100 percent squirrelproof as you can buy. It and the GSP feeder stand in a class of their own. I've watched for hours as squirrels attempt to leap to the perches, which offer little landing room, and fail each time. I've been amused by squirrels' attempts to reach over the top and either feed upside down or catch the perch from above—they either give up or fall to the ground. They keep falling and trying again. I've even seen adventurous squirrels try to lift the top of the feeder, which is too heavy and cumbersome. Unlike lighter feeders, they can't knock and spill seed out.

Sarah Abrams of Arlington, Virginia has this to say about her Mandarin feeder:

> I have hung it on a straight metal arm. The arm is attached to my wooden back porch, which stands several feet above the ground. This means the feeder's ports hang about four and a half feet above the ground and about thirty feet out from the porch railing. I filled it with black oil sunflower seeds.
>
> The squirrels climb out on the arm but seem uneasy when they reach the far end of the arm and it no doubt begins to bend under them. One or two of the more adventurous squirrels have tried hanging upside down from the chain (which is eight to ten inches long,) but apparently decided they cannot get down the steeply-sloped feeder roof. None of them has tried jumping to the perches. In the end, all give up and scavenge for whole seeds among the dropped hulls on the ground.

Still, the Mandarin isn't perfectly squirrelproof. Heidi Hughes reported that one of her customers brought back a Mandarin "that looked like someone had taken a sledgehammer to it. The squirrel ate through the top." Hughes surmises that apparently in the Midwest, where the Mandarin is manufactured, "squirrels aren't as aggressive as they are in the East." Fortunately, the manufacturer is working on a modified top with an additive that squirrels won't be able to gnaw through.

The Mandarin has three flaws. First, when the feeder starts to run out of seed it becomes increasingly difficult for birds to get at that seed; chickadees may go after that last seed by crawling inside. Once inside they can become trapped and die, "which is a horrible sight," reported Heidi Hughes. Never let the Mandarin get too low on seed (or make sure that you have another feeder available). Second, finches are crazy about it. Third, seed can spill from the feeder at high rates. When birds eat unevenly from one side, the feeder becomes unbalanced and high energy birds such as starlings and finches can knock seed to the ground. This seed can quickly become wet and moldy and become a source of disease for birds.

Mandarin

	Poor				Great
Squirrelproofness					X
Ease of refilling					X
Visibility of birds				X	
Seed capacity					X
Attractiveness		X			
Versatility of location		X			
Overall					X

GSP Feeder

Type: Hanging feeder
Dimensions: 13" diameter
Seed Capacity: More than 1½ gallons of seed
Attracts: Small birds such as finches, titmice, wrens, and downy woodpeckers. Peanuts will not work in the GSP feeder so peanut-loving birds won't be attracted to this feeder. Suet can be hung inside.

No other feeder has received as much attention as Dr. Stephen Clarke's GSP feeder. And deservedly so: the GSP design and abilities are innovative and a step beyond any other feeder on the market. It is the only feeder that birds fly up and into to eat. Through its shape, the GSP feeder provides complete protection from predators for birds as they eat; the GSP is also completely weatherproof. If you live in an area with a lot of rain or snow, the GSP could be the best feeder for you.

The GSP feeder is attractive, too. Its smooth curves are more reminiscent of a postmodern sculpture than a birdfeeder. It has an almost aerodynamic design. A muted aluminum cover, also curved, rests on top of the GSP and hides the opening through which seed is added. Instead of a chain, which most feeders use to hang, the GSP is supported by an aluminum pole. This simple addition gives the feeder a sense of durability and class; it also keeps the feeder from swaying in the wind.

The closest common geometry that the GSP feeder resembles is a dome. Birds fly into the expansive cavity and perch themselves on one of the two ledges through which seed is dispensed. There's room for about eight birds to eat at the same time—assuming they get along.

In his patent application, Dr. George Clarke described the GSP feeder this way:

> A birdfeeder comprising a body extending along a vertical axis, the body having an outer shell, a wall inside the shell, the shell and the wall defining a reservoir, the shell and the wall further defining a restricted chute, and a feed tray inside the shell, the chute communicating between the reservoir and the tray to provide gravity feed of seed, and a fly-in access opening in the shell, the access opening communicating between the exterior of the shell and the tray and being large enough to allow birds to fly into the shell, the extent of the shell between the opening and the upper end of the body being large enough to prevent squirrels resting on the end from reaching into the opening.

The original GSP feeder contained a minor design flaw which a handful of squirrels could take advantage of. These ultrasmart squirrels lifted the aluminum top with one paw, braced themselves with another, and stuck their heads into the rectangular opening used for refilling the GSP. As uncomfortable as it was, these few squirrels were able to feast on the GSP. Current models of the GSP feeder contain a latch that fits around the aluminum pole and over the top. Because of this latch (sometimes called the Rodney lock) you need two hands to lift the top—something squirrels don't have . . . yet.

I was one of those who encountered a supersmart squirrel. After I watched a squirrel lift the lid I wrote to Clarke Products:

March 4, 1987

Clarke Products Company
Box 301
Mansfield Depot, CT 06251

Dear Clarke Products Company:

I am enjoying your feeder. Of all the bird feeders I've used—about six different kinds—it took squirrels the longest to get into yours.

Here's how Rodney the squirrel (not his real name) did it. My GSP feeder is attached to the side of my apartment building with a two-foot long pole, angled up at forty-five degrees. Rodney quickly determined that he couldn't enter the feeder from the bottom. However, by supporting himself with his back claws from the brick building and hanging upside down, Rodney managed to raise the aluminum top high enough so that he could stick his head inside the space used to refill the feeder.

I've had the feeder for nine days. He got in yesterday.

Rodney doesn't mind eating while upside down.

Actually, it's taken Rodney the squirrel less time to figure out how to get inside than some of the birds that were customers of my previous feeder.

Perhaps I'm not being fair. After all, I labored hard devising all sorts of apparatuses and Rube Goldberg concoctions around my former feeders to keep Rodney and his friends out. I expect that he became an exceptionally clever squirrel during those trying months.

So, let me suggest a minor modification on the GSP feeder. A latch (instead of the package sealing tape I'm now using) would be helpful in securing the aluminum top to the rest of the feeder.

Sincerely,
Bill Adler

Dr. Clarke wrote back:

March 9, 1987

Rodney c/o Bill Adler
2800 Devonshire Place, NW
Washington, D.C. 20008

Dear Rodney:

I have good new and bad news. First, the good news. You have succeeded in nine days of doing something that in four years of testing the GSP in the Northeast, no other squirrel has done. With five thousand feeders sold, you have two other cousins, one in Simsbury, Connecticut, and one in Grosse Point, Michigan, who also learned the trick.

Now for the bad news. Your master will install the enclosed "Rodney Lock"—it gets your name because the other cousins of yours are nameless—and I fear this will curtail your dining.

You see, it sits on top of the aluminum cover and it takes two hands to open the feeder. One slides the Rodney Lock up to the tope of the hanger. It will stay there. Then the top is lifted and the feeder is filled. The Rodney Lock then drops back into position.

Sorry, Rodney.

Very truly yours,
Stephen G. Clarke
President

Before the GSP, no feeder designer took advantage of the simple fact that birds fly and squirrels don't.* Feeders have to be attached to

---

*One birder, however, isn't so sure about this. Walter Stolwein wrote this poem to express his concern over squirrels' abilities:

The Pest
The squirrel is a furry bird
Or thinks he is, upon my word.
It hogs the feeder's costly seeds
Ignoring feathered birdies' needs.

something—usually a pole or a hanging chain—and squirrels merely have to scale that support to reach the feed. But the GSP's principle is that the feed should be placed in a part of the feeder that can only be accessed by creatures that fly. To get to the GSP's feed, an animal has to fly *up*; there's no way to climb into the seed compartment. Squirrels do get on top of the GSP, but because the feeder curves around like a beach ball, squirrels can't climb around to reach the opening on the bottom.

The inventor of the GSP, University of Connecticut Professor Stephen G. Clarke, said, "I say let's give the birds a chance." The GSP was exhibited at the Fifteenth Annual Inventors Expo sponsored by the Patent and Trademark Office in 1987.

It's fun to watch squirrels try to get into the GSP. They can't, but they never seem to learn that fact.

You refill the GSP by first lifting the bracket, the Rodney Lock. They you lift the aluminum cover to expose a roughly one-inch by two-inch rectangular opening. You definitely need a seed dispenser to fill the GSP, otherwise filling it is straightforward. The seed spills into the cavities on both sides.

Sunflower seeds work best with the GSP; peanuts don't work at all.

Although it doesn't say so in the manual, there's enough room inside the GSP to hang a suet cake. Just attach the cake to a wire and wrap the wire around the inside bolt. Woodpeckers love this indoor dining.

The GSP's drawback is that sometimes it's hard to see the birds. After a short time, the GSP becomes dirty on both the inside and outside. There's no problem seeing birds flutter around outside, but once they decide to venture in to snack, they can be hard to see. In addition, if the GSP rotates (or a squirrel rotates it) so that one of the two seed cavities faces you, you won't be able to see birds inside at all.

GSP

	Poor				Great
Squirrelproofness					X
Ease of refilling					X
Visibility of birds		X			
Seed capacity				X	
Attractiveness				X	
Versatility of location			X		
Overall				X	

The Steel Squirrel-Proof Feeder (SPF)

Type: Fortress post feeder
Dimensions: Roof is 12½" x 12½", about 9" high
Seed Capacity: 2 gallons
Attracts: Cardinals, titmice, starlings, wrens, chickadees, finches, blue jays, and mockingbirds; mourning doves are attracted to the spilled seed.

The SPF was created by Looker Products in Milford, Illinois. Inventors Olin and Caroline Looker wanted to create a feeder that was squirrelproof and didn't waste any seed. The result was the Steel Squirrel-Proof Feeder, or SPF.

The SPF is a clever feeder, relying on the principle that squirrels weigh more than birds. When a squirrel lands on the platform, his weight causes a shield to close in front of the seed. When the squirrel leaves the platform, the aluminized steel shield opens again. Two steel springs in the back of the feeder can be adjusted to vary the weight that causes the shield to shut, so that heavy birds can be prevented from entering. The SPF looks a little like a fortress, and as far as squirrels are concerned, it is. They can't lift the shield and they can't bite through the metal.

The SPF is covered with a weather-resistant, light green enamel paint. The platform is made of cedar. Unlike plastic feeders that become scratched and cloudy over the years, or wooden feeders that get gnawed by squirrels or become water damaged, the SPF should last practically forever.

The SPF's large seed capacity means that a week can go by without your having to refill the feeder. The SPF mounts on a pole or post, and by placing a baffle beneath it you can increase its antisquirrel capabilities.

The SPF is easily refilled by lifting a latch that secures the top in place, and then lifting the hinged top. The inside walls of the SPF tilt downward, drawing the seed into the bin. Because all the seed reaches the opening in front of the platform, there won't be any leftover seed that can become moldy. Almost every kind of seed works with the SPF, including sunflower seed and shelled peanuts. By varying the seed, you can attract or discourage particular birds.

In fact, you may want to fill the feeder with exclusively black oil sunflower seeds, to discourage starlings, who don't care for sunflower seeds. If this feeder has a flaw it's that starlings can make a mess of the seed and spill a good amount of it (something they can do to most feeders). If you want to discourage birds from flicking seed to the ground, fill the SPF with one type of seed at a time.

The SPF wins the award in the "Ecologically Sound" category. Because seed stays completely dry and because when filled with a single seed type there's little spillage, there's little chance that seed will become moldy. There's also no opportunity for small birds to get inside and become trapped. For people who care about the well-being of their birds, the SPF is an excellent choice.

Up to six small birds or three larger ones can feed at a time. Because the feeder doesn't move, you will always see the birds as they eat.

The SPF

	Poor				Great
Squirrelproofness					X
Ease of refilling					X
Visibility of birds				X	
Seed capacity					X
Attractiveness			X		
Versatility of location			X		
Overall					X

The Cardinal Barn and Other Wooden Feeders

Type: Wooden hanging feeder, usually constructed out of cedar or redwood. (The various designs are all shaped like chalets, with two glass or plastic sides, a redwood roof, base, and sides. These wooden feeders can be hung or mounted.)

Seed Capacity: 3–10 pounds

Dimensions: Varies from roughly 12" x 10" x 9" to 20" x 15" x 12"

Attracts: Cardinals, finches, chickadees, titmice, blackbirds, nuthatches, wrens, small woodpeckers, pine siskins, and starlings. Considerable spillage also attracts mourning doves and juncos.

Wooden feeders are great because they are easy to fill, have large seed capacities, and when they offer bird watching, the watching is very good. But because they move while hanging, there are times when birds are completely obscured. These feeders are not so terrific in the squirrelproof department.

But they are made of wood: wood is pleasant and natural; it always looks better than plastic (at least in the beginning). Birds like it more and so do people. But there's a downside to wood: bird droppings show up more prominently. After a while you may pray for rain.

Wooden feeders are usually filled by lifting the roof and pouring the seed in. The seed spills out along troughs on the two long sides. It's easy for just about any bird to feast at the cardinal barn. Seed spillage brings in plenty of ground-feeding birds, but it can also bring deadly mold and avian pox.

When the cardinal barn becomes low on seed, birds may try to go after that last seed or two by pushing up the plastic sides and slipping inside, where they become imprisoned. As with other feeders that small birds can slip into, be careful when this feeder starts to run low on seed. The cardinal barn and other wooden hanging feeders have another drawback: they are squirrel attractors. Squirrels throughout the neighborhood know when there's a new wooden feeder around. Perhaps they can smell the wood, or perhaps they're just attracted to it as they're attracted to trees. Whatever the reason, hanging the cardinal barn is like an invitation to a party—and you are providing the goodies. Once the squirrels arrive at the feeder, they can choose to dine upright, sideways, or upside down; the wood is easy to cling to. And if the squirrels don't like the angles you've allowed them to eat from, they'll simply gnaw through the feeder in a few minutes. Wood doesn't provide much resistance to squirrel teeth. In fact, eating seed from the cardinal barn is so easy that squirrels will probably eat your feeder anyway, just to prove they're able to.

You can baffle classic wooden feeders, but unless you put your baffles around perfectly, you will have squirrels as guests. All they need to do is connect one paw to the feeder and they are in.

Cardinal Barn

	Poor				Great
Squirrelproofness	x to	x			
Ease of refilling					x
Visibility of birds		x			
Seed capacity					x
Attractiveness			x	to	x
Versatility of location				x	
Overall		x			

The Hylarious

Type: Fortress post feeder
Seed Capacity: 8 quarts
Dimensions: 9" x 12" x 17"
Attracts: Cardinals, titmice, starlings, wrens, chickadees, finches, blue jays, and mockingbirds; mourning doves are attracted to the spilled seed.

The Hylarious is similar in design and function to the SPF. Squirrels are prevented from entering the feeder by a shield that closes over the opening to the seed whenever a squirrel steps on the platform. While the SPF is green, the Hylarious is red. Both hold the same amount of seed.

There are some other differences between the SPF and the Hylarious. The seed in the Hylarious sits on a horizontal shelf, so not all the seed will be consumed. The platform that birds eat from and squirrels activate is metal, not wood.

Hylarious

	Poor				Great
Squirrelproofness				X	
Ease of refilling				X	
Visibility of birds					X
Seed capacity					X
Attractiveness		X			
Versatility of location			X		
Overall				X	

The Foiler

Type: Fortress post feeder
Dimensions: 9" x 11" x 14"
Seed Capacity: 10 quarts
Attracts: Cardinals, titmice, starlings, wrens, chickadees, finches, blue jays, and mockingbirds; mourning doves are attracted to the spilled seed.

One thing you have to say about many birdfeeders: their names get right to the point. The Foiler, another SPF-like feeder, works by using a squirrel's weight against him. As soon as a squirrel steps on the perching platform, his weight causes the seed hopper shield to cut off access to the seed. Sorry, Mr. Squirrel, no snack today. The Foiler has a larger seed capacity than either the SPF or the Hylarious. It must be mounted on a special post, however. Six holes stand between the platform and the inside seed bin; these holes are designed to prevent pigeons and other large birds from getting to the seed.

Foiler

	Poor				Great
Squirrelproofness					X
Ease of refilling					X
Visibility of birds				X	
Seed capacity					X
Attractiveness	X				
Versatility of location	X				
Overall				X	

Estate Feeder

Type: Pole feeder
Dimensions: Not applicable
Seed Capacity: 2+ quarts
Attracts: Finches, cardinals, titmice, chickadees, starlings, mockingbirds. The Estate feeder is among the newest feeders marketed by the Duncraft company. It combines simplicity, an adequate seed capacity, effective antisquirrel capabilities, and good bird visibility.

The Estate feeder is basically a two-quart bowl that holds about five pounds of bird seed, situated on a pole. The feeder is positioned between a sixteen-inch baffle on the bottom and a twelve-inch baffle on top. As long as you don't place the Estate feeder near any trees it should be virtually squirrelproof; the baffle is impenetrable. For added protection you can place the feeder on a squirrel spooker pole or grease the pole with Vaseline.

To fill the Estate feeder all you have to do is pour seed from a dispenser into the bowl. If you use black sunflower or other shelled seed, some hulls will accumulate in the feeder, which is fine if you don't want them scattered all over your lawn, and not so good if you're adverse to emptying the feeder frequently.

The feeder is well protected from most rains, but a storm that moves rain horizontally will get the seed inside wet. The Estate feeder is impervious to snow, as long as the snowdrifts don't grow taller than the height of the pole.

Estate

	Poor				Great
Squirrelproofness					X
Ease of refilling				X	
Visibility of birds					X
Seed capacity			X		
Attractiveness		X			
Versatility of location			X		
Overall				X	

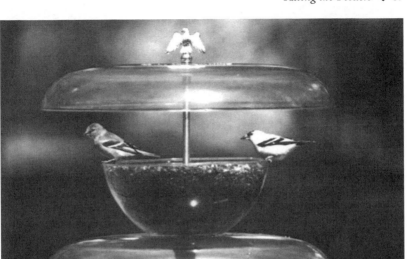

Duncraft's squirrelproof Estate Feeder attracts a variety of birds. In this photo two goldfinches are dining. Photo courtesy of Duncraft, Concord, N.H.

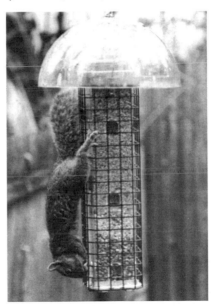

This squirrel solved the Squirrel's Dilemma by eating upside down.

Squirrel's Dilemma

Type: Hanging feeder
Dimensions: 5" square x 19" long
Seed Capacity: 4–8 pounds
Attracts: Most birds including titmice, wrens, lots of finches, chickadees and nuthatches. Cardinals and mourning doves will feed off the seed that falls to the ground.

The Squirrel's Dilemma is a long, rectangular feeder constructed of clear styrene plastic and surrounded with reinforced fox wire. Concave openings in the plastic dispense the seed. It reminds one of a medieval fortress, its forbidding shape issuing a warning to potential intruders: Do not venture near. Access to the feed is gained by sticking a beak in between the small spaces in the wire. The wire also provides a perch for little feathered friends.

The Squirrel's Dilemma lets you watch birds from three sides. If you want, you can cover the openings on the fourth side to force birds to eat only from the places where you can view them. The feeder itself won't win awards for design excellence; it's rather bland looking. However, its long shape and wire exterior keep the feeder miraculously free of droppings. The Squirrel's Dilemma can be hung from a post or tree limb.

Refilling the Squirrel's Dilemma isn't difficult, but you do have to remove the entire feeder to replenish it. Refilling is a simple matter of opening the metal top and pouring the seed in.

As for its squirrel resistance, if you *enjoy* feeding squirrels, the Squirrel's Dilemma is for you. When hung alone, without any baffles or other obstructions, it takes squirrels about ninety seconds to figure out how to dine at the Squirrel's Dilemma. Although it's true that squirrels "cannot chew on the feeder or get their head through the wire," as one bird supply catalog insists, they can get their mouths through, and that's all squirrels care about. No squirrel was ever scolded by its parents because it brought its face to the food instead of the other way around. And I've never seen a squirrel forsake a one-sun-flower-seed-at-a-time meal, especially when they can gobble at about twenty seeds a minute. Squirrels can also stick a paw inside and slide the seed into their ready mouths. The fox wire grid lets squirrels arrange themselves on the outside of the feeder in the position that's most comfortable to them. What a deal! While squirrels may have a hard time draining the Squirrel's Dilemma because they can't gorge themselves, they will hang around this reliable food source.

The Squirrel's Dilemma is a tough feeder to baffle because all a squirrel has to do is get one paw anywhere along any of the feeder's nineteen-inch sides to gain access. So even with a baffle, an agile squirrel can maneuver itself so it reaches some part of the feeder.

Despite the Squirrel Dilemma's attractiveness to squirrels, it is a fun feeder. Squirrels really can't empty it (at least not right away) and it does let you feed a variety of birds with a minimum of inconvenience. Some birds will even eat from the feeder on one side while a squirrel is invisibly snacking on the other. Feeders with large seed capacities and good visibility are always welcome.

Squirrel's Dilemma

Poor ———————————————— Great

Squirrelproofness	X				
Ease of refilling			X		
Visibility of birds				X	
Seed capacity				X	
Attractiveness		X			
Versatility of location			X		
Overall		X			

The Cling-a-Wing

Type: Hanging feeder
Dimensions: 6" diameter
Seed Capacity: 1 quart
Attracts: When filled with nuts this feeder will attract blue jays and red-bellied woodpeckers. Some people use this feeder exclusively as their nut feeder. Also attracts finches, titmice, nuthatches, evening grosbeaks, and wrens.

The Cling-a-Wing is a cute feeder. It's a plastic globe with four openings where birds can perch and eat. Smaller birds such as titmice, chickadees, and of course, finches, adore the Cling-a-Wing, but woodpeckers also eat from it when there's nothing else around. The globe prevents the seed inside from getting wet.

You refill the Cling-a-Wing by lifting the plastic stopper and pouring seed inside. You can use your hands to fill this feeder, but a seed dispenser works much better. The Cling-a-Wing can hold a variety of seed including sunflower seed, bread crumbs, and peanuts. In addition, a suet cake holder can be attached to the bottom of the Cling-a-Wing with bell wire wrapped around the bottom nut.

Although you can only see birds eating from one side, it's small enough so that you're bound to see birds flying around looking for a place to land. The Cling-a-Wing also rotates so that birds eating on the feeder's hidden side may come into view as they eat.

The Cling-a-Wing is only partially squirrelproof. If hung on a window bracket, squirrels can usually reach out from the wall and pull the feeder toward them. They can also attack from above by holding on to the ring on top of the feeder with their claws and munching upside down. If squirrels are having a difficult time eating the birdseed, they will eat the feeder. The Cling-a-Wing is among the most often-chewed birdfeeders around. Squirrels gnaw at the openings to make them bigger and they'll gnaw at the plastic belt around the feeder's equator. As they attack, squirrels will manage to spill a considerable amount of seed, which helps ground-feeding birds, but also encourages squirrels.

A large baffle placed close to the globe will keep squirrels from reaching the seed. The baffle will also make it more difficult to fill the Cling-a-Wing, but that's a common trade-off.

Cling-a-Wing

	Poor				Great
Squirrelproofness		X			
Ease of refilling	X				
Visibility of birds				X	
Seed capacity		X			
Attractiveness			X		
Versatility of location		X			
Overall		X			

The Spinning Satellite

Type: Hanging feeder
Dimensions: 6" diameter
Seed Capacity: About 1 pound
Attracts: Titmice, chickadees, finches, downy woodpeckers. The feeder cannot be filled with whole nuts, but can support peanut hearts.

This is perhaps the cutest bird feeder. The Spinning Satellite looks like a modern version of the spaceship on the old TV program, *My Favorite Martian*. As it hangs it spins; either in the wind or after a bird takes off from it. The feeder's diminutive size and symmetrical shape make it a pleasing feeder to look at. Chickadees think so. So do titmice, finches, and other small birds.

Unfortunately, squirrels think it's cute as well.

Cute is one attribute you shouldn't be looking for in a birdfeeder. Attractive, maybe, but definitely not cute.

Here's how this cute birdfeeder works. The Spinning Satellite is shaped like a nearly perfect globe. There's a circular opening underneath the satellite's equator, which has a little lip that serves as a perch. And the equator is a plastic protrusion that encircles the entire globe like Saturn's rings. The purpose of this protrusion is to keep squirrels from getting into the feeding hole. Amazingly, it accomplishes that objective—for about six seconds. Squirrels may, if they feel like it, reach over and feed from the Spinning Satellite from the top. From this position, feeding is more like feasting.

If you cover the Spinning Satellite with a baffle, which immediately destroys the Satellite's cute looks, squirrels can't feast from above.

So they latch on to the ring upside down and eat that way. From this position, they can empty the feeder quickly.

There's another option available to squirrels as well, one that is bound to please ground-feeding birds. It takes a little ingenuity or a dash of luck to figure out how to get the Spinning Satellite off its chain and on the ground. From there squirrels bat it around like a soccer ball. Another point about the Spinning Satellite: it holds a tiny amount of seed. And although only one bird at a time can eat from it, you'll find yourself filling and filling and filling the Spinning Satellite—probably every other afternoon. And still another point about this feeder: despite its little size, filling it is a pain. After you remove the cap, you put in the seed. Unfortunately, most seed dispensers won't fit the Spinning Satellite. As you try to fill it with your hands, you end up planting sunflower seeds.

Which brings me to yet another point about the Spinning Satellite. It only holds sunflower seeds. Peanuts clog the feeder, and other seeds don't flow easily through it. Because the opening angles upward, there's very little seed spillage.

In rare cases chickadees can climb inside the Spinning Satellite and become trapped.

So are there any virtues to the Spinning Satellite? Yes. It's a good way to coax squirrels away from your regular feeders. And it *is* good looking. If you already have a feeder or two set up, then go ahead and buy the Spinning Satellite. It's a fun feeder to watch.

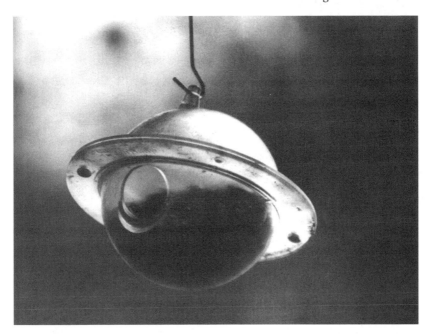

The Spinning Satellite.

Spinning Satellite

	Poor				Great
Squirrelproofness	X				
Ease of refilling	X				
Visibility of birds				X	
Seed capacity	X				
Attractiveness				X	
Versatility of location		X			
Overall	X				

The Window Chalet

Type: Window feeder
Dimensions: 9" x 6" x 4"
Seed Capacity: 1 quart
Attracts: Finches (lots), titmice, chickadees, wrens, downy
woodpeckers, and blue jays (if you fill it with peanuts). Doves and
cardinals will hang around for spilled seed.

The Window Chalet is a good-looking, chalet-style bird feeder. It attaches to your window with two suction cups, and holds a quart of seed—enough for one to three days depending on how many house finches you have. In addition to being attractive, the Window Chalet offers an excellent view of birds. You can stealthfully get within a foot of the feeder without scaring the birds away. It's an easy feeder to fill: either reach outside and fill by tilting a seed dispenser into it, or lift the feeder off the suction cups and fill it indoors. The feeder is simple to use, but can be difficult to install. When putting it on your window for the first time you'll find that the Window Chalet either ends up crooked or the suction cups keep falling to the ground, which can be a big deal if you live in an apartment building, as I did. To attach the feeder correctly you must follow the instructions carefully, because gravity has a way of defeating suction cups over time. Installed properly, the Window Chalet should stay up for about a year or until there's a hurricane. Or until a squirrel finds it.

The Window Chalet is not squirrelproof. In order for the Window Chalet to be squirrelproof one of the following criteria must be met: a) It must be high enough from any surface so that squirrels can't jump in *and* it must be positioned so that squirrels can't jump on top and crawl inside, or b) there must not be any squirrels around. Clearly the last possibility is no possibility.

There are two ways a squirrel can attack the window feeder: by jumping or climbing in, or by leaping on top and crawling over the top. Once he's inside, Mr. Squirrel can eat away. When a squirrel leaps on or into the Window Chalet it stresses the suction cups, playing directly into gravity's hands. A handful of such leaps and the window feeder is a goner. And if there's a hard surface below, hope that you're handy with superglue. If you live in a squirrel-infested area, then you may spend a lot of time running outside and looking for those semi-transparent suction cups on your hands and knees (just tell your neighbors it's your contact lens). On the other hand, having the feeder fall is better than coming home and finding a squirrel inside, wantonly feasting.

But if your feeder can be placed so that squirrels are unable to approach it, the Window Chalet is a gem. You may have to experiment to find out the perfect position to put it in.

The Window Chalet—and other window feeders—will stay on your window longer if you attach the suction cups with superglue. With superglue it will be able to resist a squirrel's weight.

Window Chalet

	Poor				Great
Squirrelproofness	x*				
Ease of refilling				x	
Visibility of birds					x
Seed capacity		x			
Attractiveness				x	
Versatility of location	x				
Overall			depends on location		

*unless in the middle of a large window

The Dome Feeder

Type: Hanging feeder
Dimensions: 7" x 12" diameter
Seed Capacity: About 1 quart
Attracts: Titmice, finches, blackbirds, chickadees, and blue jays, if you fill it with nuts and keep the opening large enough. Spillage attracts juncos, mourning doves, mockingbirds, and cardinals.

The Dome Feeder is a clever hanging feeder. A clear plastic tray that captures seed and shell and gives birds a place to perch is attached to a hexagonal hopper. The feeder is attached to a dome by a metal chain which can be raised or lowered depending on how squirrelproof you want the feeder to be, and whether or not you want to prevent large birds from getting to the seed. The feeder and tray can be raised so that it is almost entirely inside the dome, which gives pretty good protection.

You get a fairly good view of birds, except of course when they're on the opposite side of the feeder. It can be filled with a variety of seeds including hulled sunflower, millet, and shelled peanuts.

You refill the Dome Feeder by lifting the chain that connects the feeder to the baffle and pouring seed in. You cannot fill the feeder while it is attached to the baffle.

You would think by looking at this feeder that it would be completely squirrelproof when retracted within the dome. And it is—for a while. After a couple of days some squirrel will figure out the way to thwart the Dome Feeder. Beating the Dome Feeder requires not so much smarts as it does athletic ability, so usually the strongest squirrel wins. A squirrel (because there usually isn't more than one around who can do it) defeats the Dome Feeder by hanging onto the ring on top of the dome with his hind legs, stretching over the baffle, leaning underneath the baffle, grabbing onto the tray, and pulling it towards him. When he leans, seed spills out the other side and less dominant squirrels also feast. Each successive time it's easier for the squirrel to gain access to the feeder. Because the Dome Feeder has such a small seed capacity, a squirrel can empty it in a hurry.

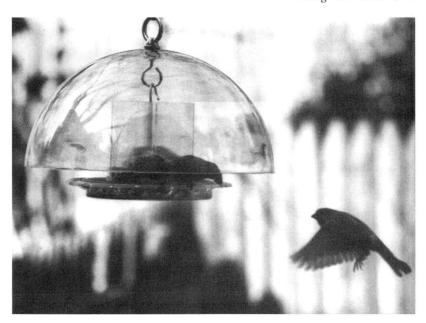

A house finch approaches the Dome Feeder.

Dome Feeder

	Poor				Great
Squirrelproofness		x			
Ease of refilling				x	
Visibility of birds				x	
Seed capacity		x			
Attractiveness		x			
Versatility of location			x		
Overall			x		

The Cardinal Classic

Type: Window feeder
Dimensions: 12" x 5½"
Seed Capacity: 1 quart
Attracts: Titmice, cardinals, finches (more than you've ever seen), chickadees, and sometimes nuthatches and mockingbirds. If you fill it with nuts you'll reduce your finch population and increase the number of chickadees, titmice, and blue jays who frequent this feeder.

The Cardinal Classic, a clear plastic feeder, is similar to the Window Chalet in application. The only differences between the Cardinal Classic and the Window Chalet is that three suction cups hold this feeder in place, rather than two, and it has a flat roof instead of an angled roof. The three suction cups are a little more difficult to attach, but they hold the feeder more securely in place. The Classic's flat roof makes it slightly easier for squirrels to enter than the Window Chalet. Some people prefer this feeder's simple design over the Window Chalet's Swiss cottage style.

Cardinal Classic

	Poor				Great
Squirrelproofness		X			
Ease of refilling				X	
Visibility of birds				X	
Seed capacity		X			
Attractiveness		X			
Versatility of location			X		
Overall			X		

The Songbird Table Feeder

Type: Open platform feeder
Dimensions: 21" x 18"
Seed Capacity: Several quarts
Attracts: Everything

The Songbird Table feeder can be a great feeder. The seed is visible to all birds. It attracts both ground-feeding birds, including cardinals and mourning doves, and birds that enjoy feeding up high, such as chickadees and titmice. You'll also see blue jays, woodpeckers, and just about everything else that flies. The Songbird Table feeder can be mounted on a deck, fence post, or on top of a pole. It's simple to fill— just pour seed into it. It comes with a "moisture draining removable screen bottom" because this feeder *will* get wet. To clean the feeder simply remove the tray.

There are several drawbacks to the table feeder. A strong wind may knock seed out of the tray. When it rains the seed is going to get wet. Birds aren't crazy about wet seed; as seed dries it rots, so after a rain you should dump the seed and replace it. The feeder will become filled with bird droppings.

Most dangerously, the Songbird Table feeder can be squirrel heaven. Mounted on a deck or a fence, the feeder is an open invitation to squirrels. In fact some people use the table feeder to draw squirrels away from their other feeders. If you put the table feeder on a pole, make sure it's exceptionally well baffled.

Songbird Table

	Poor				Great
Squirrelproofness	X				
Ease of refilling					X
Visibility of birds					X
Seed capacity				X	
Attractiveness		X			
Versatility of location		X			
Overall*					

*An overall rating is not possible given the peculiar nature of this feeder. Depending on how you intend to use it, it can either be terrific or you will be fending off squirrels all the time.

Suet Baskets

Type: Specialized hanging feeder
Dimensions: Less than 5" x 5" x 2"
Seed Capacity: 1 or 2 suet cakes
Attracts: Starlings, downies, red-bellied, red-headed, and other woodpeckers. Titmice also like suet, especially in winter, as do chickadees. Finches will gorge suet in winter, too, as will pretty much every bird.

Suet baskets aren't a particular brand of feeder, but because they are so popular and so crucial to attracting particular kinds of birds such as woodpeckers, it's useful to know how best to use them. There are a number of variations on the theme, but generally suet feeders are rectangular baskets you place one or two suet cakes in. The feeders are open and birds can feed from any side.

Suet is beef fat. You can make it yourself, buy it from a butcher shop, or purchase commercially prepared suet. Most people prefer the latter course because commercially prepared suet cakes, though more expensive, are less messy. In addition, commercial suet lasts longer than home brews, which quickly rot in warm weather. There are several different "flavors" of commercial suet cakes—plain, filled with sunflower seed and millet, and peanut filled. Suet is a high-energy food that provides many essential nutrients that birds would otherwise get from insects.

Most birders buy suet to attract woodpeckers all year round (downy, hairy, and red-bellied woodpeckers prefer suet to most other birdfeeder food) and to offer a well balanced meal to other birds. The problem with suet is that it is a favorite meal for squirrels, who will eat it all year long. (Flying squirrels and raccoons also love suet, if you're wondering why your suet disappears overnight.) To compound this dilemma, woodpeckers prefer to eat suet near a tree trunk, which makes it easy for squirrels to reach the suet; dangling suet at the end of a branch won't attract woodpeckers. Baffles are worthless when used close to the tree trunk.

What to do? There are several solutions. First, create a squirrel diverter, a platform of sunflower seeds away from your feeder. Squirrels go for what's easiest. Second, place a metal skirt around the tree to keep squirrels from climbing it, assuming that it's the only tree in the vicinity. Third, place the suet near the tree for a while. As woodpeckers become accustomed to your yard and as they begin to enjoy their free lunch, gradually move the suet further out on the branch. Now's the time for that baffle, which should cover the suet enough to keep squirrels from leaning over it, but not be too constricting for the larger woodpeckers. As you move the suet away from the tree, those woodpeckers will follow it.

Suet can solve a major problem many homeowners have: woodpeckers who drill holes in their houses. Woodpeckers damage houses because they're looking for insects in the wood. With suet you'll tempt them away from your recently refurbished siding.

Exclusively Thistle Feeders

Type: Tubular feeder
Dimensions: Varies, the most common is 16" long and about 2½" wide
Seed Capacity: About 2 quarts
Attracts: Finches, pine siskins, and red polls. To prevent house and purple finches from eating the thistle and to encourage only goldfinches, cut the perches to about one-half inch long. House and purple finches will not be able to eat from these shortened perches.

Thistle feeders are specially designed to dispense only thistle seed. They have smaller openings than normal tube feeders. Thistle seed is also called niger, and is among the most expensive seed you can buy. But because you can modify the thistle feeder by shortening the perches to attract only goldfinches, it's a good feeder to have around.

It's best to buy the kind with wooden perches so that you can easily cut them. Metal perches are hard to cut. Another advantage of thistle feeders is that squirrels don't care for thistle, and will only eat it when they are one step before starving, or to bug you. Thistle feeders are also available as window feeders, which let you see goldfinches more closely.

If you modify your feeder to attract only goldfinches, the seed may not disappear so rapidly. Replace the thistle in the feeder at least once a month to prevent it from spoiling.

This feeder can be hung from a tree or mounted on a pole.

Thistle Feeders

	Poor				Great
Squirrelproofness					X
Ease of refilling			X		
Visibility of birds				X	
Seed capacity				X	
Attractiveness				X	
Versatility of location				X	
Overall				X*	

*Remember, this is a specialized feeder.

Thistle/Sunflower Feeders

Type: Tubular feeder
Dimensions: Varies, the most common is 16" long and about 2½" wide
Seed Capacity: About 2 quarts
Attracts: Finches, titmice, chickadees, wrens; cardinals and mourning doves hang around to pick up the spilled seed (if you don't include a spill tray)

What are called "thistle feeders" are usually feeders that can be filled with either thistle or sunflower or hulled seeds. Only those feeders with very small holes are pure thistle feeders. While the advantages of pure thistle feeders were highlighted in the previous pages, there is one implicit disadvantage: thistle only attracts a limited number of species. Sunflower, on the other hand, attracts most birds. Unfortunately it brings in squirrels like an insider stock tip brings in stock brokers.

Although thistle feeders hold two quarts of feed, as the seed level drops, fewer perches become available. If you want to make all perches feeding stations, you will have to refill this feeder fairly often.

Thistle feeders have a number of good points. They hold a relatively large amount of seed, are easy to hang, offer excellent viewing of birds, and can feed up to eight birds at a time. In addition, many come with spill trays that catch shells and falling seed. Birds have an easy time recognizing that they are filled with goodies and fly directly to them. Thistle feeders have a simple elegance about them; they're unpretentious and they don't have any fancy gimmicks—all they do is feed birds. Thistle feeders feel right.

And they feel right for squirrels. Baffles are a must for thistle feeders. Because these feeders are so narrow, they can usually be hung far enough from the tree trunk to prevent squirrels from leaping to the feeder. If they do reach the feeder, squirrels can either hang upside down and eat, or stand on one of the perches—it's up to them.

If you mount your thistle feeder on a pole, be sure to baffle it below (and above if there are any trees in the vicinity).

Like all feeders, thistle feeders should be cleaned on a regular basis.

Thistle/Sunflower

	Poor			Great
Squirrelproofness	x*			
Ease of refilling		x		
Visibility of birds			x	
Seed capacity	x			
Attractiveness	x			
Versatility of location			x	
Overall	x			

*Squirrelproofness depends on how you baffle and hang this feeder; by itself, it's open game for squirrels.

The Presto Galaxy Deluxe 3 Tube Bird Feeder

Type: Tubular hanging feeder
Dimensions: Three connected tubes, each 1¾" x 24"
Seed Capacity: Approximately 6 quarts
Attracts: Titmice, chickadees, purple, house and goldfinches, wrens, cardinals, and mourning doves.

When you bought this feeder, you bought a mouthful—for the birds. The Presto Galaxy Deluxe 3 Tube Bird Feeder is a tube feeder—it's actually three tube feeders connected together. It's similar in application to the regular thistle seed feeder; the 3 Tube can hold thistle, sunflower seed, hulled sunflower seed, millet, or cracked corn. The major differences between the two feeders are: a) the 3 Tube's size—it can accommodate up to twenty-four birds at a time, and b) it cannot be mounted on a pole. This is a hanging feeder only.

But it's a fun feeder. Even if you aren't crazy about the amount of seed finches eat, you have to be amused by the way they carry on, and the 3 Tube attracts flocks of finches. If you've never seen twenty-four birds feed at the same time, it's worth investing in the 3 Tube. It may not be your regular feeder, but since the main reason for feeding birds is fun, you should have a fun feeder.

The 3 Tube is not particularly squirrel-resistant. The largest baffle only barely covers the top. There's room for twenty-four birds, which means there are twenty-four places for squirrels to eat from. All those perches make it an easy target, especially because the three tubes add up to one wide feeder.

You have to refill three separate tubes, and if birds eat unevenly from one of the outside tubes you'll need to refill it to prevent the feeder from tilting and the seed from spilling. As with all tube feeders, frequent refilling is mandatory if you want all perching stations to be open at all times.

But is the 3 Tube worth buying? Sure—if your frustration and fun levels are high enough. The 3 Tube is definitely a second feeder, not a first.

The Deluxe 3 Tube hanging feeder also comes in a thistle seed version.

Presto Galaxy Deluxe 3 Tube

	Poor				Great
Squirrelproofness	X				
Ease of refilling		X			
Visibility of birds					X
Seed capacity					X
Attractiveness		X			
Versatility of location	X				
Overall			X		

The Squirrel Baffle Bird Feeder

Type: Hanging feeder
Dimensions: 14" baffle dome with a 7" seed hopper
Seed Capacity: 5 pounds
Attracts: Chickadees, titmice, finches, wrens.

The Squirrel Baffle Bird Feeder (SBBF) is one of those feeders that you can't wait to get home to try. The picture and description on the box are tempting: "When squirrel tries to get at the food, the TILT ACTION causes him to slide off," reads the box. Finally, justice.

The SBBF can be filled with a variety of seed, including whole and shelled nuts, cracked corn, and sunflower seed. Everything fits comfortably in a bowl-like container. The bowl hooks into a baffle.

The large baffle sways in the wind, which discourages birds and may occasionally spill seed, but it does protect the feeder from squirrels. Large birds aren't crazy about the SBBF because they can't get under the baffle easily. But it is a chickadee paradise. Birds are completely sheltered as they eat.

Squirrels that land on top slip off the SBBF faster than they fall off any other feeder. They'll keep trying, but it takes an exceptionally

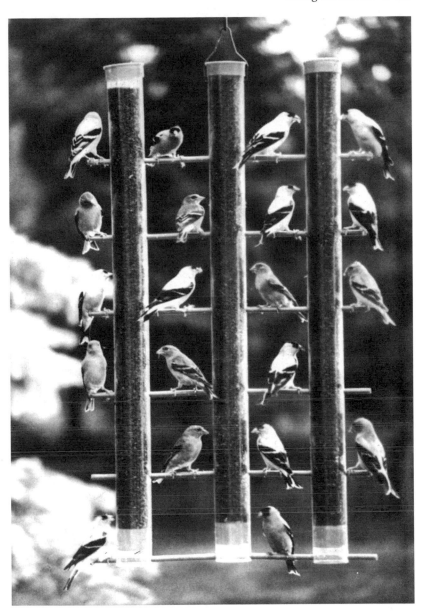

The Presto Galaxy Deluxe 3 Tube feeder may not be the most squirrel-resistant feeder on the market, but it is one of the most fun. The Presto Galaxy attracts more birds at one time than just about any other feeder. Photo courtesty of Presto Galaxy, Incorporated.

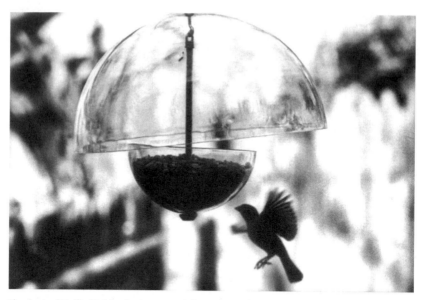

The Squirrel Baffle Bird Feeder keeps seed dry and out of squirrels' mouths.

agile squirrel to get the seed in the SBBF. I can't imagine that a squirrel would gain more energy eating the seed inside than it would expend trying to get inside.

Squirrel Baffle

	Poor				Great
Squirrelproofness					X
Ease of refilling			X		
Visibility of birds				X	
Seed capacity				X	
Attractiveness		X			
Versatility of location			X		
Overall				X	

SIX

Homebrewed Feeders

There are plenty of terrific squirrelproof (kind of) feeders on the market. Numerous inventors are sunning themselves in the Caribbean, where there are no squirrels, thanks to the sales of their feeders. Some of the most clever inventions of all time are antisquirrel feeders.

But there's no reason why you have to limit yourself to buying an off-the-shelf squirrelproof feeder. Tens of thousands of bird feeders have built their own contraptions—and they work.

Gary Wilson of New Jersey offered this home brew of an idea:

I've pretty much squirrelproofed my feeder using commercial components. By "pretty much" I mean I've had only one intrusion in the two years it's been up. The main feeder is a cedar gazebo-type platform with a central tube that holds a half gallon of mixed seed. Its mounted five feet off the ground on a short horizontal cedar four-by-four that's mounted on a vertical cedar four-by-four affixed to the ground. Tube feeders hang from the ends of the horizontal four-by-four; one with black oil sunflower and one with niger thistle. Both the main feeder and the mounting post are made by Country Home. The mounting post is called a *quick pole* and is actually two separate three-foot lengths of cedar that get connected with an internal double-ended lag bolt. The pole is affixed to the ground with a vertical length of angle iron that is internally connected to the quick pole.

Now here's the key to squirrelproofing: before connecting the two vertical pieces, I bought a twenty-four-inch long cylindrical raccoon guard from a store and placed it over the lag screw. When I connected the vertical pieces it was firmly held in place. A squirrel has to make a vertical jump of at least three feet to get to a place it can hold on. While some squirrels can jump up to five feet, most seem to get discouraged by my arrangement. The feeder is also located ten feet away from any other object to avoid assaults from above. Installation time was about one hour.

If you want to have a little fun, put your feeder on top of a pole. At the base of the pole create an opening large enough to attach a hose from your dryer. Then drill holes at frequent intervals up and down the pole. Attach the hose to your dryer, and wait. The warm air won't hurt the squirrels, but it certainly will alter the universe as they know it.

Here's another concoction that works for at least one bird feeder:

I have an arrangement that I have not seen any squirrels get by (so far). I use a standard hemispherical baffle hung from a tree branch with a hanging three-tube feeder but with an important modification. I put a ten-inch section of two-inch diameter PVC pipe over the wire and the hanging loop on top of the baffle. This keeps the squirrels from hanging over the side of the baffle and reaching a perch. They can't get a hold on the pipe with their hind feet.

Not everyone has photographs of their feeders. But some people get very creative at describing how their so-called squirrelproof feeder works. Here is how one person described it over the Internet:

Wintertime meant snow and squirrels to me as a child. I grew up in a suburb outside Boston, Massachusetts. My family lived on an acre of land with a mile of forest behind us. Needless to say, we had an abundant supply of gray squirrels who loved to get into or onto my mother's many birdfeeders. My mother refused to shoot the squirrels with the airgun we bought her. Instead, she tried several creative (and unsuccessful) devices to keep the squirrels away from her feeders. Finally, while cleaning out the attic one year, she came across a box of ancient LPs. These were the really thick, old records, made of pliable plastic, and with them she built a squirrelproof feeder.

The LP was held on the rope by tying knots in the rope on either side of the record. The record could move—the idea was for it to lay across the rope and send the squirrel sliding if he tried to climb across it to the feeder. When a squirrel came down the rope, he would find the LP. The squirrels out in our backyard were fearless, and would stretch across the LP by holding onto the rope with their back paws and would grab the rope or feeder with their front paws. Failure meant a five-foot drop to the snow, which they seemed to enjoy more than the feed. The feeder was protected about 50 percent of the time, but all this design accomplished was to create an amusement park ride for squirrels (along with Disneyland-like waiting lines of squirrels up the tree).

Mom added a second LP tied several inches under the first one. Now, when the squirrel stretched past LP 1, he encountered LP 2. The distance between the LPs caused an overlap of slick plastic. The squirrels plummeted to the snow time after time. The chickadees, titmice, and nuthatches actually got comfortable with the sight of plummeting furry forms flying past as they ate, and wouldn't even bother to fly off at the sight of an approaching squirrel. This design worked 100 percent of the time—until my mother (who now felt sorry for the squirrels) took the records down.

One advantage that store-bought feeders often have is that they are more attractive than what we can make at home. This isn't a commentary on the advantages of factory automation—it's just that many of us would rather concentrate on keeping the squirrels at bay than winning an award from *Better Homes and Gardens*. Here's one such bird feeder who subscribes to this point of view wholeheartedly:

I keep squirrels away by using a rather ugly method that seems to work. Assuming you have a pole feeder, fit a hard plastic crate with holes over the top of the feeder. If it is a rather tight fit and the squirrels don't chew through it, it will keep most big birds and squirrels out. The smaller birds will be able to fit into the holes and get at the seed. Like I said, it is kind of an eyesore. I use a similar setup under my hanging feeder to discourage pigeons. I took a larger crate and placed it on the ground under the hanging feeder. The excess seed falls through the holes of the crate but the pigeons are too big to fit through the crate to get at the seed. Little birds run right through the holes and munch away. I put a flowerpot on the crate to make it less of an eyesore but the squirrels ate the flowers. Of course, the pigeons have moved on to my other feeders, but it's a start.

I experimented with everything I could think of, including the red pepper. I tried barbed wire (it actually helped the squirrels scale the ten-foot pole) and many different kinds of feeders, before I hit on something that seems to have worked and is not too ugly.

First, you need to invest in feeders that have a wire cage around them, or at least have metal perches. The squirrels can't do too much damage to these, and it limits their seed consumption. I strung thin, vinyl-coated clothesline between two trees, about fifteen feet off the ground. I used pulleys to suspend each feeder from the clothesline, so I can raise and lower the feeders without a ladder. Each feeder hangs about three feet down from the clothesline. It seems to be hard for the squirrels to shimmy down the skinny line, and a baffle above each feeder makes it even harder.

The other thing that worked, but was kind of ugly, was putting cheap pizza pans on the line. Drill a hole in the center of each pizza pan. Use some short pieces of PVC between each pan as spacers. You should plan on three or four pans on each side of the feeder. The squirrels can jump over one or two, but seemed to have trouble with more than that.

Electricity is often a popular tool for trying to thwart squirrels. (Who among us hasn't dreamed about electricity's potential?) Here's what one clever person did:

I had one of those plastic cylinder feeders with metal perches. The squirrels were getting most of the food. I noticed that a squirrel cannot stay on the feeder without touching two or more of the perches, but that a bird cannot touch more than one. The perches are electrically isolated from each other by the plastic cylinder to which they are attached. I rigged a "shocker" circuit from a small transformer, a homebuilt "tilt" switch, and a nine-volt battery, and connected the shocker to alternating pairs of the metal perches. It worked perfectly. Whenever a squirrel jumped on the feeder, the little devil jiggled the "tilt" switch and delivered a shock to itself. The squirrel immediately dropped or jumped to the ground, sat for a few seconds, and *never* tried it again. The device eventually managed to train all of the neighborhood squirrels to stay off the feeder, so that when the battery ran down it took the squirrels several months to realize it.

And finally, these ideas:

I did, after many tries, devise a squirrelproof birdfeeder (or so I thought). It was simply a pole with a standard birdfeeder on top, but had a cone of slippery metal under the feeder, which prevented the squirrels from getting all the way to the top. It's rather standard these days, but back then it hadn't been thought of. But the resident squirrels got smart quickly: they would climb out on the overhanging limbs of the nearby trees, and jump off and land on the top of the feeder!

I thought to deter the squirrels' interest by building a birdproof squirrel feeder. This consisted of a coffee can mounted on a post, the can about six inches off the ground. The whole thing surrounded by chicken wire with maybe a three-inch space between it and the ground. I filled the can with peanuts. The idea was that the squirrel could walk under the wire, climb the post, fish out a pawful of peanuts and go on his way.

In 1834 there was a competition between two towns in Indiana to see who could shoot the most squirrels in one day. The winner bagged 900; the runner-up, 700.

In the early 1900s, because of hunting and deforestation, there was some concern that gray squirrels could become extinct.

SEVEN

Over-the-Counter Antisquirrel Structures and Devices

There was a complaint about a squirrel jumping from a tree to the roof of the Trinity Church. It has been found that the squirrel is jumping from a County tree so this is not a problem or responsibility of the Borough.

—*Rocky Hill Gazette*, Rocky Hill, NJ

There are plenty of birdfeeders on the market. Some of these have a modicum of antisquirrel abilities. Others are grazing stations for famished rodents. But even the feeders with the highest antisquirrel capabilities aren't always squirrelproof. Buying a feeder labeled "squirrelproof" usually leads to disappointment. Often a manufacturer claims a feeder is squirrelproof—and then you get it home and within two days you have the suspicion that that particular feeder must have been tested on Alaska's north slope, where there are no squirrels. Strong, persistent squirrels can figure out a way to penetrate most so-called antisquirrel feeders. Whether a squirrel will penetrate a feeder is not a matter of *if*, but *when*. Friendly squirrels teach their comrades this skill.

Even a good squirrel-thwarting feeder frequently needs to be improved. You may have to put it on a pole. Or add a baffle. Or extend the chain the feeder's hanging from. But squirrels can climb poles, crawl over baffles, and shimmy chains and cords. These traditional tools for barring squirrel attacks often fail. Instead, you have to use the one great advantage that humans have over rodents: imagination. Some bird supply companies have done the thinking for you, and offer excellent antisquirrel devices. Some of these over-the-counter devices work famously. But it may be necessary in other circumstances to let your imagination roam in your basement, garage, kitchen, or local hardware store, to find the material to construct your own antisquirrel apparatus.

Keep in mind that where you place your feeder is as important as what feeder you buy or how you reinforce it. The effectiveness of antisquirrel measures depends greatly on where you put the feeder in the first place. Trees seem to be a popular location for feeders, but popularity doesn't translate into effectiveness. Trees are not your friends; they are on the squirrel's side. Squirrels climb trees, live in trees, jump from tree to tree, eat trees, hide in trees, mate in trees. When you put a feeder in a tree you are placing your feeder in jeopardy. Baffle it well and bind it securely to the tree, or the squirrels will figure out a way to get at the feeder or knock it down. (See the chapter 5 for more on where to place your feeder.) Begin to ignore the trees in your yard and you will have taken the first step toward creating a squirrelproof structure.

A couple of safety tips are in order here. While it helps birds to feed them, not all birdfeeding practices are healthy. Moisture, for example, creates a medium for mold to grow on seed. So, as you make your feeder squirrelproof:

1. Place your feeder where it isn't likely to become soaked in a rainstorm. Baffles help keep feeders dry.

2. Discard the seed, clean and dry the feeder whenever it becomes wet.

3. Be leery about spilled seed. Although spilled seed attracts cardinals, juncos, mourning doves, and other ground-feeding birds, seed on the ground quickly becomes wet and moldy. In addition, seed beneath a feeder gets covered with bird droppings, which are vectors for diseases that kill birds.

4. Look out for your own health, too: always wash your hands after handling a feeder.

These points are covered in more detail in chapter 5, "Rating the Feeders."

If you don't consider your squirrel problem serious enough to take the countermeasures described in this chapter, just wait. Once the squirrels get a taste for things in your yard, there's no stopping them, as one birder observed in a letter to the editor of the *Dick E. Bird News*:

> I started feeding a cute little red squirrel that was hanging around my Birdsnest Boarding House. I brought him a variety of nuts and treated him royally. Now I find he is beginning to eat my new deck.
>
> —Nuts up North

(The *Dick E. Bird News* is a monthly newspaper about birds, birdseed, squirrels and related affairs. It combines facts and amusement. For subscription information, see the resources section. It's a publication no birder should be without.)

Part I: Passive Measures

Teflon

Greasing poles with oil is one of the oldest ways of preventing squirrels from climbing into feeders. All you do is coat the pole with WD-40 or other greasy stuff that's been in your basement, or let a teenager rub against it. It's entertaining to watch the grease work as the squirrels slide off. For a while. For some squirrels.

Until it rains.

Even if it doesn't rain, squirrels will persist at trying to climb up a greased pole, and eventually the slick grease will turn pebbly. When that happens they can simply climb over it.

Grease has other limitations, too. Phil Stone of Washington, D.C. said that his wife, Katharine, once greased a pole in winter. The grease kept the squirrels off until it froze one cold day, and the squirrels simply shimmied up the ice. And for anyone who doubted this story, there were claw marks in the ice.

Fortunately, technology has brought us a new weapon: Teflon. In particular, spray Teflon in a can. All you do is spray it on the pole, side of your house or apartment building, or wherever you've put the feeder, and watch the fun as the first squirrel tries to climb. (Don't spray Teflon or oil in the baffle or any other place where birds might alight.) The Teflon causes the slipping squirrel to blame its parents for incomplete climbing lessons.

Teflon is a good, temporary measure. I emphasize *temporary* because although it lasts longer than oil, when left outside Teflon will eventually come off the pole. Use Teflon when you want a way of buying time until you can think of a more permanent solution.

Nixalite

When you've reached the stage that you have to use Nixalite to keep squirrels away from your feeder, you have very serious squirrel problems. Nixalite is a dangerous-looking material. It can be a potent, almost impenetrable barrier. Nixalite is the last line of defense before you have to employ active, threatening methods like buying a big dog. Once you've used Nixalite you have surely declared war on squirrels. So before Nixalite, be warned: once Nixalite appears, squirrels will know that they no longer have to play Mr. Nice Rodent.

Nixalite was developed in the late 1940s and has been marketed by Nixalite of America since 1950 as a method for controlling—of all things—pigeons. Nixalite consists of two- and four-foot-long metal strips with 120 needle-sharp points protruding from the strips covering a 180 degree radius. The strips, which are one-quarter inch wide, and the points are constructed of 302 stainless steel.

The metal strips can be bent and shaped to conform with any surface you want to prevent squirrels from reaching.

Once installed, Nixalite doesn't need to be maintained. The points remain sharp and the steel won't rust. Should you decide to move the strips, they can be easily repositioned. Because the strips are pliable, you can use Nixalite for a variety of feeder conditions.

Nixalite looks frightening and formidable. As you approach a Nixalite-covered feeder, the spines which spin off in all directions seem to curve toward your skin. Your imagination conjures drops of blood on the Nixalite's tips; you can hear screams emerging from it. Of all the weapons in the antisquirrel arsenal, Nixalite is the one that makes you—and the squirrel—afraid. Squirrels may not have the intelligence of humans (yes, that's a proven fact), but they recognize Nixalite's dangers.

Nixalite works, that's for sure. But you have to ask yourself whether you're willing to live with a feeder that looks like a fortress.

Nixalite has another important quality. Used correctly, it won't harm squirrels (or birds). Nixalite's construction prevents animals from crawling across or over it, because they are unable to find any secure footing in the area covered by Nixalite. Nixalite is not designed to trap squirrels, entangle them, or stick into them. The spines are angled so that squirrels avoid Nixalite, rather than try to venture into it. According to the manufacturer, "Nixalite is approved by leading humane and bird societies."

Do not place Nixalite under the feeder where the squirrel might fall. A squirrel falling onto Nixalite would give you the opportunity to try your squirrel recipe.

Nixalite must be installed strategically to be effective. Properly installed, it can prevent squirrels from alighting on top of bird feeders, and keep squirrels from climbing up poles and trees.

Let's look at the on-top-of-feeder application first. One of the most enjoyable ways for a squirrel to dine is to crawl into an open feeder, such as an alpine-shaped window feeder, and munch away, sheltered from the elements. If the feeder isn't designed to let a squirrel enter, a squirrel's second preference is to hang from the feeder's roof and eat upside down. (Squirrels don't care whether they eat right side up or upside down. Indeed, squirrels would have made terrific experimental animals for the early days of the space program. Now that's an idea!)

To prevent a squirrel from entering an open-faced feeder, thoroughly cover the top and sides of the feeder with Nixalite. Nixalite should also extend over the front of the feeder to prevent the squirrel from using any surface as a platform. It's a good idea, also, to let the Nixalite stretch beyond the feeder's edges, so that there is absolutely no surface the squirrel will want to put its little paws on—no matter how hungry he becomes. There's a correlation between how terrifying your feeder looks and how successful the Nixalite is at keeping out squirrels. As you safeguard your feeder, you should have a fortress mentality.

To discourage squirrels from poaching by hanging upside down, as they like to do from baffles and tube feeders, just place the Nixalite so that the squirrels can't grip the part of the baffle or feeder they prefer. This means you may have to spend considerable time observing squirrels. Notice all the positions they grab. The Nixalite manual points out, "Installation must be handled with ingenuity and skill, so take your time . . . Effective installations don't just happen—they are planned." And remember, squirrels are tenacious: once you block a particular position, they will struggle (and often succeed) at finding another place to hold on.

Make sure you use enough Nixalite. Too little, and the squirrels will simply go around it.

Nixalite comes with metal fasteners which you can use to secure the strips to your feeder or pole. Alternatively, you can glue the Nixalite on, or use copper bell wire to hold it in position. Household cement works better than superglue, which seems to be helpful only if you want to attach Nixalite to your fingers. (Never use string to secure Nixalite. Squirrels will munch through string.)

Nixalite is most useful when you want to stop a squirrel from climbing a pole or tree. Despite their natural climbing and leaping abilities, squirrels do have to contend with gravity, and Nixalite magnifies gravity's effect on squirrels. As you lay out Nixalite, keep in mind that squirrels have great leaping ability. According to Marie Gellerstedt, president of Nixalite, "the first row must be at least four feet off the ground," otherwise squirrels can leap over it. Gellerstedt pointed out that when squirrels in her yard are being chased by her dog they can jump ten feet with a running start. Attach four or five rows of Nixalite around the circumference of the tree or pole, the first about four feet from the ground, then three or more at five-inch intervals. Do not wrap Nixalite around the tree or pole barber pole-style, because squirrels can grab hold and climb up the spiral. For the same reason, don't arrange Nixalite horizontally. If installed correctly, the squirrels will never reach your feeder by climbing up.

Currently, Nixalite starter kits, consisting of four strips and fasteners, cost $41, which includes postage. Nixalite is available only from the manufacturer, which is listed in the resources section.

Perrier bottles

You ask how Perrier bottles can stop squirrels from raiding feeders? Mere water—how can that succeed? Well, in special circumstances, Perrier bottles can prevent squirrels from getting to the spots they must launch from to reach your feeder. When leaping, squirrels need to launch themselves from particular angles. This is especially true when their target area for landing is small. Perrier bottles are especially useful when you have to position your feeder close to the ground or other surface such as a window ledge or air conditioner.

Perrier bottles work, but as with most passive antisquirrel devices, you have to apply the bottles intelligently. Before you position the bottles, pay attention to the locations the squirrel leaps from. After drinking the ninety-nine-cent water in the bottle, fill the Perrier bottles with free tap water and bunch them close together to cover the launching area. You must fill the bottle with water, otherwise Mr. Squirrel will easily knock them over. It's best if you glue the bottles together so that the squirrel will be unable to push any one of them over. Alternatively, wrap copper bell wire around the bottles. You'll need at least five bottles.

Squirrels cannot climb Perrier bottles and can't walk on top of them. The surface formed by the bottle tops contains too much empty space for them to find solid footing. No matter how much they paw at the bottles, they won't be able to get on top. For all practical purposes, you've created an area in which squirrels cannot enter—a squirrel-free zone.

Still, the persistent and knowledgeable squirrel may be able to thwart the Perrier system. Such squirrels know that although their preferred launching area is no longer available to them, they can still leap up, and although they won't land in the feeder squirrels may be able to get close enough to reach some part of the feeder, grab hold, and crawl inside. This is known as the *close-enough phenomenon*. If the squirrel can land on top of the feeder, or reach a chain, perch, or other structure . . . well, you've lost. If this occurs, you may need to combine Perrier bottles with Nixalite or grease to make life more difficult for the squirrels.

The squirrelproof habitat

Lola Oberman of Bethesda, Maryland, developed a virtually squirrelproof bird habitat. She enclosed her feeder in a wire mesh box measuring six feet high by four feet wide and long. The mesh was comprised of two-inch-wide holes—too large for any squirrel to penetrate, but large enough for most birds to get inside. The habitat worked perfectly.

You can construct an antisquirrel habitat with chicken wire, rubber-coated wire, or any similar mesh wire. Be sure to enclose the top, or squirrels will certainly climb in. Once constructed, you can place the feeder on a pole inside the habitat, or, probably more easily, suspend it from the top. With wire clippers you can construct a door to let you fill the feeder easily. If you're truly adventurous, you can construct an even larger habitat, and fill it with several feeders and a birdbath.

Woodpeckers

"Huh? Woodpeckers?" you ask. "How can woodpeckers be used as a defense against squirrels?" Well, to tell you the truth, I'm not exactly sure myself, but it appears that certain woodpeckers have it in for squirrels. According to *Animals of the World*, "One determined woodpecker will sometimes send a Gray Squirrel scampering after a few moments, for the blows from that long sharp bill of his are severe" (p. 165).

Although I know no one who's tried this technique, you might encourage red-headed woodpeckers to visit your yard. You'll either have to figure out what redheads like to eat most, or capture a few and transport them to your area. Who knows—in a little while, red-headed woodpeckers might be sold in birdfeeder catalogs along with baffles and the squirrel spooker pole.

Baffles

Baffling poles is a popular way of trying to thwart squirrels in their attempts to misappropriate birdseed. Baffles work—in theory—by creating a ledge that squirrels cannot climb around. In theory. It's like in the movies where the hero is in great peril because he is unable to climb up and over the rock ledge that extends out from the mountain. But in the movies, the hero manages to gather the energy, courage, and imagination—somehow—to get around that ledge.

Squirrels must watch the same movies, because baffles seem to provide only limited protection against squirrels. The primary way squirrels defeat baffles, according to George Petrides of the Wild Bird Center in Cabin John, Maryland, is by chewing and clawing at the surface and edges of the feeder, roughening them enough so they can grip on and pull themselves over.

There are a couple of techniques you can use to make baffles more effective. First, use the largest baffle you can find—and I mean the absolute largest. It should dwarf whatever feeder lies beneath. A gigantic baffle ensures that squirrels cannot crawl to the edge of the baffle, swing it, and catch the feeder below with their paws. Second, draw the feeder high up into the baffle. The more the feeder is near or "in" the baffle, the more difficult it will be for squirrels to jump down and in from the baffle. Third, let the baffle dangle precariously on the wire or chain it's hanging from. The more off-center the baffle's balance, the more likely squirrels are to lose their balance and fall.

Notice how squirrels use baffles. To keep from falling off, squirrels hang on to the chains, wires, or loops on the top of baffles with their back claws. They need that chain to support themselves while they try to maneuver from the top of the baffle to your feeder. Fourth, you can add to the baffle's ability to protect your feeder by making it, from the squirrel's perspective, a more complex surface. Build a super-baffle: by gluing a cone to the top of the baffle, it becomes difficult for squirrels to get on top of the baffle at all, because squirrels will have nothing to attach their back claws to.

Cone-shaped superbaffles can be constructed out of Plexiglas or aluminum; the latter is probably easier to make into a cone. The cone should be about twelve inches high and completely surround the chain. It must be as seamless as possible, or squirrels will have something to grip on to.

The cone looks like a "Coolie hat," according to Hoit Palmer of Gaithersberg, Maryland, who developed this system. "Squirrels can see the seed underneath the baffle," she said, describing how it works. "They aim for the seed, then decide to climb the tree, climb across the branch toward the Coolie hat. Then the fun begins." Some squirrels, "especially the older ones" Palmer points out, can stretch far and defeat the Coolie hat by holding on the to chain and letting gravity stretch their body, but "new squirrels can't stretch as far."

In the same vein, you can attach Nixalite to the baffle's top to make that area undesirable for squirrels. Glue Nixalite to the top of the baffle. Be sure to completely cover the baffle's top or squirrels will find a way to grasp the Nixalite and use it to their advantage.

Rating the general effectiveness of baffles is difficult. In some situations baffles provide excellent antisquirrel protection, especially if you are fortunate enough to live in an area with dumber than normal squirrels. (With certain feeders, a baffle will also protect your feeder from less desirable birds, such as starlings.) In other locales, baffles only make squirrels work harder to get their food, and, as a result, make them hungrier when they get to it. Baffles are fairly unattractive, but fortunately they don't obscure your view of birds. They also protect feeders from rain and snow, helping to keep birdseed dry.

If your feeder has a built-in baffle, such as the GSP or Mandarin, you don't need a baffle, but for most feeders they're a good idea.

Window brackets

Anytime you hang a feeder from a tree you have to deal with squirrels in their natural element. More often than not, if it's possible to hang the feeder from a tree, it's possible for the squirrel to get to it. This

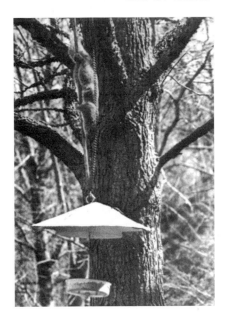

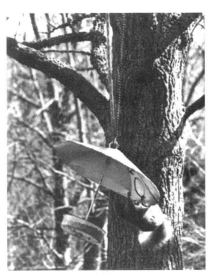

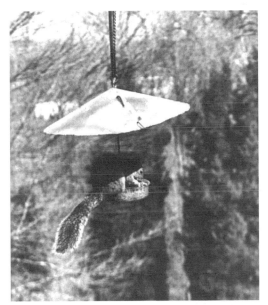

Mr. Squirrel approaches the baffle cautiously. Although his footing is never absolutely secure, the squirrel is certain that he's going to get to that birdseed. And he does.
Photos by Hoit Palmer.

axiom has something to do with the close working relationship squirrels have to trees—they know how to use them a lot better than you do.

People choose window brackets because they have no alternative. Pole feeders may not be viable for an individual's particular situation. If you don't have a yard, for example, you may need to convince your neighbors that it's OK to put the feeder in the middle of the street. Good luck. Or you may not like the look of a pole on your lawn, may not be crazy about sunflower debris destroying the grass underneath the feeder, or may not like mowing around the pole.

Window feeders aren't always practical either. They can interfere with opening the window, which may be a problem in the summer. Window feeders fall off from time to time, which is not pleasant if you live in an apartment building and have to run down seven flights of stairs to retrieve the feeder. And window feeders may easily be encroached upon by squirrels.

The solution, then, may be a pivoting arm—a steel pole that attaches to a wall and extends out several feet from that wall. Pivoting brackets come in two sizes, twenty-four and forty-eight inches The bracket can be attached to the side of a window, a fence, or any wooden or brick surface, and can be pivoted at various angles from the wall. The bracket attaches to the wall with wood screws, which are easy to use if you're putting it on a fence and very difficult if you're putting it on the side of an apartment building. To attach it to the side of an apartment building you need to a) lean out the window and turn the screws tightly, and b) have no fear of heights. Although wood screws aren't designed to fasten to brick, you can force them, but you may have to reinforce the screws with epoxy to ensure that the bracket stays in place. Because you can attach almost any kind of feeder to a pivoting bracket, it's worth the struggle—and fright—to put one up. (Masonry bits will bore through brick; anytime you drill into the side of a building make sure to get the landlord's permission first.)

As I mentioned, brackets come in two sizes: two feet and four feet. The two-foot bracket is practically useless in preventing squirrels from getting to your feeder, especially when it's attached to apartment buildings. The width of the feeder shortens the distance between the wall and the feeder, and frequently all a squirrel has to do is grab on to the wall with his back claws and stretch. If you must use a twenty-four-inch bracket, attach it to the top part of a fence or above a window so that it extends up into the air. Then the squirrel can't just reach directly out and grab it. Also consider using a narrow tube feeder so that squirrels have to reach farther to grab the feeder. Remember, once they get hold of the feeder they can pull themselves onto it. Remember also to put a baffle on top of whatever feeder you attach to the bracket, because squirrels can run up the arm with the greatest of ease. In apartments, avoid placing the bracket near a window screen—squirrels can easily climb up screens. Glass, on the other hand, foils squirrels every time.

The four-foot bracket gives you added distance between the wall or fence and the feeder. However long, brackets are not foolproof, and it may be a good idea to coat the bracket with Teflon and put Nixalite on the top of your feeder.

Pulleys

Sold in your favorite hardware store is an elegant apparatus that can stop squirrels: the pulley. A pulley enables you to place a feeder in remote locations, such as under an eve, between two distant trees, or between a house and a tree. The pulley lets you place feeders in locations that both you and squirrels have a lot of trouble reaching. Once set up, you just have to tug on the rope to retrieve the feeder to refill it, and tug again to put the feeder back in its squirrelproof place. There's no universal best place to locate your feeder, so you'll have to improvise.

35 mm film cans

Just about everything can become an antisquirrel device, 35 mm film containers included. Marlene Couture of the Duncraft Company suggests using film containers when you hang your feeder from a line that's stretched between two trees (or a tree and a pole). Punch holes in the bottom of the film containers and string between six and twelve containers through the line on either side of the feeder, just as you might string popcorn. When the squirrels reach the film containers the containers revolve around the string, and the squirrels lose their footing and fall.

Record albums

Record albums are also a successful tool in the arsenal against squirrels, especially 33 rpms. They're best used on feeders that are hung from wires strung between two trees. Before you complete the connection between the trees, string the cord through several albums on either side of the feeder. As long as the feeder and wire are high enough so that squirrels can't reach them by jumping, you should have a fairly impenetrable barrier. Squirrels will have a difficult time getting over and around the albums. They may be angry with you, but they won't get access to the birdseed. Some people say that Frank Sinatra albums work best, but field surveys have discovered that any plastic album works fine. Needless to add, you shouldn't plan to play those albums again.

Sleds

For those bird feeders whose children are passing into adulthood, there are a couple of toys that can be recycled into antisquirrel devices. Among the most common (in the northern states) and easiest to employ is the metal sledding saucer. If you've ever gone sledding with your kids you know how hard it is to stay on one, and if you have that much trouble just imagine what a squirrel's going to go through. A sledding saucer makes a terrific baffle, particularly because it's so large and so precariously constructed.

Squirrel spooker pole

The squirrel spooker pole consists of a pole with a movable sleeve that encases the pole. The sleeve, located near the top of the pole, is designed so that when a squirrel grabs it, the squirrel's weight causes it to slide down. A counterweight brings the sleeve back to its original position. Every time a squirrel tries to climb the squirrel spooker pole, he falls to the ground. Tube and flat-bottomed feeders can be easily mounted on the pole.

The squirrel spooker pole isn't foolproof, however. In every yard there's probably one squirrel who's figured out the system and has beaten it—by climbing faster than the sleeve slides. You can enhance the pole's ability to thwart squirrels by baffling above and below the feeder and by greasing the sleeve section of the pole. Although not 100 percent effective, the spooker pole gives you an edge over a regular pole.

If there was ever any doubt about the cleverness of squirrels, the ways in which some squirrels overcome the spooker pole will destroy that doubt. Peg and Paul Finn of Bedford, New Hampshire, said this about their experience with the squirrel spooker pole:

> We no sooner had a feeder attached to the top of the pole when along came Mr. Squirrel. Up the pole he climbed, clawed onto the sleeve, and down he came. We thought that was about the slickest thing we had ever seen and were in hysterics watching as three more attempts were made, all ending with the perplexed squirrel on the ground.
>
> Five minutes later he was back with a friend. They both sat under the feeder chatting and looking up. Mr. Squirrel demonstrated one more time while his partner took notes.
>
> As Mr. Squirrel was lowered to the ground he did not release his hold on the sleeve. Instead he held it in place at the bottom of the pole and his partner then climbed up the pole to the feeder without any problem. Then they reversed positions until they both had their fill.
>
> Each day was the same routine: a two-squirrel team would arrive, one to hold and one to eat.

Chemical warfare

It may sound awful, but it hasn't been proscribed by the Geneva Convention or the ASPCA, so chemical weapons are allowed in your arsenal against squirrels. Coating the surfaces of the feeder with Ben-Gay, cayenne pepper, or menthol cream will encourage squirrels to attack another feeder. In many instances you can use chemicals in the same place you would apply oil or Teflon. Squirrels hate the smell, texture, and taste of these substances. They will still work at attacking your feeder, but they will scrupulously avoid coming into contact with the noxious materials. Ben-Gay and menthol come in creams so they can be readily applied; cayenne pepper is available in various liquids in the spice department of your supermarket. Asian specialty food stores sell several different kinds of hot pepper sauces. Red pepper mixed with epoxy makes a fine deterrent and is actually used with radio transmitters placed on squirrels so they won't chew the electronics. The combination of Vaseline and red pepper works, too. You may have to experiment a little to find the best substance for your particular brand of squirrel. Birds don't like these materials either, but they can fly around them.

Avoid using ammonia. It doesn't keep squirrels away and it makes your yard smell like the New Jersey Turnpike.

Part II: Active Antisquirrel Measures

Finally, of course, they won. I came out one morning and saw that the feeders had been knocked down and were nowhere in sight. I found them later; the squirrels had hidden them in the ivy.

—Mary McGrory, *Washington Post*

Moving squirrels

It's the scheme of last resort and it is the most effective: moving squirrels. Transporting squirrels isn't difficult either—just bait a trap with peanut butter, leave the trap out for ten seconds, and voila—there's a squirrel. Then move the squirrel several miles and that squirrel won't be around to bother you any more.

Although that's just about all you have to do to evict squirrels from your property, there are some tips you should follow to make the task easier and safer. First, never stick your finger inside the cage after you've trapped a squirrel. Remember, the squirrel entered the cage to get a bite to eat, and if you put your finger within striking range, that's exactly what it is going to do. If you think you can pull your finger out before the squirrel gets to it, just remember this: you thought you could keep that squirrel away from your birdfeeder, too. Thick gloves are a good idea when moving squirrels.

Second, keep in mind that where you relocate the squirrel is important for several reasons. A distance of *at least* two miles is crucial if you don't want that squirrel to return. Farther is better, and very far—ten miles—is best, because that squirrel may beget baby squirrels who will leave their range in search of food and return to your property. A typical squirrel has a range of between one to seven acres; but we know that your squirrel isn't typical. So unless you move that squirrel a considerable distance, you may find yourself confronting her children in a season or two. Placing barriers between you and where you move the squirrel is a good idea. Superhighways work best, but if you can't get one constructed, fast-moving rivers (remember squirrels can swim), open areas (squirrels don't tread too far away from trees), rocky areas, houses with cats, a zoo, and a couple of shopping malls will do the trick.

Because you're taking the trouble to move a squirrel rather than convert it into squirrel stew, you probably care what happens to that squirrel. The health and happiness of the squirrel, once you move it, depends entirely on you. Do not put the squirrel where there are plenty of other squirrels, although this may run contrary to common sense. An area with plenty of squirrels probably is at its peak carrying capacity or even beyond it. The newcomer will have to establish her position or be banished. When there are too many squirrels in a given area, some squirrels must be driven out. Because squirrel ranges overlap, your ex-squirrel will then shift into another range where she will have to establish herself or again be banished. Remember, the squirrel you've just moved has led a cushy life thanks to your generous feeder and probably won't be as assertive as "wild" squirrels. There are a couple of exceptions to this rule, however. City parks in which people feed the squirrels may be OK for transported squirrels. Many parks, such as Washington's Lafayette Park, contain six times the number of squirrels that it would be able to support if no one fed them. The same goes for the White House lawn, where squirrels are fed by members of all political parties. The other exception is transporting squirrels during hunting season. Although it may not be wise to wander around carrying an animal in your hand during hunting season, hunting depletes the squirrel population. By transporting a squirrel to a populated range you are actually helping the species.

After you capture the squirrel, move it as quickly as possible. Squirrels do not like to be kept in small cages and will let you know about it. If they become too upset, squirrels can go into shock and die. When in shock their body temperature drops and their heart rate either increases or decreases markedly. Be sure to put newspaper or some other material between the trap and the floor of your car—squirrels have several ways of expressing their displeasure. Don't leave the squirrel cooped up too long without water, and don't leave the squirrel in your car with the windows rolled up because your car will become so hot that the squirrel will bake. Check your traps several times a day and especially around nightfall to make sure that squirrels aren't left inside for long periods. For good measure, cover the trap; it gives the squirrel a sense of security.

Peanut butter is the best bait. It's easy to apply and the smell attracts squirrels from great distances.

Not every trap will do. Have-a-Hart and Tomahawk Live traps catch squirrels safely and humanely for relocation. Squirrels wander in through a spring-activated door that opens forward and downward under their weight. The door can only be opened from the entrance side, so once inside there is no escape. Be sure to use the correct size trap. If the trap is too large, the squirrel may escape. Traps are, of course, reusable, and cost about $20. Many local conservation organizations rent traps, too.

It can take a while to trap squirrels, according to Joe Barteleme, who lives in Westchester, New York. He wrote:

> There were cages in the patio, cages on the balcony, under the big spruce, near the woodpile. After five days the catch included a raccoon, the neighbor's cat, and two squirrels. But not my squirrels. The overhead morning aerobics continued.

It took Mr. Barteleme so long to get rid of one squirrel that he had named him. When he finally caught "Henry," Barteleme had a horrible premonition:

> Just the other day I was driving Henry to his new home—a park in Greenwich—when I noticed a gray, unmarked van approaching in the opposite direction. We did not acknowledge one another. But I am certain, positively certain, that in the back of

that gray, unmarked van were countless cages of Connecticut squirrels, eagerly awaiting their destination in my backyard (from "In Wily Pursuit of Squirrels," Joe Barteleme, *The New York Times*, June 30, 1985).

Dart guns

I know what you're thinking and I want to tell all the animal welfare people out there that dart guns are entirely harmless to squirrels. In fact, your chances of hitting a squirrel with a dart gun are pretty slim.

So why bother to discuss dart guns as antisquirrel weapons? Well, everyone who attempts to thwart squirrels will eventually think of dart guns, so I might as well dispel some myths about them. If you're tempted to buy a rubber-tipped dart gun because you remember the pain you suffered—or inflicted—when using one as a kid, you'll be surprised to discover that squirrels virtually ignore being hit. I blasted one at point-blank range and it didn't even seem to know it had been shot.

If you can't discourage squirrels with dart guns, why bother? There's no really good reason, so here are some fair reasons: while you can't hurt them, squirrels aren't crazy about these darts. They'd rather you didn't. Second, it improves your aim, speed, and timing for other antisquirrel measures. Finally, it gives you something to do other than yell and flail your arms: it's easier on the neighbors.

There's only one thing your should know about dart guns (other than don't aim the gun at your little sister). Don't remove the little red tips from the darts. If you remove the red rubber tips you still won't be able to hurt the squirrels, but you most certainly will not be able to find the darts on the ground.

Robots

One advantage humans have over squirrels is technology. Squirrels may be masters of speed, dexterity, and acrobatics and have sharp teeth, but you have the technological edge over them. I'm not talking about hundred thousand-dollar laser systems, though that isn't a bad idea, but several inexpensive, high-tech devices are available for the price of a new birdfeeder (which you may have to buy anyway if you can't get rid of the squirrels).

To recognize which devices are the most appropriate, you have to see the world from a squirrel's perspective. To squirrels everything is large. Other creatures for which the world is large include, of course, birds and children. Toy robots look gigantic to squirrels and small children. Look for antisquirrel robots at toy stores and Radio Shack. Countless toys designed for little boys simulate weapons of war firing all sorts of missiles. A toy tank won't make a 220-pound man wince, but a 1½-pound squirrel has to take this "weapon" seriously.

The best kind of antisquirrel toys are remote-controlled robots because squirrels aren't going to let you get close to them. Some robots are remote-controlled by wire, others by radio—the latter is best.

In addition to tanks, there are a large variety of robots that can work against squirrels, including radio-controlled planes with which you can "buzz" squirrels as they try to escape by running over telephone lines. Think war and you'll do all right.

Some of the best robots are the "mechanical claws." These robot-toys were designed to let kids pretend they are scientists and are remotely operating a "hand" that holds dangerous material. The hand is attached to an arm that can rotate around almost a full three hundred and sixty degrees Some of these mechanical claws come on robots with wheels and can travel about.

The best way to use these claws is to leave them on the ground near your birdfeeder. Sprinkle a couple of nuts near the robot. As the squirrel approaches, instruct the robot to grab the squirrel. These robots make excellent feeder guards.

Squirrel diverters

The most effective antisquirrel measure is a squirrel diverter. It is also the simplest. Squirrel diverters are actually squirrel feeders. Filled with sunflower seeds, peanuts, and peanut butter, they keep squirrels happy, fed, and most important, away from your feeder. (Some people feed squirrels not just to keep them out of their birdfeeder, but because they like squirrels. See chapter 12.) There are only four points to keep in mind when using a squirrel diverter. First, make it easy for the squirrels to get the seed. Squirrels are notoriously lazy and are at-

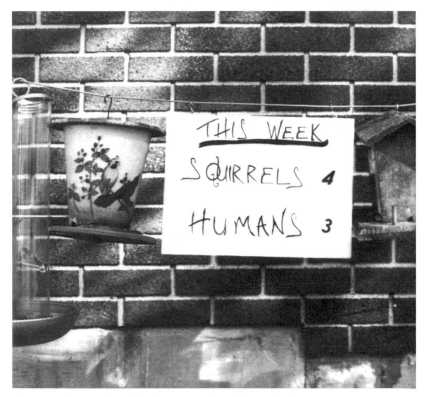

The scorecard kept at the Wild Bird Center in Cabin John, Maryland.

tracted to whichever feeder is easier to eat from. Platform feeders work best as squirrel diverters; the Cardinal Barn and other feeders with openings on the bottom work well when placed on the ground. Second, keep the diverter as far away from your birdfeeder as possible. You want to remove temptation. Third, keep the squirrel feeder full. If empty, squirrels will go back to doing what they do best—attacking your feeder. Finally, don't relax your squirrel defenses. Make your feeders as difficult for squirrels to break into as possible. Food is food to squirrels, and some will attempt to reach your feeder no matter what you do.

Diverters are a necessity if you have a handmade, designer feeder. Any feeder that you want to protect from being mauled and chewed by squirrels must be accompanied by a diverter.

Camera flashes and noise

These are only temporary measures. Firing flashes and making noise will momentarily stun or scare squirrels (and your neighbors, depending on the hour) but in the long run they won't keep squirrels away. A flash will blind a squirrel for a handful of seconds, giving you enough time to aim and fire a dart gun. These methods will help you relieve your frustrations.

Mass migrations of squirrels have been reported. In 1882 an estimated 250,000 squirrels migrated across Ohio.

Squirrels can live up to twelve years in captivity.

EIGHT

101 Cunning Stratagems

About the only mammals it is impossible to avoid feeding are the squirrels that get into birdfeeders.

—The New York Times

Finally, 101 cunning stratagems to reduce dramatically the egregious misappropriation of seed from your birdfeeder by squirrels. Some of these stratagems will be more useful than others for your particular environment. Good luck.

1. Hang your feeder from a tree. Make sure the feeder is eight feet away from the nearest branch, at least six feet off the ground, and completely covered with a baffle.

2. Dig a moat around your feeder. Fill it with piranha.

3. Fill your feeder with marbles and buy a parakeet to keep indoors.

4. Rent a guard cat.

5. Play Frank Sinatra songs on outdoor speakers, very loudly.

6. Tame a very strong, fast squirrel. Give it plenty of food and teach it to keep other squirrels away.

7. Never sleep, never play, only send out for food, and maintain a constant vigil at your feeders.

8. Read this book to the squirrels so that they understand who's in charge.

9. Fire camera flashes at them.

10. Bury rubber acorns—confuse and confound them.

11. Move to Antarctica and enjoy watching penguins.

12. Move to southern Florida and enjoy flamingos.

13. Paint your feeders to look like owl habitats.

14. Trap squirrels and send them to Antarctica.

15. Convince your neighbors that squirrels are cute and that the neighbors should feed them.

16. Let the Pentagon practice their *Star Wars* technology on the squirrels in your backyard.

17. Make your yard into a mirror maze.

18. Place a highway through your yard.

19. Electrify your feeder.

20. Construct a customized antisquirrel robot.

21. Capture the squirrels, dress them in deer costumes, and release them during hunting season. Alternatively, paint the word "DEER" on their sides.

22. Dig deep holes in the ground, and cover them with straw.

23. Encourage your neighbor to take in stray cats.

24. Take up falconry and keep the falcon untethered.

25. Breed aggressive, sterile squirrels.

26. Contact a genetic engineering firm and introduce a gene that changes squirrels' appetites to a preference for mosquitoes.

27. Coat your birdfeeder with chewing gum. That'll teach 'em.

28. Encourage your friends and neighbors to buy squirrel coats.

29. Place two half-sphere baffles around your hanging feeder, one above and one below. Leave a one-inch opening for chickadees.

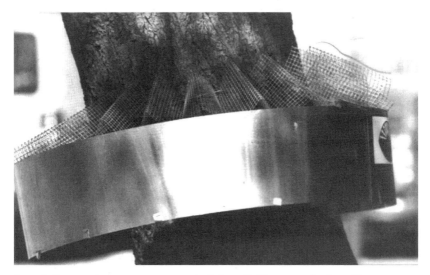

A metal skirt around a tree can prevent squirrels from climbing to your feeder and keep cats from reaching birdhouses.

30. Run outside yelling and waving your arms every time a squirrel appears. Not only will you scare squirrels away, but you'll get terrific exercise. (Before attempting this technique, check your local noise ordinances.)

31. Put your feeder on a pole and place that pole in the middle of a swimming pool. If you don't have a pool, dig an artificial lake.

32. Use a window feeder, making sure that there is at least four feet of window around the feeder and that the feeder has a roof.

33. Enclose your yard with a twenty-foot tall Plexiglass fence.

34. On the off chance that stratagem 33 fails, add a top to that fence. Angle the top up forty-five degrees and leave an opening for birds to fly through. If you have trouble with birds flying into the clear fence, paint it with stripes.

35. Capture squirrels and move them to your neighborhood dog run.

36. Tell your neighborhood butcher that you've discovered a cheap supply of meat. Tell him that he can call it chicken and nobody will know the difference.

37. Rattlesnakes are a major predator of squirrels. Acquire some for your lawn. (They also help keep solicitors away.)

38. Dig up their nuts during the winter.

39. Put a truck horn next to your feeder and use it whenever a squirrel appears.

40. Hang your feeder 100 feet down from a 200-foot-tall tree.

41. Buy a squirrel costume. Parade around your yard wearing the costume. Squirrels can't figure out what in the world is going on and it drives them away.

42. Install a windmill generator in your yard. When it's off put corn cobs on the ends of the windmill arms. Wait for a windy day, and when the squirrels climb on board release the clutch.

43. Import red squirrels. They're territorial and aggressive. Unfortunately they eat nuts, too.

44. Import red-headed woodpeckers who will vie with squirrels for nuts.

45. Import squirrel-eating hawks. (They may, unfortunately, enjoy eating birds, too. If that's the case buy the hawk-proof GSP feeder.)

46. Import blue jays or mockingbirds; they dislike squirrels.

47. Place a feeder on top of a pole. Put the pole in the middle of your yard, at least twenty feet away from any tree. Put no less than four baffles beneath the feeder and grease the pole with WD-40.

48. Put your feeder on a pipe and coat the pipe with Vaseline. Wrote George Dye to Audubon's *Naturalist News*: "I watched one venturesome squirrel shinny up the pipe until he hit Vaseline. He was surprised, and I was highly amused to see him hit the dirt. Now I Vaseline the pipe all the way to the ground. The squirrel smells the pipe and leaves."

49. Feed birth control pills to squirrels. The city of Venice uses birth control pills for pigeons, so they probably can be made for squirrels, too.

50. Place a giant Clint Eastwood poster in your yard.

51. Use radar-tracking laser-sighted guns. Originally designed for the Department of Defense, a handful of these may be available on the black market for $265,000 a piece.

52. Try sonic rodent repellers. Sold in catalogs, these devices are supposed to repel mice and other rodents by emitting a peculiar ultrasonic sound. You may have to boost the power to make it effective against squirrels.

53. Record squirrel warning sounds on a continuous loop tape and play them over and over again.

54. Practice hitting squirrels with golf balls. Your chances of making successful contact are about one in three billion, but your golf swing will improve.

55. Reprogram Soviet ICBM computers to target your backyard. Initiate an action that starts World War III. (This is an extreme measure, but it's guaranteed to eliminate your squirrel problem.)

56. Leak the news that your backyard is a training ground for Contra rebels.

57. Invite Fred the Furrier over to your house to "take care" of your problem.

58. Build a special cannon. It'll be about ten feet long and six inches wide and will fire cats. Aim this catgun directly at squirrels.

59. Feed the squirrels caramel apples. They'll love them, but won't be able to open their mouths for days afterwards.

60. Buy some lasers and set up a hologram show in your yard. Make holograms of cats and hunters.

61. Hire a hypnotist to modify squirrels' minds so that they no longer desire nuts, or think they're geckos.

62. Make use of patent 4,712,512, awarded on December 15, 1987, for a birdfeeder made from a plastic bottle, invented by Bernhard Schreib. Here's the patent as described by Mr. Schreib: A method and apparatus components for converting a plastic carbonated beverage bottle into a birdfeeder. The apparatus components include pointed feeder trays for insertion into the bottle through

specially formed slots cut in the side wall of the bottle, and a decorative sleeve with corresponding cutouts is secured around the bottle side wall. An umbrella-like cover made from a flat piece of flexible plastic is clamped atop the bottle by the bottle closure cap of the bottle to protect the seed from rain and to prevent squirrels and the like from taking the birdseed. A piercing and cutting tool is provided to pierce the bottle side wall and sleeve to create the slots for the insertion of the feeder trays and is also useful for making an opening in the bottle cap for the receipt of a support line. A reinforcing cap washer is nested interiorly of the bottle closure cap for added strength and attachment with the support line. A support hook is provided for connection to the support line and for the support of the birdfeeder made by the apparatus and method steps.

63. Employ patent 4,637,164 for a squirrel guard by inventor Harold O. Brown: An animal guard for tree trunks comprising an annular flexible plate having a central circular opening and a skirt portion completely around the central opening; at least one slot extending through the skirt forming the plate into a separable member having abutting edges; a pair of spaced fastener holes in the skirt radially aligned and positioned adjacent to one abutting edge of the slot; an inner and an outer spaced parallel arcuate slot in the skirt radially spaced from one another and positioned so that the fastener holes and the slots cooperate with each other when the plate is positioned in a truncated conical position about a tree trunk; the inner slot and associated fastener hole being a substantial distance closer to the inner periphery of the plate than the outer slot and associated fastener hole is to the outer periphery so as to not provide a gripping surface for an animal attempting to pass the guard.

64. Employ patent 4,541,362, a squirrelproof selective birdfeeder, invented by Allan W. Dehls of Bridgewater, New Hampshire: A squirrelproof selective birdfeeder includes a metallic hopper having integral side walls and a back wall defining an open front face, an open top, and a feed portal, a translucent window fastened in water-resistant sealing engagement to the open front face, a top

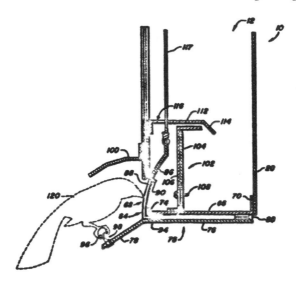

Employ patent 4,541,362.

having a sandwiched metallic plate slidably mounted in and frictionally retained by the confronting walls of the open top of the hopper, and a spring-loaded perch having an adjustable tension pivotally mounted to the bottom of the hopper and adjacent to the feed portal.

65. Employ patent 4,523,546 for a squirrelproof birdfeeder, invented by Peter A. Latham of Rye, New Hampshire: A device for squirrelproofing birdfeeders includes a flexible covering sheet mounted above or to the upper end of the birdfeeder. The sheet is dimensioned and located with respect to the feeder so that when a squirrel attempts to walk on the sheet, the sheet will flex and bend downwardly under the influence of the squirrel's weight. The squirrel will slide off the sheet and with no means or opportunity to grab onto any portion of the sheet or the feeder which it covers.

66. Employ patent 4,498,423 for a birdfeeder invented by Leon Gainsboro and Peter A. Latham: A birdfeeding device is provided with a perch which can be adjustably positioned with respect to the feeding opening to selectively accommodate different sizes of birds. The perch is movable toward and away from the feeding

opening so that for larger birds the perch is positioned farther from the feeding opening than for smaller birds. The disclosed embodiment also includes a simultaneous heightwise adjustment for the position of the perch so that it is lowered when in its more extended position. Also disclosed is an improved arrangement for attaching the perch and feeding device to the container of the birdfeeder. Another aspect of the invention relates to a birdfeeder having a storage and feeding tube which is detachably connected to an overhead support by a quick disconnect device which provides for quick and simplified filling of the feed tubes as well as an arrangement which minimizes spilling or loss of birdseed.

67. Employ patent 4,462,337 for a birdfeeder with a rotatable cover, invented by Peter Kilham of Foster, Rhode Island: A birdfeeder having a generally planar seed tray and means for mounting such in a generally horizontal position. The birdfeeder further includes a cover, generally of dome-shaped configuration, and having a lower peripheral edge frictionally supported on an upstanding peripheral seed tray rim. The cover is capable of rotational movement with respect to the tray such that a bird access opening in the cover may be adjustably positioned downwind of the feeder in its use position.

68. Employ patent 4, 434,745 for a birdfeeding device, invented by Noel Perkins of Northwood, New Hampshire: A birdfeeding device is disclosed which can be accessed by birds and not by squirrels. The device comprises a container for holding feed and a wire mesh enclosing the container. An O-ring supports the container within the wire mesh and spaces the mesh away from the container such that the mesh is not directly in contact with the container whereby squirrels are prevented from accessing the container.

69. Employ patent 4,389,975, a dual purpose birdfeeder invented by James B. Fisher, Jr. of St. Louis, Missouri: A dual purpose birdfeeder for use mounted upon a post with a squirrel baffle preventing climbing upon the feeder or for use in a free-hanging relation where it is supported on a chain. The birdfeeder is comprised of a frusto-conical hollow feeder housing with a tray at the bottom

and flat shallow roof at the top. In the freely supported relation the feeder tray has a radius not exceeding about 55 percent of the radius of the roof and the outer periphery is positioned underneath the upper portion of the housing. The depth of the tray beneath the roof also does not exceed about one-half of the radius of the roof. This relationship prevents or discourages squirrels or large undesirable birds from using the feeder tray. In the post-supported version the squirrel barrier baffle is of the same frusto-conical construction as the feeder housing for ease in manufacture and is positioned underneath the tray. A cylindrical baffle may depend from the tray to which the frusto-conical baffle may be removably attached. Means are provided for a central post to connect to the feeder. The inverted upwardly flaring baffle and its spacing of the bottom wall from the central support post effectively prevents squirrels from climbing the post on the feeder tray.

Employ any of the following patents:

70. 4,327,669, May 4, 1982, Multiple birdfeeder, Morton Blasbalg, Warwick, Rhode Island

71. 4,323,035, April 6, 1982, Squirrelproof birdfeeder, Abraham Piltch, Silver Spring, Maryland

72. 4,188,913, February 19, 1980, Birdfeeders, Norman M. Earl and Alexander M. Brown, Stafford Springs, Connecticut, and Daytona Beach, Florida, respectively

73. 4,171,463, October 16, 1979, Rodentproof cable, David Watkins, Arleta, California

74. 4,031,856, June 28, 1977, Squirrelproof post, Russell L. Chester, Fontana, Wisconsin

75. 4,030,451, June 21, 1977, Birdfeeder, Isobel Miller, Greenville, New Hampshire

76. 3,977,363, August 31, 1976, Birdfeeder, James B. Fisher, Jr., St. Louis, Missouri

77. Use the fact that squirrels are either right- or left-handed against them. I'm not sure how you can use this to your advantage, but there must be a way.

78. Idea from Bill Avery of Springfield, Virginia: "Feed them unmercifully. Get them so fat that they can no longer sit on the edge of your birdfeeder."

79. Squirrels hate the smell of naphthalene (mothballs).

80. Copper naphthenate in linseed oil is an excellent squirrel repellent.

81. Plant exotic trees, or small-seeded evergreen or deciduous trees such as birch, willow, or elms. The squirrels don't go for them.

82. Remove trees that have squirrel dens in them.

83. Follow squirrels as they gather twigs and leaves to build nests. Destroy the nests as they build them.

84. Clean and bone the squirrel. Soak the meat in egg for about twenty minutes. Coat with bread crumbs, oregano, paprika, cumin, and mustard seed. Bake at 400 degrees for forty minutes. Remove from the oven and cover with Cheddar cheese. Continue baking for another ten minutes. Serve with wild rice.

85. Place your feeder on a squirrel spooker pole. Grease the sleeve with oil. Place a baffle beneath and above the feeder. Cover the top and bottom baffles with Nixalite. That should do it.

86. Attach a motor to a pole. Set the pole to rotate at thirty revolutions a minute. Between the pole and the feeder place a ball bearing so that the feeder stays in place.

87. Try Edward F. Vigezzi's Ziploc bag technique: Normally the squirrels rummage through the debris on the deck after they attempt to get to the birdfeeders. While they are searching, I get a one-quart Ziploc bag and fill it approximately two-thirds with water. After sealing it, I then go upstairs to the third floor guest room and open the window very carefully. I palm the baggy in my hand so that when I throw it, the bag will land on one of the sides. After I get a good angle, I toss the bag at the squirrel below. (You have to make sure the squirrel is not watching you.) When the bag hits, it is a double whammy. The noise of the impact against the wood and the wall of water will startle the squirrel and he will quickly retreat to the woods. Depending on the distance the bag

lands from the squirrel, I can determine the length of time they will stay away. In addition, this method leaves the deck wet for the birds to enjoy. You always want to get close, but you should not try to hit them directly.

88. Cry. Maybe the squirrel will feel sorry for you and go away.

89. Buy toy rockets with solid fuel engines—the kind that hobbyists play with. Fire a dozen off from your yard every day. No creature enjoys eating in a launching center.

90. Kidnap baby squirrels and hold them for ransom.

91. Replace the sunflower seed with plastic seed. The squirrels will become confused and go away; the birds aren't smart enough to be confused and will return as soon as you put regular seed back in your feeder.

92. Place a television and VCR in your yard. Rent and play documentaries of owls and hawks. (Again, the birds are too dumb to be confused by the video.)

93. Go to tree climbing and take direct, offensive action against squirrels.

94. Hire a lawyer.

95. Sick the IRS on them.

96. Place a drop of superglue on either side of a peanut. Set in your back yard.

97. Import killer bees.

98. Strip the insulation off the power lines that run through your neighborhood. The next time a squirrel tries to run along the line will be his last time doing that.

99. Place several automatic lawn sprinklers in your yard and run them all the time. Squirrels don't like to come out in downpours.

100. Acquire squirrel essence. Dab the stuff around and hopefully your squirrels will become hopelessly confused.

101. Decide that squirrels aren't so bad after all.

According to Dr. C. Hart Merriam, pre-World War II experiments with squirrels showed:

They were extremely fond of music, and it affected them in a peculiar manner. Some were not only fascinated, but actually spellbound, by the music-box or guitar. And one particularly weak-minded individual was so unrefined in his taste that if I advanced slowly whistling, "Just Before the Battle, Mother," in as pathetic a tone as I could muster for the occasion, he would permit me even to stroke his back, sometimes expressing his pleasure by making a low purring sound.

When listening to music, they sat bolt upright, inclining a little forward (and if eating a nut, were sure to drop it), letting their forepaws hang listlessly over their breasts, and, turning their heads to one side in a bewildered sort of way, assumed a most idiotic expression (*Animals of the World*, 165–66).

NINE

Advanced Antisquirrel Stratagems

Over the past ten years it appears that squirrels have undergone an evolutionary change. They have gotten smarter. Not by a lot—but certainly by enough. Many squirrels are able to bend feeder doors in a single day, are faster than a speeding peanut, and are able to leap tall feeders in a single bound. Amazingly, squirrels seem able to teach their tricks to their children. The main reason I think this is happening is that squirrels are living longer than before. Not much longer, perhaps a year or two thanks to the abundance of water and food, but long enough to learn and pass this knowledge on.

In the original *Outwitting Squirrels* I proposed digging a moat around your feeder. One bird feeder had this to say about my suggestion: "A moat? Seems a bit drastic. I was planning on a small pond next year but not all the way around the yard. Besides, they'd probably build a raft to spite me." I guess what I thought was a drastic step was an underestimation of squirrels' abilities.

So we must learn advanced antisquirrel techniques. Not just your regular, old squirrel-thwarting strategies, but high-tech, advanced psychological stuff. That means spending more time—much more time

than you spent in 1988 when *Outwitting Squirrels* first appeared—
trying to look at the world from the squirrel's perspective: Get down
on all fours, as low to the ground as possible, and look at your birdfeeder
from the squirrel's perspective. Look with squirrel eyes. It does no
good to watch at your feeder from the vantage point of 5' 9" because
that's not what a squirrel does. So what if your neighbors think that
you're just a wee bit odd—thwarting squirrels isn't just a job, it's a
mission.

But merely looking at the world from the squirrel's perspective and
thinking like a squirrel isn't enough. We have to be willing to adapt
our advanced technologies and war-fighting stratagems (many culled
from the cold war era) against squirrels. Our object is to create what
one person I interviewed called an SFZ (Squirrel-Free Zone). That is
what this chapter is about.

You have to work at disrupting squirrels' supply lines, attacking
their defensive positions, and going after their bases. This means that
in addition to defending your feeder, you also have to defend your
house. It's a pretty safe bet that if you have squirrels at your birdfeeder,
they are going to be taking advantage of your home, too. They'll do
this in any number of ways, including using your attic to stay warm,
visiting your basement for snacks, and running across your roof for
the sole purpose of making that *tap-tap-tap-tap-tap* sound that drives
you crazy.

As with many strategies having to do with squirrels, there is sometimes a direct relationship between how aggressive and extreme you
are and how effective you will be. To help to squirrelproof the house
and disrupt the squirrel's supply base, one antisquirrel person put siding on his house. "Seems the new siding was too smooth for them to
climb," he said, and the squirrels slid right down. He reported that
previously, "Our house had been their house."

Squirrels go to bed before we do. There's nothing diabolical about
it—they just do. This is a biological trait that we can use to our advantage. How? Notice that houses with teenagers have fewer incidences
of squirrels in their attics. That's because squirrels aren't crazy about
loud music. In fact, loud music can help drive squirrels away. The
louder the better, and the longer the music plays the better. Led Zeppelin works quite well in this regard. (I think I've just given away my

approximate age.) Consider placing stereo speakers in your attic and blasting away from sundown until when you go down. (If your neighbors complain, just tell them what you're doing and that you'd rather use noise than poison.) In about a week you will have driven the squirrels away. If your neighbors hate you, that's a small price to pay for protecting your birds.

Sometimes the most advanced strategy is the most straightforward. Here is what one bird feeder wrote to me:

> I take the simple approach to squirrel-free feeding. My feeders are all mounted on wrought iron posts, with the simple, flying-saucer shaped guards halfway up. I keep the feeders close enough to tree cover for the birds' comfort, but far enough away so the squirrels can't jump to the feeders. My squirrels *never* get my birdseed, but every once in a while one will run up the pole and bump into the guard—this craftiest of creatures looking really dumb. Once in a while, we see a squirrel run out on the limb of a western hemlock with the clear intent of jumping to the feeder, only to come to a screeching halt when he discerns he won't make it. My squirrels do K.P.—cleaning up dropped seed off the ground.

Another advanced strategy is to erect an amusement park for squirrels. Seriously. One birdfeeder thought that rather than fight squirrels, it would be a good idea to entertain them. So here's what she did:

> I've found that when dealing with nature it's often better to "go with the flow" rather than fight an unfightable fight. Squirrels have been here a long time and will be here long after we're gone. Yes, the little furry creatures (eight at last count) were wreaking havoc in my yard—eating the birdseed, rampaging through the hanging feeders, and driving my springers crazy. So, I decided to try to help them at their own games—I put out "squirrel toys." Squirrels are really very, very bright and curious. If there's something smart and fun to do in the yard rather than something boring the squirrels will head straight for the fun thing. I've set out a squirrel swing, a squirrel corncob bar, and a squirrel

pine cone trapeze. It keeps them busy and gives me hours of amusement and entertainment, and they leave the rest of the yard alone. At least it has worked for me.

Some people would consider this consorting with the enemy. It's all a matter of definition. If your objective is to spare some seed for birds, then playing games with squirrels might be OK.

The first thing any bird feeder notices about squirrels is that these critters like to climb. And they're good at it. Better than your or me, and better than your average house cat. If you could hang your feeder in midair, some ten feet above the ground using antigravity supports, then you would have a great advantage over squirrels. Unfortunately, such technology doesn't exist in our solar system so we have to rely on other technologies.

One alternative to the tradition of hanging tube feeders from a metal line is to use fishing line. While fishing line is something that squirrels can easily chew through, it's generally invisible, and squirrels are not going to climb down what they can't see. To a squirrel, this succulent tube filled with sunflower *is* hanging in midair. "It's too high to jump up and reach," a squirrel thinks (after trying to jump and get at the seed for several days in a row). "And there's no way to climb down," the squirrel concludes after viewing the feeder from above. Of this method one birdfeeder said, "I hung my tube feeders up with fishing line, testing the theory that the squirrels might be foiled by the clear and apparently invisible line. The entire summer has seen only one squirrel make it to the hanging feeder—and moving the feeder from a nearby branch has stopped even this clever fellow."

Whatever advanced strategy you follow or develop, winning won't come easy. As one contributor to rec.birds, a favorite spot on the Internet for swapping squirrel stories, wrote:

You have to see it as a game between you and the squirrels. You have to plan to spend a great deal of time observing the reaction of the squirrels to your attempts. You need to remember that your repeated efforts are in fact training your set of squirrels.

But even more importantly he added, "The only way you can stop a fanatic is with another fanatic headed in the opposite direction."

The Vermont Department of Agriculture reported in March, 1981, that there is "no pesticide registered with the Environmental Protection Agency for the control of red squirrels in maple orchards."

The average number of squirrel roadkills is one every ten miles.

TEN

Protecting Gardens and Flowers

When squirrels aren't gobbling down your birdseed, they are exploring your garden for bulbs, seeds, nuts, and other delectables. Never mind that the squirrels may not find anything to their liking—their searching alone can turn a well-manicured garden into the surface of the moon. To protect gardens, it's sometimes necessary to resort to extreme measures.

Judith Dilkie of Ontario, Canada, erected a virtual fortress around her bulbs:

> It was formidable. I dug the garden, planted the bulbs, put down sturdy chicken wire and then bricks all the way around to hold it down. I took it off as the first crocus appeared. My *first*! I have never been able to get the crocuses past the squirrels before.

There are several good reasons behind the fortress strategy. First, it encourages squirrels to go elsewhere. Of all the emotions I've seen in squirrels, spite is not among them. Squirrels don't dig up gardens—or raid feeders for that matter—because they are mad at you. No matter how angry *you* get at squirrels, they will feel exactly the same way toward you: You're the guy who plants the bulbs, or puts the seed out. Your neighborhood squirrel isn't going to dig up your garden for personal reasons.

But while they're not spiteful, squirrels are generally lazy. Given the opportunity, squirrels would prefer to have their food brought to them. They are not hunters, and are not interested in a challenge for the sake of a dare. If your tulips are hard to get to, then the squirrel will probably go somewhere else.

Which brings me back to chicken wire. If you encase your bulbs in a cage before you plant them, even if the squirrel is able to dig them up, he won't be able to eat them! (Spite and holding a grudge may not be squirrel emotions, but who said that we humans weren't entitled to those feelings?) Clearly this is an extreme approach, but if squirrels dig up your garden season after season, just one year of protecting your bulbs with chicken wire may coax your squirrels to move on.

Transporting squirrels may still be the best strategy for dealing with squirrels that munch on your bulbs. How far should you move squirrels? One person I interviewed said, "I take them to a little piece of land about two miles away that is bordered by railroad tracks on the long side of a triangle parcel of land, a deep, water-filled quarry on the one side, and a road adjacent to a golf club on the remaining side." Sounds about right to me. One gardener feels that learning to like bulbs, roots, fruits, and plants is an acquired taste, which is why trapping and moving squirrels can be temporarily effective. This gardener reports:

> Between yesterday and today, I captured three squirrels in a family and took them to my traditional spot beyond a quarry, nestled against the railroad and two roads. It's ideal for getting them disoriented. When I see no squirrels after my peanuts in the Have-a-Heart trap for several days straight, I know that I've done my job well for the year and my apples will be safe. Any squirrels that roam into my yard after that are "newbys" and haven't a clue about what good tasting apples are like. They usually have formed foraging habits already—it's when they've spent a winter and raised a family in my back yard that spells trouble.

This is the general principle about transporting squirrels. While new squirrels will soon move in to fill whatever void you've created, these new squirrels will have to learn all over again about the goodies in your yard. Here's what another gardener said:

> I have only a few mature apple trees in my small suburban back-yard. Squirrels have played havoc with the apple crop in early years but I fought back and fought back hard. A neighbor had a Have-a-Heart trap that he wasn't using and gave to me for help. Every June I transport between eight and fifteen squirrels to the countryside three miles hence. This eliminates the knowledge base about my fine orchard. I've had passive, snarling, and even swearing and hissing vermin transported to new homes with little difficulty. Without the help of traps, my small crop had previously been devastated by the local family of squirrels living in tall evergreens on my property. One day I hardly had time to return home and reset the trap before another found my baited trap. The Have-a-Heart trap never failed in any year to keep the crop intact.

Gardening supply stores sell various noxious chemicals that do indeed work to repel squirrels. Mothballs work, too. Pretty much anything that humans don't like to smell also bothers squirrels. You can experiment with all sorts of foul-smelling materials, but avoid organic compounds since whatever is edible will get eaten, and the last thing you want is to attract a brand new species or two to your yard.

Another point to keep in mind when using noxious aromas to discourage squirrels is the material's staying power. Merely sprinkling ammonia around your tulips may work for a short while, but the ammonia is going to evaporate, dissipate into the soil, and get washed away in the next rain. Generally, solids are better than liquids, which is why mothballs tend to work.

Where to place the mothballs or other material? The best place is around whatever you want to protect. Not too close, but not too far away. Protect the general area rather than individual plants, because what you want to do is discourage squirrels from your garden in general. If you have time watch how squirrels approach your tulip bed. It's likely that they will be coming from a nearby tree, and it is between the tree and tulips that you should place the heaviest concentration of mothballs (or whatever you are using).

The old standby, red pepper, works well in gardens. If you elect to erect a fence around your plants or vegetables it's worth the extra trouble to coat the fence with petroleum jelly and cayenne (red) pepper. This gives squirrels added incentive to keep away.

You can also sprinkle red pepper around the perimeter of your garden—it won't last, but it does help to thwart squirrels in the interim. Put the red pepper as close to your plants as you can.

Some people use spray vegetable oil to help the red pepper stick. Spray whatever you want to put cayenne pepper on (this works for birdfeeders, too), then sprinkle the pepper on top.

Alternatively, a number of gardening supply houses sell dry blood—another thing that squirrels don't like. I can relate to that. If you're squeamish about touching dried blood, use a powdered sugar container to distribute it. Some gardeners plant their bulbs with blood meal around the bulbs, then they put chicken wire on top of the bulbs until the warm season approaches. Squirrels tend to do their digging in the winter, and by the time you're ready to remove the chicken wire, the squirrels are ready to stop digging—I hope.

One technique that I have long advocated is feeding squirrels. This tends to keep them away from gardens and birdfeeders. (Plus it tends to keep the hard-line animal rights advocates at bay.) But there are a couple downsides to feeding squirrels as a strategy for preventing them from gorging themselves in your feeder and your garden. The first, and most obvious, problem is that if you stop feeding the squirrels for a while—such as when you go on vacation or have to pick up groceries on the way home from work—they will expect food. The first day (or hour) there isn't anything around for them, they will be curious. The second day, a little confused. The third day, very angry and hungry. By then your feeder should be empty, too, which encourages them to root around your flowers and vegetables even more.

The second problem with leaving food out for squirrels is that what's to stop other critters from enjoying this feast? Chipmunks, flying squirrels, opossums, and every other varmint in the neighborhood will enjoy themselves once they've heard the news. Fortunately, only a limited number of animals are really that interested in peanuts (assuming that's the food you've put out for squirrels), but you do have to take them into consideration.

The third problem with leaving food out for squirrels, whether in a squirrel feeder or not, is that squirrels are messy. Whatever you give them, don't feed squirrels shelled peanuts or your backyard will look like the floor of Giants Stadium after the Super Bowl.

Finally, there's this somewhat surprising problem encountered by one gardener:

Someone in my neighborhood feeds the squirrels and all this does is encourage the squirrels to bury the nuts—in my garden. While feeding squirrels may keep them out of birdfeeders, it doesn't seem to solve the digging problem, and because of it I am constantly unearthing half-rotted peanuts, walnuts, and whatever other nuts these rats with furry tails find appealing.

Squirrels will be squirrels, and they're very good at doing the kind of things that squirrels are known for: tightrope walking, high jumping, raiding birdfeeders, digging up bulbs, and gnawing outdoor furniture. From a gardener's perspective, squirrels are especially good at digging up bulbs. But sometimes the results of all this squirrelly behavior are extraordinary. Here's what happened to one individual: "There's a great squirrel around that does not dig up my bulbs. Instead, he plants bulbs in my garden that he's stolen from the neighbors. I got some fantastic grape hyacinths last year." When it comes to your garden and squirrels, prepare for the unexpected.

The National Zoo in Washington, D.C., assumes that a certain amount of food it puts out for its animals is going to go to "native wildlife," i.e., squirrels, and compensates appropriately.

ELEVEN

The Feline Menace

It's such a relief to see a squirrel on a "cat watch," while eating its well-earned seed.

—*The Christian Science Monitor*

Although this book is entitled *Outwitting Squirrels*, it's not really just about squirrels. *Outwitting Squirrels* is about protecting your birdfeeder from all sorts of enemies: squirrels, anonymous malicious children, pigeons, and cats. Although squirrels are the most annoying and costly pests—one squirrel can consume a pound and a half of birdseed a week—they're not necessarily the most disruptive. That award, of course, belongs to malicious children. Since there's nothing you can do about malicious children that aren't yours, let's focus on the second most disruptive pest: cats.

Cats are bad. Very bad. They scare birds from your feeder. Those that they don't scare they kill; really not good for birdfeeding at all. When a cat kills a bird that you've fed, it's as if you're feeding the cat indirectly. That's not what birding is about. If you wanted to feed cats you would have bought a six-pack of Nine Lives, not five pounds of hulled sunflower seed. Some people say that cats are beneficial because they drive squirrels away, but what's the use if the consequence of this ecology is that the only animals in your backyard are cats?

Two Kinds of Cat Problems

There are two kinds of cat problems. The first, called *Type Y*, is your cat. The second kind of cat problem, called *Type N*, is your neighbor's cat. (There's actually a third type of cat, *Type S*, strays, but Type S cats only prowl neighborhoods with mice and I'm sure you don't live in that kind of neighborhood.) Each problem creates its own set of potential solutions. Let's look at the Type Y cat problem first.

Type Y cat problems

The Type Y cat is a common element in people's homes, running second only to microwaves as a possession that doesn't let you do anything you couldn't already do. The cat usually appears the weekend after the following is heard: "Daddy, can I have a cat please if I promise to take care of it please can I Daddy please okay please?" In the beginning, Type Ys (kittens at that stage) are tolerable, even cute. Sure they mark up the furniture, coat the kitchen floor with kitty litter, like to greet dawn with shrill meows, and confuse your leg with a scratching post. But they are soft and cuddly. Within a few weeks the kittens turn into bigger kittens and then, following nature's plan, turn into cats. Their meows become louder. Their claws become bigger and sharper. Their litter box becomes . . . . Their willingness to play when *you* want to diminishes. Their love for the pre-dawn hours accelerates.

Your patience disappears.

So you let the cat out of the house. You're a little nervous at first because the cat could get hit by a car or run away. (Not that running away would be terrible in the abstract, but you would be the one assigned to put a fresh set of size Ds in the flashlight and go hunting up and down the street yelling, "Here, kitty, kitty. Here, kitty, kitty.") But cats like it outside and who are you to argue with nature?

Until. Until the cat discovers your birdfeeder and launches into its Great Lion routine. Hunter and Protector of The Backyard. Provider of All. Yes, your cat is generous and faithful, bringing back trophies for you to see and enjoy. What is particularly upsetting (to you) is that the cat is proud and wants to make a big impression; so she deposits the bird on your pillow. If you confront your cat about this and try to discuss the problem in as normal a tone of voice as you can maintain under the circumstances, she gets upset but still brings the birds inside. Peggy Robin, who has owned several cats, discovered that if you scold cats they then hide their captured birds, usually in closets—and not so cleverly—leaving a trail of feathers along the way.

Fortunately there's a simple solution to the Type Y cat dilemma. Keep your cat indoors. This may not be ideal, but as you have already discovered, it's better than having your cat create an indoor dead bird exhibit.

Type N cat problems

Neighbors' cats are a serious problem and do not lend themselves to simple solutions. Your neighbors are not going to appreciate your suggestion that they keep their cats inside. And you can't keep their cats in your house. You could be arrested for catnapping. Even worse, everyone will think that you're one of those crazy people who fills his house with cats, and probably has willed his entire estate to them. You can't shoot the cats because that will get your neighbor mad and she may shoot your birds in revenge. (Although there is the possibility that with so many squirrels around your yard she may think squirrels are your pets and shoot them. But that's a risk you have to evaluate for yourself.)

What follows are the options available to you for coping with bird-killing Type N cats. Good luck.

1. Get the cat to wear a bell—it does the trick. You may have trouble convincing your neighbor's cat (or yours) to wear a bell, but in the long run cats will appreciate the bell because it increases the challenge of the hunt. Bells are not foolproof, but they do even out the odds. Dick E. Bird recommends the heaviest bell possible, such as the Liberty Bell. It keeps them from jumping too high.

   Some cats have learned to defeat bells, however, by pretending to be statues. They lie in the lawn, sometimes under a shrub, and when a bird hops along, they thrust their paws out and *poof*, no more bird. Birds, it seems, never learn about cat statues. (Some people say this is nature's way of removing stupid birds.) Other cats learn to walk in a way that silences the bell. When this happens, substitute a transistor radio for the bell.

2. Feed the cats. The cats may be killing and eating birds because they're hungry. Look closely at your neighbors' houses. Do they need to be painted? Are the lawns in bad shape? Your neighbors may be too cheap to buy catfood for their pets. As far as your neighbors are concerned, they let the cats out and—by magic— the cats are fed! If you can, sculpt the catfood into the shape of a starling or pigeon.

3. Talk with the cats. Explain to them about birds, bees, and irate birders. People talk to cats all the time and the cats seem to understand, although they may not agree.

4. Buy a doberman.

5. Frequently loud noises work. Of course loud noises scare away birds, but birds come back quickly. Cats are a little more rational about sound. Some favorite noises are Led Zeppelin albums, a tape recording of a cat having its tail stepped on, and a sonic boom.

6. Scare the living daylights out of them. One man wrote to the *Dick E. Bird News* that he put his feeder on top of his car and hid inside. When a cat jumped on the hood he revved the engine, blasted the horn, and hit the brights. That cat has never been back.

7. Dig moats. Cats respect that.

8. Use high-power water guns, especially the battery-operated type. This is Dick E. Bird's favorite anticat technique. He claims it is extraordinarily effective; after a few shots cats find other yards.

9. Buy mice and release them in your neighbor's yard. Cats prefer mice to birds because mice stay on the ground all the time, while birds force cats to try to fly.

TWELVE

What to Do if You Think Squirrels Are Cute

There are an increasing number of individuals who view all of this baffle-buying, arm-flailing, water-pistol-firing, and general antisquirrel hysteria as foolish. These bird feeders—yes, bird feeders—adhere to a different school of thought: not outwitting squirrels. They don't bother to bother with squirrels. Although this may appear to be a defeatist attitude, many admirers of this system believe that theirs represents a holistic approach toward wildlife. Birders who believe in feeding squirrels instead of acting out vengeful fantasies toward them, arrive at this philosophy for several reasons. First, their attitude is that all wildlife should be treated equally. Birds, squirrels, flying squirrels, gazelles—they're all wild creatures and deserve to survive. Second, these birder-squirrelers feel that squirrels are cute, too. (There's no coincidence in the fact that many are myopic.) The way squirrels shinny on a branch, their furry faces, the way they scratch their heads with their paws—all of this is fun to watch, they say. Third, these people have usually become exhausted trying to defeat squirrels. They're pooped.

I think we all know that feeling.

Actually, there's nothing wrong with this approach toward squirrels. While not outwitting squirrels may be giving in to the enemy, it can save a lot of time and money, as well as lower your blood pressure. "People who feed birds spend more time feeding and talking about squirrels than they do about birds," said Tom Post of the Audubon Workshop. It's only a tiny step further to actually enjoying feeding squirrels.

One proponent of this point of view is Dick E. Bird, publisher of the *Dick E. Bird News*. (Dick E. Bird's real name is Richard Mallory, but all his friends have been calling him Dick E. Bird, so he figured, well, if that's what people call him, that's what he should be called. Currently, he's trying to get his name trademarked.) Dick Bird created the *Dick E. Bird News* as a way of promoting his company's birdhouses. After some time, he decided that publishing the *Dick E. Bird News* was more fun and rewarding than selling houses, so the house business is dwindling, while the *Dick E. Bird News* is becoming more popular. Bird tries to combine pure facts and fun facts in the *Dick E. Bird News*. He devotes considerable attention to squirrels because wherever you find feeders there are squirrels. Bird says that he could spend even more time writing about squirrels, but birders, he found, do want to read something about birds every once in a while. Bird's considerable expertise with feeding birds and the resultant squirrel problems has led him to a single conclusion: "There isn't anything that's going to keep squirrels away. My philosophy is to feed squirrels and birds and enjoy."

Dick Bird has seen just about every conceivable antisquirrel measure:

> I've heard everything—from baffles to grease. One guy had an electric fence charger hooked up to his feeder so that squirrels got jolted. I had a Droll Yankee feeder that I tested and I thought that there was no way a squirrel could get in. I hooked the feeder part way up high into the baffle. The feeder was hanging on monofilament line far away from any branch so there was no way a squirrel could climb or lean on to it. I watched one squirrel fly down onto the dome and go crashing off onto the ground. Then one day—I don't know how he did it—there was a squirrel sitting inside that feeder.

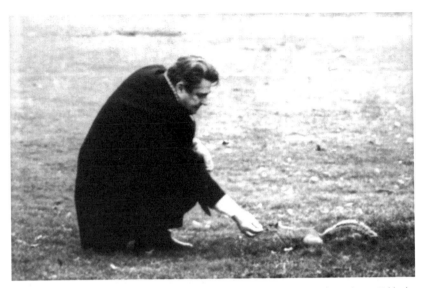

Soviet security chief Mikhail Dokuchayev fed squirrels on the White House lawn during Mikhail Gorbachev's visit to Washington in 1988. Photo by Peter Heimsath.

His conclusion? "Squirrels must have suction cups on their feet."

Bird knows that squirrels aren't smarter than humans. It's just that "What else is there for squirrels to do other than try to break into feeders? The squirrels don't know that you're putting out birdseed for birds. They think it's for them."

There's another advantage to providing food for birds and squirrels. It keeps them from eating birdfeeders. "Basically, as long as a gray squirrel can get the seed he wants, he won't chew on a feeder," Bird observes. "But if he can't get to the seed—he's dynamite. He'll chew through whether it's plastic or metal."

But on this score, Bird does offer some advice. "Ben Gay or hot pepper—apply them when you spot a squirrel starting to chew on your feeder. That stuff will keep them from eating away. But how long it lasts, I don't know."

How does one manage to feed squirrels and birds? "We have a separate feeder for squirrels," says Dick E. Bird. "In the fall we forage around and collect acorns and other nuts, put them out for squirrels, and the squirrels go crazy. Collecting nuts works well. Squirrels will only find 20 percent of what they bury. The other nuts become lost or trees or something. What we do is provide the squirrels with what they've buried." It's easy to do this, Bird maintains: "A lot of people who feed birds are already into nature and hiking. Foraging works. On one walk you can collect about a bushel of nuts."

You'll find squirrel-lovers just about everywhere you find bird feeders. They're not as plentiful, but they are as vociferous. Julie Gillisipie of Bethesda, Maryland, is one such person. She said about the bravery of her squirrels:

> For five years I have fed a host of birds and an average of three to seven squirrels. I never tried to discourage squirrels and never seem to suffer from them. I instead have enjoyed their antics, play, and the remarkable way they trained our three cats. The squirrels fed mainly on the driveway and the cats learned they couldn't catch them, so the squirrels allowed the cats to within three feet.

After the *Wild Bird News* featured my article about outwitting squirrels, the publisher received a letter from a prosquirrel person who expressed her sentiments about feeding squirrels. Mildred Raitala's letter sums up how many squirrel lovers feel about thwarting squirrels:

Dear George,

I am disappointed at Mr. Adler's attitude in regard to squirrels. I have fed and studied birds most of my life, however that does not keep me from buying roasted peanuts, sunflower seed, and filberts in season and feeding the squirrels. The only reason they get in the birdfeeders is that they are hungry. In the fall of 1987 there were not many acorns. We have cut down so many trees that squirrels depend on us for food. So why torment these cunning little acrobats by trying to starve them out?

How would Mr. Adler like to be stuck in a snow storm in a tree without a supply of food? If you give them food they will leave the birdfeeders alone, as well as the bulbs in the yard. If I were hungry I would try every means I have available to get food.

Mildred Raitala

Squirrel lovers offer their friends more than mere affection. When Clarence Shilling died in August, 1982, at the age of 78 he left his entire estate of $90,000 for an endowment to feed birds and squirrels. Shilling was a retired mathematics professor who taught at North Dakota State University. Foundation officials said, "He spent many, many days coming up with language to include in his will that would provide a perpetual endowment in Fargo-Moorhead to care for squirrels and birds."

When Good Squirrels Go Bad

This is the story of Ken Gorelick, Cheryl Opacinch, and Seymour the Squirrel. It's a story about a couple who befriended a squirrel, became close compatriots of this squirrel, and then suddenly found that this squirrel abused their trust. It's a story about happiness and disappointment. It's a happy story with a sad ending, but one that shows that sometimes you can love a squirrel too much.

Ken Gorelick and Cheryl Opacinch live near the National Zoo in Washington, D.C., an area whose native wildlife consists of squirrels, raccoons, piliated woodpeckers, hawks, orphaned poodles, and escapees from the Zoo. Trees fill the streets, alleys, and parks in the area. There's "a stand of maples out back that the squirrels frequent," says Gorelick. A squirrel which Gorelick and Opacinch named Seymour began appearing at the bedroom balcony of their four-story townhouse during the winter about five seasons ago. Long branches from the maples, a telephone wire that comes into their house, and balconies with railings on every floor provide ample access for squirrels.

Gorelick and Opacinch admired Seymour. Not long after he appeared they began supporting his heavy nut habit. It was an arrangement that benefited both parties: Seymour got his nuts and Gorelick and Opacinch got to see Seymour. "He was a striking squirrel," Gorelick said. "Seymour was large with long fur and a long bushy tail. He would run to the balcony door like he had known us for a long time. Seymour would wait outside, sit on his hind legs, crane his neck, and ask 'Where are the nuts? I know they're here somewhere.' And he was right," Gorelick said in tones of admiration, love, and bittersweet melancholy. He spoke as if conjuring the words from deep memory. "One of us would have to distract him by tapping on the glass of the window, so he would go in that direction. After we distracted him from the door, we would open the door a crack and toss out the nut," Gorelick continued. "He would thank us and then go off with the nut. Seymour would then come back in a few minutes for another nut. Then he would send over a lady friend and two or three cousins."

Gorelick and Opacinch fed Seymour through the winter. They become fond of him and thought that he was one of the most beautiful squirrels they had ever seen. "This ritual exchange would occur every day. He knew that we were interested in seeing his tail and he would flick it for us. He could fold it right back to the base of his ears. He would flick his tail for us because he knew that we enjoyed it. We developed a relationship."

As summer approached, Gorelick and Opacinch changed their routine slightly. Gorelick said, "In warm weather we tend to leave the glass door open and the screen door shut." From the balcony "Seymour could see the bowl of nuts sitting on the dresser beside the bed" that they would feed him with.

This is when their relationship deteriorated. "Seymour knew that the nuts were his," Gorelick said softly. "One day we failed to show at the regular time. Finding the glass door open, he took it upon himself to come in on his own. He ate his way through the screen door—he gnawed a hole through the metal screen.

"He cleaned out the bowl and exited.

"Seymour didn't get into anything else," Gorelick added, as if defending Seymour from misplaced allegations.

"He didn't think twice about it, I believe. Seymour was back the next day at the usual time. He figured that we wanted him to have those nuts.

"I was very angry," Gorelick reflected. "I would say we had a huge falling out and I never felt the same after that. He could tell. He came around a few more times and I just glowered at him. He came around a few more times and stopped. He just left because he wasn't wanted."

Gorelick's had time to think about what happened between him, Cheryl, and Seymour. Other squirrels have come by, including

Seymour's grandsquirrel, Gregory, but "there has never been another Seymour. He was a uniquely gorgeous creature."

Still Gorelick doesn't regret what happened. "I just felt that we could not continue the kind of hospitality that he was growing to expect," Gorelick said.

But Gorelick and Opacinch don't fault Seymour. "I can't blame him really. He just went for his nut bowl. That's why he didn't understand and was hurt. Perhaps I should have explained, but perhaps I couldn't trust him anymore. And he may have felt the same way after I turned on him so viciously.

"It was a classic case of misunderstanding," Gorelick concluded.

Attracting Squirrels

"Are you kidding?" you ask. No, absolutely not. There are plenty of people who like squirrels and want to coax them into their yards, and there are others who've reconciled themselves to the fact that they are going to feed squirrels no matter what. Attracting squirrels is a much easier task than attracting birds. Indeed, all you have to do is put out a birdfeeder and squirrels will flock to your house. So why bother to make any extra effort? The reason is that with a little effort you can increase the squirrels' pleasure in dining and your pleasure in watching them.

Some birders prefer that squirrels eat from their birdfeeders, because it's fun to watch squirrels scramble, climb, and stretch to get to them. These people have found that one feeder serves all. That's fine.

Chapter 7 talks about erecting squirrel diverters to keep these mammals away from your feeder. Squirrel diverters have two attributes that make them work. First, they are kept as far away from the birdfeeder as possible, and second, diverters are easy for squirrels to get to. A bowl with sunflower seeds or nuts will work well both as a diverter and as a squirrel feeder. Alternatively, there are plenty of commercial squirrel feeders. The Audubon Workshop, for example, sells a "corn grabber" that coaxes squirrels to "jump, swing, hang upside down, pull the chains up to themselves, and fight for turns." Another product, a Squirrel-a-Whirl, lets squirrels spin on a windmill-like device as they eat.

If you're serious about keeping squirrels in your yard, you'll need two other elements: water and squirrel boxes. For water any birdbath will do. Just remember to clean it regularly. Build a nesting box and the squirrels in your yard will be your friends forever. Squirrels prefer human-made nesting boxes to squirrel-made nests because they are sturdier and offer greater protection from the elements. A nesting box should be about fourteen to sixteen inches tall, four to six inches deep, and four to six inches wide. Make the entrance hole about two inches in diameter and place it about two inches from the top of the box. Finally, securely fasten the box to a tree, between one-half to two-thirds of the way up the tree. A couple of words of caution, however: As Gorelick and Opacinch learned, befriended squirrels decide that being inside your house is a lot more pleasant than staying outdoors all the time. Don't leave nuts or other food inside where squirrels can see or smell them—they'll get to them, and if you're extra unlucky they will decide that the stuff in your sock drawer makes wonderful nesting material. The second caution is on a slightly more serious note. If you start to handle squirrels or feed them by hand, eventually you will get bitten. As one author noted, the fastest way for a squirrel to get access to a nut is to bite the hand holding it, which then promptly drops the nut. Squirrel bites are not generally serious—although they are painful—if you've had a tetanus vaccination or booster within the past ten years. As a matter of safety, all biologists who regularly handle squirrels receive boosters. So if you start to get close to squirrels, make sure you get a shot first.

Peter Jenkins and His Pet Squirrel, Mad Max

Not all squirrel stories involve theft, intimidation, and agony. Some people like squirrels. A few have pet squirrels. It's not my purpose to encourage readers to adopt squirrels, nor do I necessarily believe they are cute pets. But those of us who are firmly in the outwitting squirrels camp can learn a great deal about squirrels from those who have an owner-pet relationship with them—even if it's not clear who owns whom.

Peter Jenkins found Mad Max, a gray squirrel, about four years ago when he was climbing a tree. Jenkins, a tree surgeon and co-founder of Tree Climbers International in Atlanta, Georgia, spends a lot of time in trees and comes eye to eye with squirrels on a regular basis.

"Max is a refugee from a dead tree," Jenkins told me. "The deader the tree the more wildlife is in it. A dead tree is easier to carve. Anyway, we were removing a large white oak. I'd climbed up the tree and stripped the branches. While up there I was keeping my eye open for nesting sites. If I come upon an animal's nest and there's a baby in it, the parents will run away from the nest, but will return later. I will evacuate the babies before I drop the tree." Jenkins always carries a cardboard box with him when he's dropping trees. "If there's a nearby tree, you can get a cardboard box and tack it to the tree. It makes a great new nest."

Jenkins continued with Max's story. "In this case there was no tree to tack a box to." Jenkins had combed the tree carefully. "I didn't know there were any babies in the tree. After the tree hit the ground, I started to cut it up in different sections. About halfway through I heard that pitched whistle. Baby squirrels have a high-pitched distress signal. Buried inside a sawdust pile was a squirrel. This squirrel was about as young as you can find.

"Mad Max still had his umbilical cord. He was about one and one-quarter inches long. But despite his size, he was yelling his head off."

I asked Jenkins how Max got his name. "I was driving down the freeway with both doors open—it was in the summer, real hot. A semi truck came by. Mad Max was in a cardboard box, and the truck just sucked the box out of the car. I was doing about fifty-five. I ran out and got to the box and Mad Max was still in it. I couldn't believe he was alive. So I called him the Road Warrior" (after the character portrayed by Mel Gibson in the movie, *Mad Max*).

After some time, "I tried to release him. He literally walked over the neighbors' cat who was snoozing. Mad Max never saw a cat before and wasn't afraid of it."

Jenkins and his wife had to fulfill the role of mother squirrel. They had to prepare a special milk formula ("not cow's milk; it'll kill them") and feed Mad Max every three or four hours.

Squirrels in captivity do differ from those in the wild (if you call a birdfeeder-filled backyard "wild"). "Mad Max was raised alone," Jenkins said. "If you raise squirrels in pairs they're half wild. Mad Max will chase females a little bit, but he pretty much doesn't pay attention to other squirrels.

"Mad Max is in a cage inside our screened-in front porch. We let him out there. He's gotten completely out several times but always goes back to the screened porch. He's totally uninterested in the wild."

Max is as good a climber as any squirrel, but not as daring. "Mad Max can run up and down trees, but doesn't go up super high."

Max lives well, too. "Mad Max has a steady diet of pecans. We have four pecan trees in the yard. Once in a while he gets almonds. He has a bad addiction to chocolate and we try not to give him too much because it's so rich."

Max isn't perfect, however. "Once and a while he slips in the house. He's always trying to turn the doorknob to get in. If he has a pecan in his mouth, there's no way you're going to catch him. He's in the hiding mode.

"You have to watch him inside. Sometimes he likes to take a bite out of an antique piece of furniture. If you keep him in the house for three or four hours he gets into the mode of having to make a nest. The first place he goes is the Kleenex box. He takes some Kleenex in his mouth and bunches it up into a wad. Then he runs to a cardboard box. He keeps going back and forth between his box and the Kleenex box. It's very funny.

"Mad Max makes clicking sounds. A lot of clicking sounds. Once and a while he scolds when a neighborhood cat comes around, but not too often."

Jenkins has had some close encounters with squirrels in trees. "I was attacked once. When a squirrel reaches adolescent stage, the parents become protective. I was deadwooding a tree" when it happened, said Jenkins. "I had one dead branch left and the branch came out on a nest. I swung over and started cutting. Then I looked, and two yards over saw two parent squirrels in the next tree. They ran down my tree and were gnashing and lunging at me. I started barking at them but it didn't do any good. Then I started swinging my rope to scare them.

They backed away and kept scolding me. Then the parents ran to the three adolescents."

Jenkins thinks squirrels are wonderful. "I love squirrels. They are much more intelligent than birds. I don't think they're trainable to do tricks, but Max knows certain things. He knows my tone of voice. If I lower my voice he cowers down. If he bites too hard I hit him on the top of the head with my knuckle—he knows he's bitten me and cowers."

Max knows Jenkins and his wife, but "reacts differently to strangers." When Jenkins comes home, Max will "jump on me and go through my pockets. He likes to hug my elbow." But Jenkins adds, "he's not good around strangers. I found that out the hard way. He bites. Two or three of my friends were jumped on and bitten.

"Max knows exactly who's who.

"After I've been out trimming and working different trees and I come home, he sniffs and sniffs me. I bring him branches from the trees I have been cutting. He'll spend fifteen minutes sniffing me."

Jenkins has had time to reflect on squirrel behavior. "Different squirrels have different personalities. I have a friend whose pet squirrel loves French fries. But Max won't touch them."

In the original Norman-French version of the fairy tale *Cinderella*, her slippers are made of squirrel fur.

Washington, D.C.'s first wild black squirrels were said to be escapees from the National Zoo. Twenty-eight black squirrels from Ontario, Canada, were brought to the zoo between 1902 and 1906.

THIRTEEN

Quitting

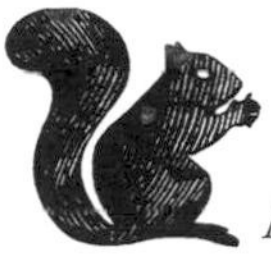

A lot of people really do like squirrels. One such individual is Gregg Bassett, president of the Squirrel Lovers' Club. If you are genuinely prosquirrel, then by all means join:

The Squirrel Lovers' Club
318 West Fremont
Elmhurst, IL 60126
(630) 833-1117

Another such person is Iris Rothman, whom I've know for years. Iris and I get along well, despite our differing views of squirrels. (It's kind of like one of us rooting for Kasparov, the other for Deep Blue.) Here's what Iris says about squirrels:

Humans have a hard time outwitting squirrels because, ounce for ounce, squirrels are smarter. Squirrels are ambitious and in-genious—they willingly tackle any antisquirrel device you rig up and, more often than not, they figure out a way to defeat it. And while they're not as pretty as birds, they have far more per-sonality. They are endlessly entertaining, whether soaring from

179

tree to tree in heart-stopping leaps or tackling yet another obstacle course set up to keep them from reaching the sunflower seeds.

Like most people, I started out feeding birds and fending off squirrels. But one day, in the words of Henry Mitchell, gardening writer for the *Washington Post*, "I saw that I would have squirrels forever and therefore resolved to love them. Things have gone smoothly since." With a little ingenuity, some safflower and thistle seed, and a lot of dried blood spread around my plants, I have managed to have more birds, more flowers, and more squirrels than anybody else in my neighborhood.

A few years after *Outwitting Squirrels* first appeared, I realized that many of the people who profess a love for squirrels aren't entirely sincere. Their love for squirrels does not stem from a natural affinity for furry tails or cute little ears, or even for the way squirrels wrinkle their noses. Liking squirrels has nothing to do with appreciation and amazement for the way they jump and climb and perform all manner of acrobatics. No, for many ex-birdfeeders turned squirrel-lovers, being prosquirrel is simply a matter of giving up.

I think that a lot of prosquirrel people are actually quitters. They are tired of what they consider to be a losing battle; tired of constantly having to wave their arms back and forth; tired of throwing things; tired of building barriers out of sharp metals; tired of transporting squirrels across state lines; tired of digging moats; tired of mixing waxy, noxious chemicals; tired of running to the local rent-a-cat. A lot of former bird feeders turned prosquirrel would rather take the afternoon off and nap.

Here's what one such person I spoke with via the Internet had to say:

I don't know how to defeat squirrels at the feeder and have given up. I throw my seed on the floor of the deck and feed the birds and squirrels together. The first year, I tried knocking on the window—the squirrel ran away. Five minutes later it was back. I ran outside and yelled at it and it ran away. Five minutes later it was back. I went outside and yelled again, and the squirrel yelled back. We got almost nose to nose and I blinked first. He even ignored my fifty-pound dog.

As for squirrel antics, if all the seed gets eaten and a squirrel is hungry, it sometimes comes and knocks on my kitchen window. This sends my four cats ballistic, but the squirrel just sits on the other side of the glass and smirks.

To these people, I say: there is hope. After millions and millions of years of evolution, we are still ahead of squirrels. Consider all those things we can do, but squirrels cannot: we can walk into a store and buy sunflower seed, we can coat the poles in our yards with various gooey substances, we can read about squirrel physiology and psychology, and we're not afraid of vacuum cleaners.

I have high hopes for civilization. We have survived world wars, the cold war, devastating plagues. We have gone to the moon, and sent probes past the outermost edge of our solar system. We have eliminated major diseases, and we have invented *Wheel of Fortune*.

But only if we keep up our struggle to outwit squirrels can humankind expect to progress towards the next level of development, whatever that may be. So if not for the birds, then for ourselves: let us continue to outwit squirrels.

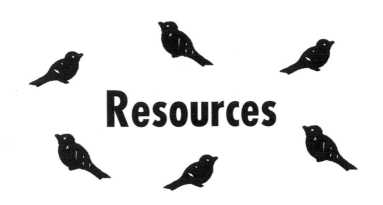

Resources

Bird and Outdoor Publications

The Dick E. Bird News
PO Box 377
Acme, MI 49610
Subscription price: $15 bi-monthly

The Dick E. Bird News is subtitled "The Best Darn Bird Stories Ever Told." And that's just what it is. *The Dick E. Bird News* is a bi-monthly eight-page tabloid that contains useful and fun information about the bird world. In it you'll not only learn how to attract birds, how to keep pests away from your feeder, how to take pictures of birds, ("You can't go through the woods like General Patton and hope to come out with an enjoyable experience, let alone a few good pictures"), but you'll find out about strange laws, such as the New Jersey law "making firecrackers legal by permit for the purpose of scaring birds away from cornfields," and the Connecticut statute that makes it a crime punishable by fine or imprisonment for "enticing of a neighbor's birds." *The Dick E. Bird News* is filled with photographs and drawings.

Bird Watcher's Digest
PO Box 110
Marietta, OH 45750
Subscription price: $15 a year

Bird Watcher's Digest, a bimonthly magazine, is the oldest and most popular birding magazine. Its *Reader's Digest* form makes it easy to take along on trips. And it's comprehensive. Anything you want to know about birds will be in *Bird Watcher's Digest*. A typical issue contained the following features: "Feeding Wild Turkeys," "Feeding the Birds," "SnowGeese at Brigantine," "FDR: Bird Watcher," and more. There's also verse and short fiction. The journal's regular departments include "The Behavior Watcher's Notebook," "Letters," book reviews, bird puzzles, and "The Backyard Bird Watcher's Question Box." The latter is one of this magazine's most valuable features—it's where readers can receive answers to their questions about birding. Because *Bird Watcher's Digest* has the largest number of readers of any bird magazine, it also has the most display and classified advertisements, which are frequently the best way to find out about new products and birding adventures. Each issue is filled with color and black and white photographs.

Bird Talk
Audubon Workshop
1501 Paddock Drive
Northbrook, IL 60062
Membership/subscription fee: $15 a year

Bird Talk is a bimonthly newsletter published by the Audubon Workshop for the members of its Helping Hand Bird Club. The Audubon Workshop is a mail-order bird supply company, and the Helping Hand Bird Club provides discounts and other services to its members. This four-page newsletter contains well-researched articles about particular birds, how to attract birds, birds and acid rain, bird nests, and other topics.

The Potomac Flier
Fairfax Audubon Society
PO Box 82
Vienna, VA 22180-8310
Subscription: $10 a year for non-members, free to members

The Potomac Flier is published eight times a year by the Fairfax Audubon Society, part of the National Audubon Society. The eight-page newsletter contains articles about local events, bird migrations, new books, seabirds, and Audubon Society activities.

Audubon Naturalist News
Audubon Naturalist Society
8940 Jones Mill Road
Chevy Chase, MD 20815
Subscription: free to members (membership is $30 for an individual, $40 for a family)

Published ten times a year by the Audubon Naturalist Society of the Central Atlantic States, the *Audubon Naturalist News* features articles about conservation, bird tours, and book reviews. *The News* comes in tabloid form and usually runs eight pages.

Wild Bird News
7370 MacArthur Boulevard
Glen Echo, MD 20812
Subscription: free

Published by the Wild Bird Center, which is located in Washington, D.C., along the Potomac River, *Wild Bird News* is one of the most interesting newsletters. It's published four to six times a year, and contains both articles about birding in the Washington area and features about birds in general. One of *Wild Bird News'* most interesting features is "Ask George," in which publisher George Petrides answers questions about birding.

Sierra
85 2nd Street
San Francisco, CA 94105-3441
Subscription: free to Sierra Club members (membership is $35 a year for an individual membership, and $120 a year for a contributing membership)

Although not a birding magazine, *Sierra* frequently contains articles about birds and birding expeditions. *Sierra* is among the premier outdoor and conservation magazines. Its photographs are spectacular. In addition to its regular features, *Sierra* regularly publishes articles about nuclear waste, recycling, Congress and the environment, outdoor books, and travel spots. Several times a year the magazine lists Sierra Club trips.

Stores and Catalogs

Below are listed companies that sell wild bird supplies. Call or write these companies for their catalog or to order specific products.

Duncraft
102 Fisherville Road
Concord, NH 03303
(603) 224-0200

Audubon Workshop
1501 Paddock Drive
Northbrook, IL 60062
(847) 729-6660

Wild Bird Center
7370 MacArthur Boulevard
Glen Echo, MD 20812
(301) 229-3141

Noel's Bird Feeders
PO Box 1
Northwood, NH 03261
(603) 942-8390

Hyde Bird Feeder Company
56 Felton Street
PO Box 168
Waltham, MA 02254
(617) 893-6780

Droll Yankee Bird Feeders
27 Mill Road
Foster, RI 02825
(401) 647-3324

Audubon Naturalist Society
8940 Jones Mill Road
Chevy Chase, MD 20815
(301) 652-3606

Bird Watcher's Digest Store
PO Box 110
Marietta, OH 45750
(614) 373-5285

Nixalite of America
1025 16th Avenue
PO Box 727
East Moline, IL 61244
(309) 755-8771

The Barn Owl Gift Shop
2509 Lakeshore Drive
Fennville, MI 49408
(616) 543-4175

Carey's Farmers Market
5651 Virginia Beach Boulevard
Norfolk, VA 23502
(804) 461-1580

Wild Wings
2101 S. Highway 61
Lake City, MN 55041
(612) 345-5355

Further Reading

America's Favorite Backyard Birds, Kit and George Harrison, Simon and Schuster, 1983.

The Bird Feeder Book, Donald and Lillian Stokes, Little Brown, 1987.

How to Attract Birds, Ortho Books, 1983.

"The Natural History of Squirrels," John Gurnell, *Facts on File*, 1987.

The Biology of Ground-Dwelling Squirrels, Jan O. Murie and Gail Michener, eds, University of Nebraska Press, 1984.

Building Birdhouses and Birdfeeders, Ed and Stevie Baldwin, Doubleday, 1985.

The Backyard Bird Watcher, George Harrison, Simon and Schuster, 1979.

About the Author

Bill Adler, Jr. is the president of Adler & Robin Books Literary Agency. He is the author of over a dozen books including *Outwitting Critters*, *Outwitting Toddlers*, *Outwitting the Neighbors*, *The Home Remodeler's Combat Manual*, and *Baby English: A Dictionary for Interpreting the Secret Language of Infants*. When not outwitting squirrels, Adler flies a Pitts Special, an aerobatic airplane, because "squirrels can't tolerate five gs, so I can be sure that there aren't any around when I fly." He lives in Washington, D.C., with his wife Peggy who is also a writer, and their two daughters, Karen and Claire.

Also from Chicago Review Press

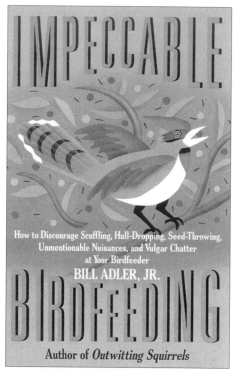

IMPECCABLE BIRDFEEDING
How to Discourage Scuffling, Hull-Dropping, Seed-Throwing, Unmentionable Nuisances, and Vulgar Chatter at Your Birdfeeder
Bill Adler, Jr.

This book is for all those who delight in the higher pleasures of birdfeeding and would like to attract the well-mannered of the avian species while keeping the vulgar element at bay. It includes insider tips on mess-free nuts, seeds, and other foods along with the culinary preferences of over 50 different species. Other ways to woo a warbler included here are knowing their nesting habits, the trees and shrubs they love, and where they like to bathe. Learn which feeders encourage neat dining and how to customize any feeder to curb messy, noisy behavior. An excellent companion to *Outwitting Squirrels*.

160 pages, 5⅜ x 8½
15 b & w photos
paperback, $9.95, 1-55652-157-X